The Mind of a Murderer

DR RICHARD TAYLOR

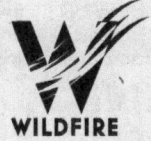

WILDFIRE

First published in 2021 by
Wildfire
an imprint of HEADLINE PUBLISHING GROUP

First published in paperback in 2021 by
WILDFIRE
an imprint of HEADLINE PUBLISHING GROUP

4

Cataloguing in Publication Data is available from the British Library

ISBN 978 1 4722 6820 4

Offset in 11.61/13.76 pt Garamond MT Std by Jouve (UK), Milton Keynes

Printed and bound in Great Britain by Clays Ltd, Elcograf S.p.A.

HEADLINE PUBLISHING GROUP
an Hachette UK Company
Carmelite House
50 Victoria Embankment
London
EC4Y 0DZ

www.headline.co.uk
www.hachette.co.uk

For Katherine, Louisa and Hannah

Author's Note

The details of the case histories in this book are either disguised or composites of cases, with alterations made to the biographical, geographical, temporal and cultural details in order to protect confidentiality without losing the essential elements of the case. I have used pseudonyms for homicide perpetrators and other individuals involved, such as doctors, police officers, lawyers, witnesses and family members.

Real names are only used where the information presented in the case history is already entirely in the public domain. And for those public domain cases in which I have been involved (listed below), other than describing my role, I have only used information available from detailed homicide inquiry reports, media reports or law reports. I have taken great care not to disclose any confidential interview material obtained by me unless it is in the public domain. For example, extensive extracts of psychiatric reports about Anthony Hardy, including the one I supervised, were published in the inquiry report.

Other individuals not in the public domain have consented to being named in the text. Where published research or books are quoted, the authors' names are used to reference their work and selected references are available in the endnotes. Technical terms are explained in the text.

Cases that I have been involved in where real names have been used, but the information presented is already available in the public domain are, in order of appearance: Anthony Hardy, Daniel Joseph, Maxine Carr, Nimpha Ong, Sara Thornton, Kathleen McCluskey, John Wilmot, Christopher Nudds (aka

Docherty-Puncheon), Sheikh Abu Hamza, Dhiren Barot, the 'gas limos' and 'plane bombs' conspirators, Muhaydin Mire and Robert Stewart.

The following are cases I have not personally been involved in, and thus all information is taken from the public domain: Ted Bundy, Ed Kemper, Andrew Cunanan, Aaron Alexis, Navjeet Sidhu, Louise Porton, Tania Clarence, Victoria Climbié, Baby P, 'Adam', Peter Sutcliffe, Andrea Yates, Myra Hindley, Rosemary West, Kiranjit Ahluwalia, 'Giselle Anderson', Sally Challen, Guenther Podola, Rudolf Hess, Stephen Hawking, Emile Cilliers, Robert Hansen, Mohamed Atta, Timothy McVeigh, various prisoners at ADX Florence federal supermax prison, Brenton Tarrant, Anders Breivik and Khalid Masood.

Contents

Introduction

Murder is not just a crime: it is a major public health problem. In 2017 alone there were 464,000 recorded victims of homicide globally. At a rate of well over 1,000 unlawful killings per day, deaths by homicide far exceeded the 89,000 killed in armed conflicts and the 26,000 victims of terrorism. Some 87,000 women and girls were intentionally killed in 2017, of which 50,000 were killed by intimate partners or other family members.

Some parts of the world are more badly affected than others. Across the Americas, the number of murders is consistently high. In some countries in Latin America the homicide rate is fifty times that of Western Europe and is a leading cause of death, especially among young adults. Meanwhile, there has been a significant increase in knife killings amongst the 800 offences initially recorded as murder in Great Britain and Northern Ireland in recent years, despite an overall gradual reduction in homicides in Europe.

The United Nations' definition of homicide is 'unlawful death inflicted upon a person with the intent to cause death or serious injury'. In UK law, the offence of murder – as opposed to manslaughter – is committed when a person of 'sound mind' unlawfully kills any 'reasonable creature' under the 'Queen's peace' with intent to kill or cause serious bodily harm.

Why do people kill? Most homicides involve extremes of 'normal' – or at least understandable – mental states such as anger, rage, impulsivity, fear or jealousy, but there can be a fine line between these states and mental disorder at the time of a killing. In psychotic homicide, there are mental state changes well outside the standard range. This usually involves a killer who has completely lost contact with reality and been pitched into the delusions and hallucinations of psychosis. This situation is most commonly seen in schizophrenia, a serious mental illness. Globally, around 0.5 per cent of the population live with a diagnosis of schizophrenia, but they account for somewhere between six and eleven per cent of homicides. In other words, according to one major study, this group have a nineteen-fold increased risk of committing homicide. The vast majority of people with schizophrenia are far more likely to be the victims of violence or self-harm than they are to injure others, and it's important that people suffering with mental illness are not stigmatised by the violent behaviour of the few. But the increase in risk can't be ignored as, in contrast to the overall decline in homicide numbers, the number of homicides by those with schizophrenia has risen.

London's Metropolitan Police solve around ninety per cent of their murder cases (compared to around sixty per cent solved by police forces in many cities in the USA), partly because New Scotland Yard has specialist homicide teams that are given substantial resources to investigate murder cases (although with street-based and gang-related killings, the reluctance of some witnesses to speak out presents an increasing challenge). Another reason for the impressive clear-up rate is that homicides by 'strangers' are rare. Most victims know their killers, so the police don't have to look far to find the perpetrator. In fact, one of the most common forms of homicide is when one half of a couple kills the other, often at the point of a break-up. The victims of this form of homicide are usually female (only one per cent of male victims annually are killed by a partner). However, the population group with the highest risk of being victims are infants under one year of age – and the killer is usually the mother.

Alcohol and illicit drugs are present to some degree in almost half of all homicides, but they rarely provide the sole explanation for an incident. Financially motivated homicide is surprisingly rare, comprising around six per cent of all killings in the UK and the USA (including robbery and burglary homicides). Sexual homicides are even more uncommon, accounting for less than one per cent of killings, but they receive disproportionate attention, especially if there's a series of sexually motivated murders of strangers.

As a forensic psychiatrist, it is my job to assess perpetrators of serious crime and to treat those who are found to have a mental disorder. I most often assess killers soon after their offence, writing reports and giving expert witness evidence at trial and for sentencing. But my involvement doesn't start or finish with the Crown court trial.

Once the heat and light of the criminal justice process is complete, a perpetrator of homicide needs to be contained to protect the public. But we must also try to understand their offence, not only to treat their mental disorder and rehabilitate them, but also to reduce the risk of further homicidal behaviour. Ultimately, if release is to be considered, I need to evaluate the dangers and supervise release, and later I may have to recall them to secure hospital or custody. As well as working with known killers, I also conduct risk assessments of those who may pose a threat of violent behaviour and who (very rarely) may be in danger of going on to kill. In other words, I aim to prevent homicides, although risk prediction is notoriously inaccurate.

When I started in forensic psychiatry, there was a sense of innovation and optimism. Although there are still beacons of excellence, with outstanding services in some of the secure hospitals and much-improved mental health care in prisons, for example, the optimism has nonetheless been tempered by a decimation of addiction services and a severe reduction in general psychiatric hospital beds. We are now at a point where drug-fuelled knife homicides have risen significantly and where community mental health services are so overburdened and under-resourced that the police and other emergency services are being asked to step in, in our place. In some cases, this has led to terrible consequences, including murder.

This is a book about my work. We'll explore sexual homicide; psychotic homicide; matricide; infanticide; filicide; the killing of intimate partners by men, and the killing of intimate partners by women (often victims of abuse killing their abuser); homicide as a result of alcohol and brain damage; murder followed by amnesia; murder with a financial motive and murder or mass murder through violent extremism and terrorism. And I'll go beyond the media reporting to show that, while every case is different, there are observable patterns in the different types of murder. On top of all those cases I have been involved with professionally, I have a personal connection to a homicide, and I will describe the case and its impact on my family.

Above all, though, this is a book about the state of mind of those who kill, and how we can attempt to make sense of their crimes to try and ensure they never kill again, as well as learning how to spot the warning signs in other would-be killers.

Although there is an awful lot of murder in this book, I hope that its overall message is one of understanding and, ultimately, humanity.

Sexual Homicide

Case Study: Anthony Hardy

I

His Nectar card was partly his undoing. When he bought black bin liners for the body parts of his victims, he couldn't resist claiming the points at Sainsbury's. The police caught him on CCTV.

The killer in question was Anthony Hardy, best known as the Camden Ripper. To understand how his desire for Nectar points and my work intersect, we need to go back to January 2002, when police visited his London flat on what they no doubt assumed would be a routine call. Quarrelling with his neighbour over a leaky pipe, Hardy, then fifty-one, had scrawled an obscene message on her door with car battery acid. But when the police gained entry to his flat, their suspicions were aroused by a locked bedroom. 'What's in there?' they asked. Hardy pretended not to have a key until one was found in his coat pocket. The officers opened the door.

In the room was a bed; next to it, a bucket of warm water and a camera on a tripod. On the bed was the body of a thirty-eight-year-old woman, Sally 'Rose' White.

The facts, you might think, speak for themselves. Sure enough, Hardy was duly charged with murder. However, the bite mark on Sally's right thigh and the small abrasion on her head were not fatal injuries and, having found evidence of coronary heart disease, the pathologist, Freddy Patel, ruled that the likely cause of death was a heart attack.

Given this finding, the police had no choice but to drop the murder charge. On 12 March 2002, Hardy pleaded guilty to criminal damage of the neighbour's door, was sectioned on a hospital order under the Mental Health Act and moved from HMP Pentonville to a local open psychiatric unit, St Luke's in Muswell Hill. Under the care of a general adult psychiatrist, he received treatment for a 'mood disorder'. In psychiatry, the term 'mood disorder' refers to a range of disturbed mental states, including depression, which can vary in severity from a two-week period of depressed mood, loss of interest, fatigue and feelings of worthlessness and so on, to a severely depressed state of mind with suicidal thoughts and psychotic experiences. Mood disorder also refers to bipolar disorder, in which there can be distinct 'manic' episodes of persistent irritability and mood elevation, with reduced need for sleep, a tendency to speak in a rapid manner (known as pressured speech), grandiosity and so on.

In Hardy's case, the issue was a mild to moderate lowering of mood, made worse by heavy drinking, with some suggestion of previous mood swings. But because of the unusual circumstances, a risk assessment was requested from a forensic psychiatrist.

Which was where I came in.

Forensic psychiatrists are a select and secretive bunch. We make up around 350 of roughly 330,000 doctors registered with the General Medical Council in the UK, and our work is little known. We are medically qualified (unlike our clinical psychologist colleagues). Doctors, in other words: specifically psychiatrists first, and forensic experts second.

My own route into it was tortuous and unplanned, via six years of medical school and three years as a junior doctor, including A & E and overseas aid work. I then joined the Maudsley psychiatry higher training 'rotation', a six-year programme with placements in specialities like psychosis, addictions and child psychiatry, finally latching on to forensics for reasons I would only really reflect upon later.

'Do you deal with dead bodies?' I'm often asked. Well, I have, in the past, starting with day three of my medical training at UCL, when we were introduced to our cadavers to begin months of dissection. But while forensic pathologists use their training to determine the victim's cause of death, there are also forensic accountants, forensic odontologists, forensic toxicologists and forensic anthropologists, all applying their expertise to the court of law, or 'forum' – hence the term 'forensic'. In forensic psychiatry, we're only interested in the dead body for what it may reveal about the perpetrator's state of mind. Ours is the interface between psychiatry and law. Most commonly, this involves treating mentally disordered offenders: that is, psychiatric patients who have committed serious offences. We evaluate and write reports about our patients and, as independent experts, give evidence in criminal and civil courts about someone's psychiatric status and criminal responsibility. Our role can be pivotal in murder cases where the defence is Not Guilty by Reason of Insanity (NGRI), or when one of the partial defences of diminished responsibility, suicide pact or provocation (now called loss of control) are put forward. All these, to a greater or lesser extent, depend on psychiatric opinion, which can be fiercely contested.

Not for us the 'whodunnit' (well, not so much, although we might get involved in a detainee's fitness for police interview or in disputed confession cases, where the mentally disordered may confess to things they haven't done). We're more interested in the why, and our focus is on the perpetrator in custody. What were they like before the offence? Why and how did the murder come about? Are they fit for detention? Are they fit for trial? Are they partially or wholly criminally responsible, or are their actions explicable in terms of mental disorder?

Then we must decide what should happen to them after conviction. Secure hospital or prison? Mad or bad? Or a mixture of both? If they come to hospital, what level of security do they require, and can we treat them? Will they recover? Have they, and we, made sense of their offence? Can we develop a relapse prevention plan? Are they safe for release?

These questions all arise after arrest. Although we don't usually get involved in profiling unknown suspects, we do get asked to perform risk assessments on those who have not yet committed a serious offence. One such risk-assessment case was Anthony Hardy.

I remember Hardy's assessment well. It was 28 August 2002 when I interviewed him. There were a number of unusual details in Hardy's background. Psychiatric interviews are confidential, but Hardy's background history and extracts of his psychiatric reports are already in the public domain in the independent inquiry report, so I can discuss them here. Hardy was born in Burton-on-Trent, in Staffordshire. He was said to have worked hard at school and wanted to escape his somewhat deprived origins. He met his wife, Judith, while studying Engineering at Imperial College, London, and they married in 1972, going on to have four children and spending a period of time living in Australia. Despite instances of domestic violence, and Hardy not bothering to conceal his extra-marital affairs, his wife agreed to several attempted reconciliations.

While living in Australia, he had been investigated for a serious assault on Judith in 1982. He'd hit her over the head with a bottle of frozen water and then tried to drown her in the bath. Hardy had chosen the shape of the bottle so that it might plausibly suggest Judith had slipped and hit her head on the bath itself, while the idea of freezing may have come to him via the Roald Dahl short story *Lamb to the Slaughter*, in which a woman bludgeons her husband to death with a frozen leg of lamb and then serves it to the investigating detectives. (There's much talk in the media about the pernicious effects of video games and rap music – not so much about the corrupting influence of Roald Dahl's short stories.) Either way, the charges against Hardy were dropped and the marriage fell apart, although it was another four years before the couple would divorce for good. He lost his job in engineering and drifted downwards socially, going from minicab driving to unemployment.

Back in the UK, Hardy was diagnosed with bipolar disorder, abnormal personality traits and alcohol abuse. He spent short periods in prison for criminal damage to his ex-wife's house, as well as stealing her new partner's car during what would nowadays be seen as a campaign of harassment. He had short stays in psychiatric hospitals as well as living in various hostels in London, and picked up convictions for theft and being drunk and disorderly. In 1998 he was arrested when a prostitute accused him of rape: charges that were later dropped due to lack of evidence. By 2002, living on benefits, drinking heavily and with badly controlled diabetes, he was leading a largely reclusive existence in a dreary low-rise council block just off Royal College Street in Camden.

He was a physically imposing man, heavy-set and over six feet tall. At interview, his speech was measured and he seemed to give considerable thought to his answers before responding. He denied any manic or depressive symptoms, and was giving little away in terms of emotional expressiveness, which in psychiatric terminology is called a 'flattened affect'. He gave a minimising account of the harassment of his ex-wife, even though he had once driven all the way to Bury St Edmunds just to lob a rock through her window. I remember that he made me feel uneasy. He was a reluctant interviewee and his internal world remained very much a mystery, although he said that he had always been easily bored, impulsive and a thrill seeker. He accepted he'd committed the criminal damage to his neighbour's door, painting 'fuck off you slut' on it, then pouring the battery acid through her letter box using a cut-off cider bottle as a funnel. He said he had been drinking heavily at the time. He also claimed he couldn't remember how Rose White came to be in his flat, although he thought he might have invited her back there and admitted openly that he had picked up prostitutes in the Kings Cross area before. According to one of the nurses working that day, Hardy told her he was very upset I'd asked him about Rose and my questioning on that subject had made him have suicidal thoughts.

While still at St Luke's, he took up the offer of an alcoholics' day programme outside the hospital and was given leave during the day to spend time at home in his flat, with no reported problems. He expressed remorse about his behaviour towards his neighbour, and there was no further sign of animosity towards her.

We compiled our report (unusually, both my trainee psychiatrist and I had interviewed him to compare notes). In it, we noted his history of hostility towards his ex-wife and, with the details around the dead woman, Rose, making us uncomfortable (especially the camera and tripod), we recommended that the local Multi-Agency Public Protection Arrangements (MAPPA) panel, an inter-agency forum run by police and probation to monitor risky individuals, be informed, so a plan could be put in place before his discharge. Our conclusion was that he could pose a risk of serious violence to women, independent of disturbed mental state and alcohol use, but we also had to work on the basis he'd had no hand in the death of White, given the post-mortem findings.

I had no more involvement with Hardy, and the following months were taken up with other cases. Until the events of New Year's Eve, 2002.

I carry two phones: a personal one and a work one. That night I had my personal phone in my trouser pocket, while my work phone was in a jacket hanging in the hall just outside the kitchen, at the bottom of three small, uneven stairs.

Our two children were then aged three and one, and going out for a New Year's Eve party was not on the agenda, so we were having guests over for dinner. The weather was wet and windy so, frankly, I was pleased to be staying in; moreover, I was cooking, and thus in my element.

With both parents being full-time doctors, home life involved a complicated division of labour, each of us taking turns to pick up our boys from nursery depending on who had to work late. Like any young family, we had a pretty exhausting schedule, but I happily traded laundry duties and childcare scheduling for the role of chief cook. It is easy to slide into convenience options like putting a piece of breaded fish in the oven. But at the weekend, time spent making fresh seafood pasta was an effective diversion from the day job. What's more, I'd found a way to take advantage of my visits to prisons and obscure psychiatric oubliettes as an opportunity to drop in on suppliers of interesting ingredients, from Salvino's Sicilian deli near Holloway prison to the Spice Shop on the way back from Wormwood Scrubs and Coastline Galicia, one of the surviving old-school fishmongers.

Our guests that night were another two psychiatrists. I'd splashed out on a decent bottle of full-bodied red and was cooking an ambitious menu. Preoccupied as I was, it took a few moments for the sound of my work phone in the hallway to cut through Miles Davis's 'Max is Making Wax' from *Live at the Pasadena Civic Auditorium,* and by the time I'd wrestled it from my jacket pocket, I'd missed the call.

I looked at the screen, feeling the first stirrings of disquiet. It was from our police liaison psychiatric nurse, Doug Cardinal. As his job title suggests, Doug acted as a go-between for us and the police. The mere fact he was ringing meant something bad, an SUI – 'serious untoward incident' – had occurred. The fact that he was ringing *me* – when I was not on call – was cause for very serious concern.

I tried to call him back but got his voicemail. *He's probably underground in the custody suite*, I thought, and went back to Miles Davis. But the calm of pre-dinner food prep was fading, replaced by a nagging concern. The fact is that, while all doctors worry about a wrong decision harming their patients, we forensic psychiatrists have two other fears. The first is that a patient may take their own life. The number of suicides every year is estimated to be around 800,000 globally – double the number of homicides. In England and Wales, there were 6,507 suicides in 2018, a typical year. That figure was almost ten times the number of homicides that year, and dwarfed the 1,770 road deaths. Of those suicides, around 1,700 are by mental health patients; so this is a tragic but relatively frequent feature of psychiatric work. But worse still is the fear that a patient could take someone else's life. Homicides by psychiatric patients number roughly seventy-five cases out of around 800 total killings annually in the UK (around ten per cent). Of those, about two-thirds may be committed by a patient who is being treated by a psychiatrist.

In other words, homicides by patients are relatively rare. But when they do happen, they're catastrophic, and they're a forensic psychiatrist's worst nightmare.

At this stage, I was of course mulling over the killers on my list and wondering which of my cohort might have 'gone off'. I considered Gavin Faulkner, a Glaswegian with schizophrenia who had knifed a stranger and shoved him in the Regent's Canal after apparently hearing the victim whistling 'David Watts' (Gavin had a long-standing delusion that Paul Weller was stalking him). Or perhaps it could be Paul Kennedy, a cheerful Irishman who had lived in a council flat next to a pub. He had beheaded a member of his Scientology church group over delusions that his fellow congregant was having an affair with his girlfriend, acting in a state of morbid jealousy ('morbid' in medical and psychiatric terms being any state that is affected by disease or outside what we call the realm of normal mental states).

Half an hour later and another two calls had gone straight to Doug's answerphone. Our guests arrived and a glass of wine did little to stop my mind drifting back to work. I slipped out to the kitchen again and pressed the green call button to redial Doug's number. This time – at last – he picked up and confirmed my fears: something serious was afoot. A murder hunt, to be precise. Human body parts had been found in a bin. There were a number of lines of investigation, but a former patient was being sought 'to assist police with enquiries'.

That patient was Anthony Hardy.

This came as a surprise. As far as I knew, Hardy was subject to civil commitment (section) under the Mental Health Act on a six-month treatment order and should still have been in St Luke's. In fact, it would later transpire that he'd been released in November, having been discharged by a review panel without my knowledge, but at the time I was floored by the revelation that he was out, much less being sought as part of a murder enquiry.

Even so, there was a ray of hope. He might just have been added to the list of usual suspects as a matter of routine, since a young woman had been found dead of a heart attack in his flat earlier that year. The fact that police wanted to talk to Hardy might – just might – mean nothing. I clung to that hope for all of an hour or so, before Doug rang back, this time as I was slicing the slightly undercooked and bloody haunch of venison.

'Hardy's definitely the prime suspect, I'm afraid, Richard,' he said.

'Okay.' I felt my heart sink. 'And what makes you say that?'

'They've found a headless torso wrapped in bin liners in his flat.'

Well, that would do it, I thought, feeling the hairs on my neck stand up.

'Is he in custody?' I asked.

'No, he's on the run. They're declaring a major incident.'

I started to develop a strange dissociated feeling, as if this were not happening. A homicide – no, a *double* homicide – by a man we'd assessed just a few months previously. I thought frantically about how this could have happened. My mind went to the case of Christopher Clunis, a man with schizophrenia who had killed Jonathan Zito at Finsbury Park Station in 1992. Although there was initially little attention paid to the story, a long campaign by Jonathan's wife, Jayne, prompted a searching public inquiry. It turned out that Clunis had spent time in nine psychiatric units in five years and had attacked fellow patients and nurses with knives. At the time of his fatal encounter with Jonathan Zito, he was being seen by a number of psychiatric care teams around London, had been discharged from hospital not long before, and was living alone in a bedsit, not taking his medication.

Published just after I started in psychiatry, the Clunis inquiry heralded a major shift towards risk awareness and defensive practice, as evidenced by a hushed conversation I witnessed in the hospital canteen between two senior psychiatrists about a colleague who had been named in the report. The overhaul of supervision arrangements meant we had to rigorously plan, discuss and document all discharges and follow-ups. But risk assessments – such as the one my team had done on Anthony Hardy – were an entirely different kettle of fish. These were often patients who were not subject to detention but were presenting signs of worrying mental states or behaviours. I had always thought that risk assessments were the greatest hostage to fortune. Nowadays we use more structured and evidence-based tools, which combine actuarial and clinical approaches, but these were not in widespread use in 2002. Our prediction skills have improved but remain poor, a bit like trying to do a long-range weather forecast in September for July 1st of the following summer: you can talk about likely climatic patterns, but you can't predict rain on a particular day with any more than a vague categorisation into low, medium or high risk.

If we cannot predict risk with any reliability, then we must at least try to manage it. So unless immediate detention and transfer to Broadmoor (a high-security psychiatric hospital) was recommended, there was always a chance of an unexpected tropical storm – a fatal outcome that could call our judgement into question. As my old consultant mentors used to say, 'Cover your back . . . lay a paper trail', or 'Start at the homicide inquiry and work backwards.'

In the case of Hardy, as with any other such assessment, we had looked at risk history. This was based on the conclusion that Rose White had died of natural causes. Thus, while Hardy's risk history suggested a potential for violence, threats and harassment towards prostitutes or intimate partners, it didn't include homicide. The camera on the tripod had been a troubling and unnerving detail, and had led to some speculative thought as to what else might have been going on. But – in the absence of any film in the camera – there was nothing in the information we had about any use of bondage and sado-masochistic sexual practices, and we were hardly qualified to challenge the findings of a Home Office pathologist, so we'd put those suspicions away.

Now, though, my mind returned to the body of Rose, and how she must have been far more significant than we had originally thought. What had really happened to her?

Much later, our guests departed, with 2003 having officially begun. I found myself alone in the kitchen, loading the dishwasher, these thoughts rattling around my head. I struggled to sleep that night.

*

On New Year's Day, I awoke with a feeling of dread in the pit of my stomach. Putting on a brave face, I helped get the boys up and ready for their day. My eldest was munching boiled eggs and soldiers in his high chair.

There was a light drizzle and a grey sky. Looking through our north-facing French doors into the garden, I could see the green turtle paddling pool filling with rainwater. I tried to take my mind off morbid ruminations with mundane tasks, such as cleaning last night's candle wax from the dining table. It had not been the relaxing New Year's Eve I had planned.

A coffee addict, I rinsed out the pot and spooned in some grounds from my favourite coffee shop, the Algerian in Soho, and sparked up the gas hob. My wife was trying to stop me catastrophising about the likely fall-out, accustomed as she was to my bouts of forensic anxiety.

'It never turns out to be as bad as you think,' she said, no doubt referring to a homicide that had happened two days before our delayed honeymoon trip a few years before. I was grateful for her words of comfort, even though I had a feeling it would actually turn out to be worse.

I thought of Craig, my trainee. Conscientious and thoughtful, he was one of the better trainees I had had, but right now he'd be blissfully unaware of the events of the night before. I waited until 10 a.m., pacing around the kitchen, three cups of espresso doing nothing for my nerves, before I called him to share the bad news.

'I'd really like to re-read our report,' I told him. 'I don't think he can have been manic, do you? From what I've heard of the crimes so far, he sounds too organised for that.'

By 'manic' I mean a period of time during which the patient has elevated levels of either expansive or 'irritable' mood, as well as abnormally and persistently increased activity or energy. For it to be mania, it needs to occur for most of the day for at least a week, and to not be related to the direct effects of drugs or alcohol.

Neither of us knew, of course. Details at that point were sketchy at best. Nevertheless, I could sense Craig's discomfort. 'Don't worry,' I assured him, 'I'll have to carry the can. You were under my supervision.'

No question about it. The buck stopped with me.

A further call to Doug Cardinal helped clarify some details: the police major incident had begun when a homeless person looking for food found human remains in a council wheelie bin near Hardy's home in Royal College Street, Camden, on the day before New Year's Eve. The homeless person had opened a green refuse sack and, having been assaulted by a foul smell, found that it contained a pair of human legs. He reported it, and the area was cordoned off while the police made a search. The human remains they discovered were subsequently identified as belonging to two women, Bridgette Maclennan, thirty-four, and Elizabeth Valad, twenty-nine, both of whom were known to work in the Kings Cross area as prostitutes.

The day after, police obtained a warrant to search Hardy's flat, on the basis of the events that had occurred there earlier in the year, but it turned out they needn't have bothered. When they arrived, they found the front door open.

Inside, a light was on but the flat was empty. The bedroom was locked, and a cloth laid along the bottom of the door did nothing to prevent a revolting smell emanating from within.

When the door was opened, an upper torso was found inside, partly wrapped in black bin liners and duct tape. This torso was Maclennan's, while two pieces of leg belonging to Valad were also discovered.

In an industrial bin outside, police found Valad's arms, as well as her left foot, and the lower torso of Maclennan. Other parts had been disposed of in various Camden locations and were subsequently discovered. The heads and hands of the two women were never found.

To me – thinking again of the camera and tripod – this had all the hallmarks of a sexual homicide, and a serial one at that. I was familiar with the typology of sexual homicide crime scene analysis developed by Robert Ressler and John Douglas[1] of the FBI in the 1980s, and knew that such murders had been conceptually divided into 'organised' and 'disorganised' (although David Canter, a UK criminologist, has subsequently challenged the validity of this over-simplified dichotomy[2]). In any event, an organised crime scene didn't help determine the presence or absence of active mental illness, since even those with bizarre delusions are capable of purposeful planning. Even so, wrapping up torsos seemed a step too far for someone acutely manic.

I used my dial-up modem, and once the familiar squelching sound of the connection had subsided, I entered the encrypted passcode from my security fob and opened Craig's email containing our report. As I read through it, I felt relieved that it was very thorough. That, at least, was a minor consolation.

2

The next day was grim and grey. It matched my mood as I made my way to the medium-secure psychiatric hospital, my main place of work.

Medium-secure psychiatric hospitals are tucked away on the outskirts of London, and if you don't know their function, you wouldn't know they're there. My base at that time was on an old Victorian-era district general hospital site, just where the green belt starts, within the M25. You drive around the one-way system, past a multi-storey car park and then – before reaching the mortuary – you turn left down a slope to the back of the site, going past the mental health unit, a low-rise building housing inpatient wards containing around fifteen patients each. In those days, these patients were on short-term hospital admissions lasting a few weeks, but now it's sometimes only a few days. Many non-secure units of this type have been closed since, with even more patients shunted into the community. (The rhetoric is about least restrictive care, but the reality is about cost-cutting.)

At the bottom of the slope is a series of brown-brick, pitched-roof, two-storey buildings from the early 1990s. This is the medium-secure unit. After the asylums were closed in the 1970s and 1980s, it became clear there was a small group of patients who could not be managed in the community. Our local asylum decanted over 1,000 people into various forms of community care, but a hard core of challenging and aggressive patients were moved into what was known as an interim secure unit. These purpose-built units were designed to provide a halfway house between high security at Broadmoor and local psychiatric services. They were also part of a policy to divert the mentally disordered out of prison custody.

This was a more liberal and optimistic era, inspired by the cutting-edge and well-funded Dutch forensic centres, like the Van der Hoeven Clinic in Utrecht. In the Netherlands, criminal responsibility is graded on a sliding scale, with time spent in hospital for treatment and in prison for confinement apportioned accordingly. The pioneers in our field had been inspired by the Dutch to be more ambitious in planning our medium-secure service, a beacon of high standards and good funding in a cash-strapped NHS.

Sadly now, twenty or so years on, despite huge advances in the evidence base of forensic psychiatry, the quality of forensic services, and better patient and carer involvement, the impetus is in the other direction. We have moved to a more punitive – and, at the same time, risk-averse – approach. Crown court judges are more reluctant to send mentally disordered murderers to hospital rather than prison, and this has been reflected in the case law. In addition to this shift in legal and judicial attitudes, there are concerted efforts underway to reduce spending on inpatient and forensic psychiatric care in the NHS.

Travelling to the secure unit on that rainy morning, I parked my car in the half-empty car park. I had finally scrapped my old red Alfa Romeo 164 after numerous repairs and was now driving a more sensible hatchback with two child seats in the back.

The entrance to the secure unit was an airlock: two sets of electronic doors controlled by a receptionist. This was 2002, and we were still a few years off the fingerprint biometric technology we would come to use.

Then, as now, the clinical areas consisted of individual patient bedrooms to which patients were given their own key. This degree of relative freedom requires more staff than prisons, where the whole wing can be banged up with one officer on duty. In contrast to prison, all patients, once stabilised, are offered a bespoke range of treatments: medication, addiction groups, individual psychology and all kinds of occupational therapy.

Generally, the atmosphere is settled, but when things do kick off it can happen very quickly, and alarms will summon the rapid response team to de-escalate or restrain or, *in extremis*, seclude any acutely disturbed and violent patients.

Unlike those in an old asylum, the purpose-built wards were clean and well-lit, their double-height ceilings creating a sense of space and the illusion of freedom. The perimeter, with its 5.2-metre close-mesh fencing topped with anti-climb Cobra Spikes, was a different matter. Security searching, and staff trained in martial arts-based 'control and restraint' techniques – as they were called at the time – completed the package.

I attached my keys and personal alarm to my belt and entered the unit, joining the subdued discussion in our clinical director's office. In the meeting were the Clinical Director, two of my colleagues – both forensic psychiatrists – plus Doug Cardinal, as he'd been on the ground when everything kicked off. Later on, we'd have a legal adviser, but at this point we were thinking about eliminating any further risk to others. Damage limitation would come later.

Hardy's mental health records had been sealed to prevent any retrospective tampering, so I summarised the case history for the benefit of those present. Most pressingly, Hardy was still at large, so we discussed what information we needed to share with the police.

'I'm certain they must know about the incident with his wife, but I'll make sure,' I said, worried that he might even be on his way to see her. A final act of revenge, perhaps.

Any journalists would be referred to the communications department. As was standard procedure with high-profile cases, we would neither confirm nor deny that Hardy was known to our service at this stage.

Talking about Hardy, of course, meant the discussion moved on to other well-known homicides by psychiatric patients, and here I couldn't help but recall the Luke Warm Luke inquiry. The patient, Michael Folkes, who'd changed his name in a bizarre tribute to the Paul Newman character in the film *Cool Hand Luke*, had been under psychiatric supervision after a less serious offence some time before.

Folkes had turned up in a distressed state at the Maudsley psychiatric hospital, but was allowed to leave by clinical staff. The next day he stabbed Susan Crawford seventy times and beat her with a fire extinguisher, just eight hours after he had been earmarked for emergency re-admission. He was convicted of manslaughter at the Old Bailey in 1995 and sent to Broadmoor.

The subsequent inquiry, which dragged on for four years at a cost of £750,000, recommended supported accommodation for those with mental illness and criticised the decision that had allowed Folkes to switch from compulsory treatment with a long-acting injectable medication to self-administered tablets. The consequences for the senior forensic psychiatrist who had overseen this decision were serious.

Not long after this case, the decision was taken to beef up aftercare arrangements for forensic cases, with specialist teams monitoring more closely those patients leaving secure hospital – especially those who had killed before.

After a homicide inquiry, it is inevitable that forensic psychiatrists become more risk-averse and cautious about granting leave outside hospital and discharging patients, but it is important not to let these instincts affect the liberty of patients. These days, 'positive risk-taking' and 'patient flow' have become catchphrases used by managers when pushing us to discharge more cases and save money. It's just as glib as it sounds: at the end of the day, it is the psychiatrist who will have to answer for their decision if it all goes wrong.

None of this was doing much good for my already fragile state of mind. There were muttered words of sympathy from colleagues, but everyone knew the reality was that these homicides could be potentially career-ending. A poor assessment – even if that assessment was based on incomplete information – could mean being suspended, dismissed or publicly humiliated; it could mean facing clinical negligence proceedings or investigation by the General Medical Council. Inevitably it's all about process. You're entitled to make an error of judgement unless your actions were too far away from what colleagues would have done, but the real issues include whether you formally recorded your findings and shared information with other appropriate agencies.

In the event, it would be months before I gave evidence to the SUI panel and over a year until the public homicide inquiry.

After the meeting, there were a number of important tasks. Risk of serious harm overriding any concerns about patient confidentiality, I rang my police contact and he suggested I speak directly to the SIO (senior investigation officer). I called the mobile number, and it was answered by Commander Andy Baker, head of Metropolitan Police Homicide. 'How can I help you, doctor? I'm rather busy this morning – looking for human heads in a landfill site.'

My breath caught in my throat. *Could I have prevented this?* Should I have transferred Hardy to our secure unit and asked for a Broadmoor opinion? I described Hardy's harassment of his ex-wife, and Commander Baker confirmed that the investigation team were aware of this and that uniformed officers were posted at Hardy's ex-wife's house.

Meanwhile, Hardy remained at large for around a week. The CCTV which captured him buying black bin liners in his local Sainsbury's, and claiming the Nectar points, suggested a calm and purposeful behaviour around the time that he was dismembering the bodies in his flat.

It also emerged that, earlier in December 2002, Hardy had telephoned Frances Mayhew, a twenty-five-year-old Camden resident, to tell her he'd found her handbag. She had mislaid it after an evening out at a Camden pub not far from Hardy's flat. Mayhew later said that when she went to his flat to retrieve the bag, Hardy tried to entice her in, but she refused. She said, 'I started to get frightened and said, "Listen, you can keep the bag, I don't want it anymore" . . . As I tried to run, he said, "Fine, you may as well keep it." And then he flung it at me.' Three days later, she received letters and a Christmas card from Hardy. She left the city over the Christmas break but on her return to Camden she discovered that Hardy was wanted by police and so she came forward to tell the story. 'Had he been at all violent and tried to drag me into the flat or something, the likelihood of me being in small pieces right now is very high,' she said. During searches of Hardy's flat, a drawing was found of Frances Mayhew with a noose around her neck.

With Hardy still at large, there was a very real fear he might find another victim before he could be caught.

After a tense few days, an off-duty police officer spotted Hardy in a cafeteria in Great Ormond Street children's hospital. GOSH was about one-and-a-half miles from Hardy's flat, and Hardy had gone to the NHS pharmacy there to collect his insulin prescription (perhaps to avoid being seen at a Camden chemist). When arrest was attempted, a fight ensued, during which one police officer was knocked unconscious and another was stabbed in the hand and received a dislocated eye socket. Back-up arrived and Hardy was, at last, safely detained.

After the arrest, a detective who searched him changed his forensic examination gloves for a fresh pair and Hardy laughed, saying that he preferred Marigolds. And indeed, Marigold gloves were found when police searched his flat, along with devil masks, which he used to put on the victims' faces before he photographed them. There were huge quantities of pornographic videotapes. Police recovered fantasy letters he had written, intending to send them to magazines, illustrating various sexual encounters he claimed to have had. He had marked 'Rose White RIP' on a glass bottle.

During their seven-week search of the flat, police found numerous cruciform graffiti and weird satanic drawings. Hardy had also sent film negatives to a friend, which were developed at a laboratory in Soho. The photos included forty-four photos of his victims (already dead, as confirmed by the forensic pathologist, who noted the post-mortem skin lividity, a gravity-related redness caused by the settling of blood after death). They were shown with masked faces and posed with sex toys, and the lab that developed them had assumed they were consensual photos, untrained as they were in post-mortem skin changes. In the case of Ms Valad, Hardy had dressed her up in a pair of Mr Happy socks that he'd bought on 6 December.

Analysing behaviour before, during and after an offence is always important in trying to determine state of mind at the 'material time' (a technical legal term used to refer to the immediate period around the killing). Hardy's pre-trial assessments were to be conducted by others, previously unconnected with the case, but I had to start thinking about how this might play out at trial. Although Hardy had a history of depression as part of a suspected bipolar disorder, there appeared to be no evidence, so far, of a mental state disturbed by active symptoms. But his double (or triple) murder had all the emerging hallmarks of a sexually motivated killing by a likely psychopath or sexual sadist.

It is very common in forensic psychiatry to have limited information from an interview of the subject. With Hardy, it was necessary to try and piece together a formulation based on what we knew from the available records, attempting to fill in the blanks of his account, given the known outcome. He had described being a thrill-seeker in childhood, and the description of his marriage suggested an egocentric or narcissistic and callous man, who had treated his wife appallingly while pursuing self-gratification through extra-marital affairs. We had evidence of extensive pornography use, as well as prostitutes, and now two bodies, killed sequentially by what was later thought to be crush asphyxiation. In other words, having killed the first, he must have lured the second to his flat in what probably started as a consensual transactional encounter but then became homicidal once he was in control. The posing and humiliation of the bodies seemed to suggest a sadistic element, with Hardy enjoying his sense of control over his victims. The likelihood of diabetes-related impotence fuelled the speculation that this domination had replaced an overtly sexual act.

Sexual homicides are rare and include the compulsive or organised subtype, where, as suggested by New York forensic psychologist Louis Schlesinger, 'a fusion of sex and aggression results in a powerful internal drive' such that the killing itself is sexually gratifying.[3] Alternatively, sexual homicides may be explosive and disorganised as a result of a breakthrough of underlying sexual conflicts. Both subtypes can be planned or unplanned; for example, a sex killing may be opportunistic if the killer happens to encounter a suitable victim. Some murders with a sexual element may be a panic killing after a sexual offence, in a vain attempt to evade detection. Every crime is different and the above divisions are to some extent simplistic, but I was guided by certain questions. Was Hardy a compulsive and organised sex killer? Was he a sexual sadist? Was he also a psychopath?

In the 1886 forensic classic, *Psychopathia Sexualis* – also a favourite in fetish bookshops – Richard von Krafft-Ebing noted the fact that lust and cruelty frequently occur together, writing, 'sadism . . . may also consist of an innate desire to humiliate, hurt, wound or even destroy others in order to create sexual pleasure . . . [and] may become an unlimited desire for subjugation.'

Of course, many paraphilias – or 'intense and persistent' sexual preferences – like certain fetishes which may involve sexual arousal to inanimate objects such as clothing and shoes, or consensual sexual practices like bondage, domination or sadomasochism, are not abnormal or criminal. But when they involve 'psychological distress, injury or death' to others – for example paedophilia, or secretly filming voyeuristic images of women in public places through 'upskirting', then they cross the line to sexual deviance or what we now call 'paraphilic disorders', and can become criminal offences.[4] This distinction has proven to be a contentious but important one.

It became the central issue, and led to a bizarre and uncomfortable experience for me, at the trial of a fetish-obsessed murderer, Michael Wenham, at Reading Crown Court. He had killed a prostitute while depressed as a result of a botched penis-extension surgery, paid for with £15,000 that he and his wife had been saving to buy a caravan. There was a dispute at his trial about whether anyone was distressed by his sexual perversions, as exemplified by extreme pornography found on his computer. So, despite my protestations that a psychiatrist has no expertise in judging the mental state of actors in porn films, the judge decided he would rather the two experts resolved this issue in a side-room. You can understand his reasoning, as the alternative would have been to turn the courtroom into a sleazy cinema. So while the jury were given a break, I found myself with a fellow psychiatrist and my junior psychiatrist-in-training in a conference room full of lawyers with wigs on, as we watched the pornographic footage found on the killer's laptop. Were the people in the footage enjoying themselves or were they distressed? In other words, was this paraphilia or paraphilic disorder?

I suggested that subjugation and humiliation was part of the overall theme of the pornography. My opposing expert, a distinguished professor, gave the opposite opinion, namely that everyone seemed to be enjoying themselves.

Wenham was, as you would expect, convicted of murder regardless of the forensic analysis of his porn collection. As I joined the commuters on the train from Reading back to London, I found myself wondering, not for the first or last time, how I ended up in this highly idiosyncratic branch of medicine.

Park Dietz, a high-profile American forensic psychiatrist, and technical adviser to the TV show *Law & Order*, had described an escalating pattern of 'paraphilia' as following a series of stages. Stage one: sexual fantasies and masturbation. Stage two: enticing a sexual partner to act out the paraphilia. Stage three: paying prostitutes to act out the paraphilia. Stage four: abducting or coercing victims to act out the paraphilia.[5] Wenham's escalation had clearly followed this pattern, as he had cajoled his wife into participation and had hired various sex workers, including a dominatrix.

At Broadmoor high-secure hospital, Malcolm MacCulloch, in a study of sixteen psychopathic sexual offenders, noted that there was a progression of sadistic fantasies, which continuously changed to maintain arousal and pleasure. He noted that 'behavioural try-outs' were very important in organised compulsive sexual crimes.[6] So it seemed plausible that Hardy had been developing fantasies of domination and killing. But had he also been enacting 'try-outs' by getting prostitutes, before Rose, to agree to being tied up? New Jersey-based psychiatrist Eugene Revitch wrote that, contrary to popular belief, erection, ejaculation and intercourse do not necessarily accompany a violent (sexually motivated) assault or murder, since the brutal act may be a substitute for the sexual act.[7] This could well have been Hardy's way of achieving gratification now diabetes had rendered him impotent.

Dr Reid Meloy, forensic psychologist and professor at the University of California, has interviewed many serial sexual killers and has consulted with the FBI, assessing Timothy McVeigh, the Oklahoma bomber, and Ted Kaczynski, the Unabomber, among many other high-profile cases. Meloy has written influential works on the psychopathic mind,[8] predatory violence and threat assessment.[9] It occurred to me that Hardy was starting to fit into patterns of sexual sadism and psychopathic violence noted by Meloy.[10] A psychopathic person is someone who has an elevated score on the Psychopathy Checklist – Revised (PCL-R) – or psychopath test – an extensively researched measure developed by Canadian psychologist Robert Hare that is widely used in forensic settings, although the reliability of scoring remains controversial.[11]

The test measures personality traits and behaviours including callousness, lack of empathy, pathological lying, impulsivity and having a parasitic lifestyle. A high score on the test has been linked to violent behaviour, abnormal brain function[12] and impaired moral reasoning.[13]

The cut-off for being a psychopath is thirty out of a possible forty points in the United States, but a lower cut-off is often used in Europe (as a 'glib and superficial charm' is said to be more common in the US).

To call a person a psychopath is problematic. Forensic psychiatrist John Gunn argues that the label is stigmatising because of the associations, in common usage, with cruelty and monstrous behaviour.[14] There is also the danger of reification: that is, by giving a tentative hypothesis (here, psychopathy) a fancy name, it sounds as though psychologists and psychiatrists have discovered a new condition, when in fact it is merely a description. However, since those with high scores on the checklist are frequently found among those who commit sexual homicide, I will use the term psychopath as it is pithy, albeit imprecise and pejorative. I will do so on the basis that, when used in this book, it implies an individual with personality traits and behaviours commensurate with a PCL-R score above twenty-seven out of forty.

Meloy pointed out that the 'wish' to kill the object of one's sexual desires is 'peculiarly understandable' in some disturbed and aggressive males, arising from a combination of sexual longing and aggressive devaluation of the female object of desire – perhaps because of previous rejections by women. But the 'act' – rather than merely the 'wish' – of intentionally killing the object of one's sexual desire, is the most extreme form of sexual aggression and is a relatively rare event, accounting for fewer than one per cent of homicides in the USA. However, this progression from a 'wish' to kill a sexual object to a homicidal 'act' seemed to apply to Hardy's depraved offences.

Meloy also argues that serial sexual homicides are examples of predatory violence, which is planned, purposeful and emotionless. The evolutionary basis of predation is hunting.[15] In Hardy's case, the targets were vulnerable young prostitutes and the goal was to sexually assault, kill and dominate even after death by posing the bodies in a humiliating way, and then by dismembering them. A more common type of violence much more often seen in murder cases is impulsive, reactive and emotional, often referred to as 'affective' or 'self-preservative' violence, and I will return to this later.

Research has shown that psychopathic individuals are much more likely than other criminals to engage in predatory violence and appear to be particularly suited to doing so.

Cat behaviour is a good example of this distinction. When

a cat is cornered by a dog, its hair will stand on end and it will hiss, in warning mode, with an arched back, wide eyes and teeth and claws exposed. This is 'affective violence', an instinctual behaviour designed for survival against an imminent threat. However, I once observed a cat in my back garden stalking a nesting blackbird and its chicks. It was crouched low to the surface of the wall, making no sound, with teeth and claws retracted. During predation, the animal needs to inhibit arousal to be successful in killing its prey. This lack of emotion has been noted in both adolescent and adult mass murder cases, examples of criminal violence that are virtually always predatory.

Meloy suggests that psychopaths are better at predatory violence thanks to their low levels of arousal and reactivity, as well as the fact that they are grandiose and self-important, emotionally detached and lack empathy with their victims' suffering.

Did this apply to Hardy, given his killing and dismemberment of his victims, or was he merely a sexual sadist? There is technically a distinction, but both sexual sadists and psychopaths tend to inflict pain or injuries on others while being emotionally detached from the suffering they cause.

Sexual sadists and psychopaths use extensive fantasy preparation before they engage in predatory violence, and it seems likely that Hardy's pornography use may have taken him from a more benign predilection for consensual bondage and sado-masochism to an extreme form of sadism; namely, pleasure through dominance to the point of power over life and death, with a remorseless disregard for the rights and feelings of his victims and their families.

All of this leads to the question of whether sadists and psychopaths are made or born. A small proportion of behaviourally disturbed children have been found to have callous and unemotional traits, and these fledgling psychopaths are more likely to engage in serious violent behaviour when they grow up. Research by Essi Viding at UCL confirms that violent behaviour can be genetic: that is, inherited.[16] But a genetic predisposition to psychopathy and violence may be aggravated if the child experiences significant abuse.[17]

Hardy may well have been callous and unemotional, and his admitted thrill-seeking may have been a way to try and self-stimulate given a lack of arousal, but had he been mistreated in childhood, could he have turned out even worse?

With the evidence of sexually sadistic behaviour – which had not been identified before – it was becoming clear that Hardy's bouts of high and low moods, which psychiatrists had diagnosed as bipolar disorder, were of little relevance to the killings.

Hardy was assessed by a psychiatrist appointed by his defence team and it was expected that all these issues would be teased out in a high-profile Old Bailey trial, but Hardy pre-empted this with an unexpected late guilty plea to the three murders.

So the barristers for prosecution and defence had to prepare for sentencing, with each presenting aggravating and mitigating factors accordingly. Not much mitigation here, you may well think, and with mandatory life imprisonment, the only question became the minimum prison term before possible parole.

From a moral, philosophical and legal perspective, to what degree does the different neurobiology, reduced arousal level and impaired empathic abilities of a psychopath, or a sexual sadist like Hardy, limit or enhance their free will? Generally in the legal context, and especially in the United States, sexual sadism disorder and psychopathy are seen as aggravating rather than mitigating factors, viewed as more of a defect of character punishable by law, rather than a mental disorder worthy of reduced criminal culpability.

Hearing about brutal multiple murder cases such as this one, people ask me why we don't still have the death penalty. Of course the return of hanging in the UK would be popular with some. I saw protesters with a noose outside the Old Bailey when Lee Rigby's killers were being sentenced in 2013. Let's hope we never have a referendum on the subject. There are a few arguments in favour of the death penalty, namely the enhanced retribution of 'an eye for an eye' and a greater deterrence factor, which populist politicians – trading on their hard-line law-and-order credentials – occasionally endorse (including Home Secretary Priti Patel). But there are also many arguments against: the unconstitutional 'cruel and unusual punishment' of a prolonged death-row experience, the breach of human rights, and the difficulty of obtaining the drugs required for lethal injections being just a few. Perhaps the most cogent argument against is to ask, can we always be one hundred per cent certain we are hanging/shooting/electrocuting/poisoning the right person? We had better be sure there's been no cross-contamination of DNA at the crime scene or in the forensic lab because if so, there won't be much comfort in a successful appeal.

In around fifty-eight countries the death penalty still applies – usually by shooting (China), beheading (Saudi Arabia) or hanging. In the USA, the sixty or so inmates awaiting lethal injection raise all sorts of questions for my forensic psychiatrist colleagues. For example, I'm glad I don't get asked to medically certify that a prisoner's mental competence is now restored enough for their death sentence to be carried out. Can a doctor treat someone to make them fit for execution? Believe it or not, in the USA it happens.

These days, a UK judge has no sentencing discretion after a murder conviction. Introduced following the abolition of the death penalty in 1965, the mandatory life sentence is there, in place of the hangman's noose, to reassure the public that murderers will not get off lightly after avoiding the drop. A murderer will automatically become a 'lifer', which means that, after an extended period in prison custody, they can only ever be released on a 'life licence' (parole). This means they will be supervised and liable to be recalled to prison for the rest of their natural life, even if later paroled. However, the judge sets the minimum term. That is the period of time that must be served for retribution and punishment before any application for parole can be made. Life sentence minimum terms for murder nowadays start at fifteen years and go up to thirty years or whole life, depending on how serious the aggravating features are. Years are added or subtracted depending on aggravating or mitigating factors.

Hardy had pleaded guilty.

Murder (three times over) – Life sentence (three times over).

Hardy's tariff was later upgraded to a whole-life-term sentence, one of only seventy in the UK, but not the last that I would see.

An expert who saw Hardy before trial – referred to as 'Dr K' in the public inquiry report – also opined that, for Hardy, the onset of diabetes was an enormous blow.

'His distress, anger and frustration at the diminution of his sexual prowess has been expressed in increasingly sadistic sexual activity . . . I believe the offending is linked to the defendant's sadistic personality, his intoxication with alcohol and his rage at his sexual dysfunction induced by diabetes.'

I think that sums it up pretty well.

In the meantime came the issue of how and why Hardy had been released from St Luke's in November. It turned out that our detailed risk assessment report had lain unread in a post-room tray, but the review panel had gone ahead anyway. Our recommendation to inform the police via MAPPA had of course not been followed up.

MAPPA[18] was in its infancy then and its role was not well understood. In any event, psychiatrists were wary of sharing information with the police. Later I would become involved in trying to improve that, and our forensic service would pioneer working jointly with the police force, but in 2002 Hardy had been released by an appeal panel back to his own home. He had been offered supervised accommodation but had objected to this, saying it was too strict and that he wanted somewhere more liberal. This was his choice to make, as the legal mechanism to enforce staffed accommodation was not enacted until 2007. He had attended one of the psychiatric wards on 27 December to collect some medication and it was noted that he appeared stable. By then it is likely that both of his victims already lay dead in his flat.

Some months passed and the local SUI panel began to hear evidence. Three members of the board grilled witnesses about the case and went on to draft a report. Over a year later, after much press coverage, the independent homicide inquiry would convene. Fortunately, I was never named in the press – although I am outing myself now. There were five of us who had seen Hardy during 2002, and several more had seen him in the years before that.

As you might imagine, the inquiry was a sword of Damocles hanging over me, thoughts of which had to be suppressed while my work continued. I questioned my judgement about every decision that year. No surprise there. It was the same tendency to risk aversion that is inevitable after a homicide. As forensic psychiatrists, we do society's dirty and difficult work and are caught in a daily dilemma between two unhappy positions: the rock of the coroner's court after a serious further offence, and the hard place of contested review tribunal over a patient's detention. Damned by lawyers, pressure groups and the media for detaining, restraining and medicating our patients, and also pilloried by professional bodies and independent panels for releasing them when it all goes wrong.

The full public inquiry was to be chaired by well-known solicitor Robert Robinson, a mental health specialist, with two professors of psychiatry contributing to the review: Professor Tom Sensky on the panel and Professor Tony Maden, then running the new DSPD or Dangerous Severe Personality Disorder unit at Broadmoor as independent expert adviser. I had written a detailed statement, which was sent to my malpractice insurers the Medical Protection Society for comment, and we spent a day preparing with solicitors instructed to represent the forensic service.

Finally, on a bright sunny day in 2004, I took the tube to Victoria and made my way to the modern glass offices of NHS London. Professor Sensky and Robert Robinson asked me probing questions about all aspects of the case, from assessment and diagnosis to risk assessment and information sharing. I don't remember the precise wording of the questions I was asked that day, but I do remember that I had that strange feeling of derealisation that goes along with anxiety (or exhaustion after a long night on call). It feels as if the floor is tilting against your feet, as if you are not really in the room and this is not really happening, a mildly dream-like state. I must have snapped back to reality as Professor Sensky asked, 'Did you consider the possibility that he was a sexual sadist, a potential serial killer?'

'No, I didn't,' I replied. 'He was clearly misogynist, aggressive and perverse, but we had to base our assessment on the assumption that the first death had been from natural causes. His depression and bipolar were relatively minor compared to other cases, plus he'd been agreeing to take medication and engage with his team. In short, he was not detainable under the Mental Health Act.'

By this time, of course, the flaws in the original post-mortem on Rose White had emerged. When Freddy Patel's evidence was later reviewed by Nat Cary, a more experienced and highly respected forensic pathologist, it was noted that – incredibly – Patel had not taken the crime scene into account in his report. Also, given the blood on the back of Rose's head, the brain should have been sent for neuropathology. Subsequently, likely cause of death was amended to asphyxia.

Patel was later struck off the medical register after the infamous Tomlinson case (a newspaper seller who died after being floored by an over-enthusiastic riot police officer), and it transpired that Patel's sloppy practice involved perfunctory post-mortems routinely diagnosing cardiac deaths. The tragic consequences of his actions had not been limited to the Hardy case and the General Medical Council concluded that his work was 'not of the standard expected of a competent forensic pathologist and liable to bring the medical profession into disrepute'.

I don't recall exactly the rest of the questions I was asked by the panel, but they went something like this: 'Do you think the police should have been notified of his discharge?' This in reference to Hardy's release in November 2002.

'Absolutely,' I told them. 'We had recommended that he be referred to MAPPA.'

'But that didn't happen, Dr Taylor. Can you explain that to the panel?'

'MAPPA is very new. The mental health teams are not familiar with how it is supposed to work. Psychiatrists and police are not used to talking to each other.'

That was about to change and this case was influential in that regard.

'Do you have any other comments to make?'

'Only that in all honesty, I understand an appeals panel will have to discharge if the detention criteria are not met, but a notification to the police via MAPPA might have allowed a discussion to take place between agencies. Our assessment was based on incorrect information from the start. We had no way of knowing that he was a sexual sadist.'

The reality is that even if police had known about his release, the only certain way to prevent the offences would have been twenty-four-hour surveillance, and however concerned the police might have been, it is very unlikely this would have been carried out.

My points were noted and, released from my duty, I emerged on to the sunny street. Office workers were enjoying their lunchtime sandwiches but I had no appetite, and I didn't feel any relief. Oblivious to the sunny weather, I trudged to the tube station at St James's Park, not able to face the crowds at Victoria. As I walked, the tragic faces of Hardy's victims played on my mind.

It was another year before the inquiry published their findings – a whole year of that sword still hanging over my head. Meanwhile, my day-to-day work continued: review meetings of inpatients, every decision to grant community leave considered and recorded in detail, every recommendation and risk assessment a source of corrosive anxiety. For me, the thought of another homicide inquiry was too much to contemplate. The work went on and the cases rolled in: ward rounds and tribunals, wounding with intent and arson.

But then came another sexual homicide case that dragged my mind away from thoughts of Hardy.

Case Study: Lee Watson

3

It is sometimes said that you don't choose forensic psychiatry, forensic psychiatry chooses you. Attributes required for the profession include having the stamina for long journeys to remote prisons, a strong stomach, and steady nerves in the face of violent patients. Add to that an understanding of the detailed nuances of psychiatric and legal language, as the liberty or otherwise of a defendant can hinge on the precise wording of a phrase or two. You also need a thick skin for cross-examination by the Middle Temple and Lincoln's Inn's finest. And that's just for starters. It differs from standard medicine. To be a doctor, you have to be ready at the end of a blue-light ambulance ride to deal with whatever emerges; to be a forensic psychiatrist, you have to be ready at the end of a secure van ride from Belmarsh to manage those arrivals too disturbed for a high-security prison.

We forensic psychiatrists tend to fall into three subtypes. First, the so-called 'surgeons of psychiatry' – brash and confident types who wear suits, pride themselves on being decisive and don't listen to their colleagues. These types tend to have more of a prosecution-leaning approach, coupled with a refusal to accept there might be any chink in their armour. At the other end of the spectrum you have what you might call the halo brigade. They are not interested in taking on extra murder cases as an expert witness; they wear oatmeal wool jumpers with elbow patches and see themselves as treating deprived and unfortunate members of society – no matter how wicked they've been – and always with a rehabilitation focus and patient care at the centre of their work.

Somewhere in between, where I and most of my colleagues like to see ourselves, are those who are a mixture of both: psychiatrists with an attraction to clear-cut thinking and detailed analysis, but also the ability to empathise and communicate with troubled men and women, and their victims.

No matter what stripe, all of us need to be able to formulate complex interactions of brain, mind, social relationships and behaviour. We take the lead in our teams, knowing that we are responsible for detention and the prescription of mind-altering psychotropic drugs. We have to carefully translate all of this into legal language for the court and then, in the event of a trial, convert it further into plain English for the jury.

So it is not a job for the faint-hearted, and just as many trainees are put off by the pressure as are attracted by the challenge of it.

Most crucial of all, in my view, is an understanding of your own psychological make-up and cultural preconceptions, so you can monitor your reaction to a diverse patient group and challenging scenarios and think and reflect before acting. It was only some time after I became a consultant that I began to ponder, as have many of my colleagues, on the tragic impact of mental illness on my very own family – something I'll go into greater detail on later. This reflection and awareness of vulnerability is what gives us, I think, the tolerance for madness and self-destruction, setting us apart from other medics and surgeons.

I needed all of these essentials for the case of Lee Watson.

One Friday afternoon in March 2003, while waiting for the Hardy case to work its way through the system, my secretary alerted me to a four-inch-thick envelope bearing the frank of the solicitors Motts Lewis. I'd intended to leave work slightly early, but curiosity got the better of me, so I tore it open and began to thumb through the contents.

The opening pages bore the familiar scales of justice logo of the Crown Prosecution Service. Treasury tags in the top left-hand corner held the various sub-divisions of papers together: indictment, witness statements, custody record, ROTI (record of taped interview), exhibits, unused material and prosecution case summary. I cleared two dirty coffee cups and some unopened journals from my corner desk and set out the papers in separate piles for an initial read-through, sticky notes and highlighters at the ready.

The first few witness statements were from police officers describing the discovery of a young woman's body in woods near an underpass of the A2 close to Dartford. Locals, interviewed about what they'd seen, talked of spotting a young man with cropped dark hair, wearing a green or brown short jacket.

I skipped on to the crime-scene photographs. You can tell a great deal from looking at the evidence of behaviour at the crime scene. Exasperated by a defence expert who hadn't considered the crime scene – and with the gallows humour common to cops – a homicide detective once asked me, 'How can you comment on Picasso without admiring his handiwork?'

The pictures were presented in sequence, beginning with innocuous images of a sparsely wooded area covered in autumn leaves. The ground was on the other side of a low fence away from the path, where the only indication that something was amiss were the usual signs of 'forensication' of the scene, with police tape in the background and plastic stepping plates to avoid disturbing possible footprint evidence.

The body had been discovered by a dog sniffing around, leading the owner to some fingertips protruding from the undergrowth. Police photographs showed the makeshift coverings being removed in sequence: leaves were brushed aside and then old timbers of a rotting pallet were removed. Finally, the naked body of a young, dark-haired woman was revealed.

This was twenty-three-year-old Chiara Leonetti, a Bond Street sales assistant from Milan.

Looking through, I was already starting to formulate an impression. This appeared to be chaotic, impulsive behaviour, conducted in broad daylight, probably a tragic chance encounter rather than the calculated predatory behaviour of, say, Hardy, who had lured his victims into his flat before overpowering them.

The crime scene photographs then continued with the transport of the body to the mortuary, through to the post-mortem, a sequence which began with the victim's body lying supine on the forensic pathology slab. There was a terrible injury to her left leg – a foot mangled – and although this would turn out to be the work of a fox, other wounds were evident, especially catastrophic injuries to the left side of the skull and face, later said to be consistent with being hit with a heavy rock.

Subsequent photographs showed the pathologist, Dr David Green, cutting through the ribcage, taking out the vital organs for weighing and for dissection in order to exclude death by natural causes. Then the scalp and facial tissues were cut away to examine in more detail the injuries below the skin. A further series of photos showed the victim's body being gradually dismantled in the pathologist's meticulous search for evidence to explain the cause of death.

In the event, Dr Green concluded that the victim had indeed died from those terrible head injuries. These had been sustained during repeated blows to the head, including several with a hard-edged object. Noted was the fact that a blood-stained brick was found near the body. There were pre-mortem bite marks on the left ear, left breast and on the pubis, and several post-mortem abrasions suggested the body was dragged to its final position.

Worst of all, though, was the evidence of severe sexual assault. The victim's lower clothing and bra were not present and Dr Green found injuries consistent with severe mutilation of the abdomen and genital area. Blessedly, these injuries had been inflicted after the victim's death. But there was no DNA evidence to suggest rape or ejaculation by the killer.

When the case later went to court, Dr Green told the jury that of over 20,000 post-mortems he'd conducted, he'd only seen one other case with such severe post-mortem genital mutilation injuries. Had the killer returned later to the scene of the crime to further mutilate his victim's body? I would have to ask him.

Time had got ahead of me, so I decided to brave the Friday evening traffic and head home. As I drove, I wondered if I'd regret having read the papers just before leaving work on a Friday. The following day, I took the children to the local park, saw piles of autumn leaves beneath the trees and sure enough, I couldn't help but think of the crime scene, while that night, in bed, my wife's dark hair was a troubling reminder of the corpse. At every turn, it seemed, were the images from the papers I had read, polluting what should have been happy family moments.

By Sunday evening I'd given up even trying to put the case out of my mind and began reading some of the witness statements.

The young man who had been spotted in the area turned out to be Lee Watson.

Watson's sister, Candice, described how his behaviour had become strange in his twenties. She said that he lied about his work and talked of being arrested for an assault she believed he'd invented. She also said their mother found photographs of women in his room who looked like prostitutes in sexual poses.

Elsewhere, numerous witnesses including family, his former girlfriend, and acquaintances reported his habit of repeated deception in the form of what we call self-aggrandising lies. It would later emerge that his workmates referred to him as 'a phony' for his tendencies to invent stories about fictitious girlfriends and cars, and and to fabricate excuses for his poor timekeeping. In fact, his GP counsellor – whom he had gone to see for depression – confirmed that he had begun to acknowledge his lying and felt bad that it had led to the break-up of his relationship. (I felt for the GP counsellor – this case was a bit beyond what she must have been trained for.)

Meanwhile, various witnesses who saw the defendant around the time of the attack described him as 'crazy', 'nutty' and 'loony'. He claimed to one that he had a gun, and that someone had just beaten up his girlfriend. They said he was 'pretty racist' and was 'jumping around, acting funny, drunk or on drugs'.

Meanwhile, the police had linked him to other attacks on women in the North Kent area, all of which had occurred on the same day. First, he had approached forty-four-year-old Shireen Noor from behind, grabbing her bag and arm and pulling her hair so hard that a large clump was torn out. Noor was dragged for about fifteen metres in the direction of a wooded area before Watson ran off.

Twenty minutes later, a seventy-eight-year-old victim, Denise Wallace, was attacked from behind. When Watson put his hand over her mouth, she bit his fingers hard, which caused him to let go and run off. Later, at 5.25 p.m., fifty-one-year-old Tina Harris was also attacked from behind before being punched in the face. Watson escaped with her bag and was seen running off in the direction of the nearby roundabout.

A short time later that same day came the murder itself. Chiara Leonetti had travelled home on the 492 bus from Bexleyheath to Foots Cray but had disembarked early. By a cruel twist of fate, she'd taken a different bus to normal because of the warm weather. At 5.51 p.m. a friend telephoned her mobile from Milan. The call was answered and her friend heard cries of distress, sobbing or wailing, along with the noise of buttons on the receiving phone being pressed.

Chiara Leonetti's body was found the following day.

Everything I learned reinforced my initial impressions of the murderer as chaotic and impulsive, rather than calculated and considered. A man who took advantage of random encounters instead of planning in advance. I was already formulating questions for an interview.

The following week I travelled to interview Lee Watson at HMP Belmarsh, which is one of the UK's eight high-security prisons, built on former marshland next to the Thamesmead estate and near the Crossness sewage treatment works on the edge of south-east London. A grim and imposing but modern brick building, it had been copied from an American model, no doubt to save money on architects.

Some of the more hardened prison officers – and Belmarsh has its share – view visiting psychiatrists with disdain and suspicion. We're there to help both prosecution and defence make sense of these cases, but even though we may well be instructed by the 'good guys', officers see us as potentially 'nutting off' prisoners to a cushy hospital when they should remain behind bars.

All of which means we often don't have the warmest of receptions, and it's not uncommon for our journeys to be in vain. 'Sorry, Doc,' we'll be told, 'he doesn't want to see you, won't come out of his cell,' only for us to hear later, from a concerned solicitor, that their client had been waiting anxiously for the expected visit, and nobody had ever knocked on their cell door.

These days I am more assertive in such circumstances, insisting on being taken to the cell and asking to speak to a

Governor grade if not. Circumstances change all the time, of course, and I have to adjust – adaptability being another quality needed for my profession. More than once I've interviewed highly paranoid and aggressive prisoners through a cell wicket, or over the shoulders of prison officers kitted out in riot gear. Other times an interview is simply not possible. If the prisoner won't cooperate, or is so acutely psychotic they're unresponsive on the cell floor, smeared in their own faeces, then an opinion must be based on observed and reported behaviour alone.

Having checked in at the front gate of Belmarsh with my faxed booking confirmation, I left my watch, keys and wallet in a locker, keeping only paper and two pens (no paper clips or treasury tags). The checks, a notch up from airport security, involved metal detector walk-through, electric wand and thorough pat-down searches, having removed all items including cufflinks, belt and shoes. I then had to wait patiently for my escort, the prison healthcare nurse, before we crossed a yard patrolled by dog handlers wearing black paramilitary fatigues and radio earpieces, Alsatians straining at their leashes.

It's a place that instils fear and paranoia. My first time there I found myself wondering if I'd ever get out, if they'd detain me on a trumped-up charge or maybe for some long-forgotten minor transgression.

As usual, prison vans stood waiting for inmates, like a high-security taxi rank. Although people imagine that a prison with a population of around 1,500 is largely static, a London remand prison will have up to a hundred movements every day. These include prisoners going to court and coming back again, those being transferred to training prison, and fresh detainees from court.

Each prisoner is checked in and logged, and personal possessions have to be bagged and recorded. Prison-issue clothing is handed out, usually oversized grey or red tracksuits depending on the prison. There is a cursory health screening examination by a nurse. Forms are filled in and a prison GP will see anybody with more severe medical problems. Up to a third of prisoners will be withdrawing from illicit drugs, such as heroin, or from alcohol, and will need some kind of detoxification regimen to prevent them from having seizures or other problems on the wing.

Typically, severely psychiatrically disturbed patients and high-risk offenders will be escorted straight to a single cell in the healthcare centre for closer observation. This is recorded along with the 'inmate medical record' in a special orange-coloured file, which in 2003 could also be accompanied by a second file called a '2052SH' (SH for self-harm). The healthcare centre consists of a couple of dormitories with about ten beds, housing some patients with minor mental health issues needing observation, as well as patients with significant physical health problems, such as legs in plaster or other medical issues. The high-risk cases are in bare single cells with CCTV monitoring. The staff are a mixture of nurses in uniform and prison officers. An alarm-bell press can summon a rapid response team of burly prison officers within seconds.

We passed through a series of heavy steel doors, each requiring either a special laser-cut key or a CCTV and verbal check with the security control centre that no prisoner was trying to 'tail-gate'.

I found myself anticipating meeting the monster who'd killed this beautiful young woman and, perhaps for this reason, I was too impatient to wait for an interview room to become available, insisting on seeing him in his cell instead. In I walked at last and there he was: Lee Watson.

I'm often asked whether I can immediately determine someone's personality on first meeting. Of course I can't; we're not psychics. But give me one to two hours with a cooperative interviewee and I'll have a pretty good idea what's going on. A standard assessment involves a thorough biographical history and Mental State Examination, which is an established but flexible template that all psychiatrists use to explore the patient's inner world.

But it's not just what the subject tells us, it's how they tell us: how they behave and interact during the interview. We record how they look, how they speak: guarded and monosyllabic or garrulous and expansive. We enquire about specific issues such as mood, any suicidal or homicidal thoughts, anxiety, obsessions and compulsions. A detailed probe for the various forms of psychosis is essential.

We are looking for abnormalities of behaviour and mental state, which will help us understand (and recreate for our colleagues, or for the court) the psychopathology or the internal world and mental phenomena experienced by the individual. This is purely a description of their thoughts and feelings, which may point to a diagnosis, and is part of the bedrock of our profession first developed by the German-Swiss psychiatrist Karl Jaspers over a century ago. Traditionally, the final questions we ask the subject are about how they see themselves: do they think anything is wrong? And if so, what? This is because the question of their self-awareness or 'insight' can be important, especially later if we are to think about treatment.

Thus, a psychiatric interview is a bit like a tailor's dummy. We start with a standard framework, but the individual responses help us build up a picture, gradually adjusting and trimming our impression as more information comes through. We ask open questions, like, 'Tell me about your family life,' or, 'Have you developed any new interests recently?' – a question which has produced some hair-raising responses. If they speak freely, we let them run, but we may have to interrupt to clarify or probe when the answers are monosyllabic or unclear, or if they drift off the topic. It's important not to show too much reaction if you want their responses to be unmodified by feedback. Expressing shock might stop them giving a full account.

Watson was a quiet and slight man, about five foot six or seven, with close-cropped hair and a bewildered look on his face. Physically he was like a frightened schoolboy, the shy one in the corner of the playground. He did not come across initially as either the disorganised psychotic or the menacing psychopath the crime scene had indicated. As is so often the case in forensic psychiatry, preconceptions of what the killer would be like had to be re-evaluated.

Right from the beginning he was happy to engage with me, and cheerful. The tedium of long days behind a heavy steel door makes cooperative interviewees of the most recalcitrant. He told me that he was going to plead not guilty to murder, but guilty to manslaughter, claiming, 'I don't really remember what went on, I didn't know who or where I was.'

Amnesia doesn't count as a defence, of course, so he'd obviously misunderstood something his solicitor had told him. Back then, the legal test to be considered was the old 1957 Homicide Act definition of 'diminished', originally brought in to save the mentally disordered from a mandatory death penalty for murder. Though it was tightened up in 2009 to require a 'recognised medical condition', in 2003 Watson would still have had to demonstrate an 'abnormality of mind' that 'substantially impaired' his responsibility.

(Of course, as I knew well from my visits to American prisons and hospitals, only an insanity defence will save a killer from the full force of US sentencing, and in some states Watson would have been facing the death penalty.)

So that was my benchmark: did Watson have an abnormality of mind? And if so, which one?

He told me he had been at Belmarsh for about two-and-a-half months, in the hospital wing (a standard precaution, as murder followed by suicide used to be a significant problem amongst murder perpetrators in prison). He said that he was spending most of the time in his cell sleeping, eating and reading and that he was feeling fine, not depressed; in fact, he was upbeat about the future. 'I can see light at the end of the tunnel,' he told me.

Discussing his family history, he told me that he was born in Dartford, that his father ran a jeweller's shop in Sidcup and that his mother suffered from depression. He said, 'When I was a kid, I wasn't the norm. Inside I had a hatred . . . I was never satisfied with my Christmas presents . . . I felt like a bomb was exploding inside me.'

Was this hindsight bias, I wondered, knowing where he had ended up?

When I asked him about hobbies, his response was alarming. 'I used to love shooting animals in the back garden with air rifles. I had a great big collection of weapons, blank firing guns, deactivated guns, cannonballs, shells and machetes.'

I had suspected a disturbed development but this was pretty extreme. I tried hard to maintain my poker face, gently encouraging him to tell me more.

He described his gun collection: a deactivated Lee–Enfield bolt-action rifle, a replica MP5 sub-machine gun, and a replica Beretta 92FS air pistol. He also owned a Gurkha's kukri, a US military Ka-Bar utility knife, a First World War-era bayonet and a selection of Buck knives and box cutters. He told me he had tampered with the rifle and succeeded in adapting it to fire blank rounds, and he would feel exhilarated handling his collection of spent ammunition, which went from small-calibre cartridges to tank ammunition. He had also adapted his air guns with special springs and washers to increase their power beyond the legal limit.

'I used to hunt for pigeons and pheasants, starlings, rabbits and rats with snares and traps,' he told me, adding that if he found an animal still alive in a snare he might observe its suffering or shoot it to put it out of its misery. One incident he found particularly amusing was when he strapped a live rabbit to a fencepost and attached a large rocket firework. Once he'd lit the touch paper, the rabbit struggled to get free until the exploding rocket 'blew it to bits'. He also laughed while describing how he had stuffed a live pigeon into a drain to 'watch it die and rot', and kicked another pigeon, next 'throwing it into the air'.

He told me he was bullied at junior school in Gravesend, that he had been very small for his age, with freckles, all of which made him an easy target for the cruelty of other children throughout his schooldays. He felt he was naive and too friendly, and would lend toys to friends which were then stolen. He was being beaten up before school on a regular basis and by the age of eight had started to truant.

He went on to secondary school in Swanscombe where the bullying continued. By now, however, he was fighting back, and his retaliatory beatings of other children were going too far. He said he enjoyed hurting them if he got the better of them.

After school he started work-based training via a National Vocational Qualification in painting and decorating and undertook an apprenticeship as a trailer fitter. He was sweeping up and steam-cleaning trucks and trailers, but was unhappy, and bullied by the foreman, who called him a 'little shit'. This bullying, he said, would carry on throughout his working life. As a result he often skipped work and spent the day sitting on the Gravesend to Tilbury ferry, going back and forth.

Dismissed from this job for poor attendance, at the age of twenty-two he enlisted in the army's 2nd Signal Regiment as a mechanic. During basic training he was once thrown out of a Bedford truck and was constantly teased by fellow recruits who would sabotage his efforts, at one point stripping down an engine he'd just fixed. The army allowed his discharge without penalty.

He used to be reckless at work, for example leaving wheel nuts loose and swanning off on the job. During time as a loader he said that the foreman had teased him when he accidentally dropped a steel bar, and so Watson 'decked him', thinking, 'I'm damned if I'll let you take the mickey out of me.' He was dismissed for that, and said, 'All I ever wanted was a job I could do without someone having a pop at me. I stood my ground once.'

After painting and decorating, injection-moulding and machine-loading, he was unemployed for about a year and 'in a right mess', drinking heavily and breaking up with his girl-friend. 'Things started going wrong,' he told me, which was something of an understatement. He was hitting 'the crack, the weed, ecstasy, coke and speed' and was frequently as 'high as a kite'.

I asked him about his sexual preferences. He denied having any interest in sado-masochistic sex or any other fetishes or paraphilias. He denied ever attending strip clubs, and when I asked if he had ever used the services of a prostitute he replied, 'I can't remember.'

He said that he had recently spent time on sex chat lines, but had lied to the women he spoke to, 'just to meet someone who was going to treat me with respect, simple as that . . . they thought I was a high-flyer; they would say, "You sound really nice."'

His attempts at restoring his self-esteem were clearly desperate if he felt he had to lie to sex chat girls (this being before the internet explosion of online content for every sexual whim).

How reliable is his account? I asked myself. He seemed disarmingly honest about some pretty negative things. However, I suspected there were even darker corners of his life that he was keeping from me. I probed further, asking about his offending. He had previously been charged with attempted burglary, he told me. He was outside 'some bird's window'.

'I was having a wee, I ran off and she opened the window.' He said there was no evidence against him and, 'I had no knives. I wasn't watching her. There was no proof at all.'

This sounded like exhibitionism, perhaps an aborted 'fetish burglary' or even a contemplated 'burglary rape', confirmed by his spontaneous denial before I had asked him.

'I never exposed myself and I didn't try to get into her flat.'

I feared he was protesting too loudly. Could this be evidence of paraphilic escalation? Fetish burglaries can involve stealing underwear and masturbation, and are found in the histories of many sex murderers. Exhibitionism, fantasies about coercive sex, a 'try-out' of a fetish burglary, sexual assault . . . rape homicide?

His lies had been exposed recently when his girlfriend went to his family, but he admitted that he lied to 'make myself seem bigger'. He'd tell people he had expensive cars such as a Audi S4 Quattro, which he said was in a garage having its head gasket repaired. 'I used to lie about everything because I felt insignificant,' he said, and explained he would do it to make him feel like he was the 'one at the party'.

He had some depression and suicidal thoughts and his parents had nudged him to see the GP, hence the counsellor, but 'while seeing her I got a hell of a lot worse'. He said that the counsellor opened up things he'd not thought of. He learned that his lying hurt his family and friends and for that reason had been unable to cope with the counselling sessions.

It was pretty clear that his lies made him feel better about himself. I started to think the well-meaning counselling might have helped push him over the edge, taking away his only means of managing his low self-esteem. This had been coupled with the drugs and his girlfriend's rejection, while the exhibitionism at the window incident was a hint at the sexual frustration and misogynistic hostility that lay within.

I was beginning to build a picture of how Watson had escalated out of control.

4

A psychiatric murder report is best approached by first constructing a timeline. Starting with family origins, it is important to work through the subject's biography and gradually approach the material time with increasing detail. This involves careful questions about the day before, the night before, the morning of the offence and the killing itself.

Some defendants can't bear to describe the actual moments of the killing and you have to push them through the time frame to get to the act in question. Asking about the offence is always sensitive. We have to re-caution them, as more than once I've found myself witness for the prosecution. If someone denies or explains involvement in a murder, but later tells the psychiatrist a different version of events to the one they gave the police, then a senior prosecution barrister (Queen's Counsel or QC) can easily use this to trip up the defendant (or the psychiatrist) at trial. So we have to faithfully and very carefully record what we are told, since interview notes can be required by the court, with defence or prosecution counsel looking for any discrepancies.

I once spent an uncomfortable two days sitting in an Old Bailey courtroom behind Bill Clegg QC, clutching my interview notes and report, waiting in case he called me as a prosecution witness in a Samurai-sword murder case where one defendant had effectively given me a confession, having previously denied any involvement in the killing when interviewed by the police.

Hardy, of course, had never told anyone what was going through his mind at the time of the murders he committed, but there was no such problem with Watson. He described how, in the days beforehand, he'd been 'drinking a lot and bombing drugs: weed, speed, seven to eight Smirnoff Ices, four to five pints of lager, wine, vodka . . . I hadn't slept properly for about two weeks.'

He then told me that on the day in question he'd been wandering around and had some more drinks, in a pub he couldn't remember. He had also been drinking pints and was using speed and puff 'right up to when they arrested me'.

For the attack on Shireen Noor, he said, 'I can't remember. I remember getting hit over the head with a dog lead.

'I had a big gash on my head and a bleeding nose. I must have jumped on a bird.

'I just have some general flashbacks . . . I remember that I got my boots muddy.'

Regarding the other attacks: 'I don't remember, although I remember giving a ring to some kids – I gave them my silver spider.'

About Chiara Leonetti, he said: 'I think she was coming out of an underground tunnel when I bumped into her.

'I was talking with her and that sort of thing, but I was out of me trolley.

'I think the intention was we were going to make love.

'She was going over this fence, either she fell over, either it was me or it was her. I can't remember.

'We were going through trees and then she threw a rock at my head.'

By now he was laughing. 'I remember me hands and jeans were covered in claret. I hit her with a rock and there was probably something bubbling from her mouth.

'She said something about HIV, she said, "I've got HIV."

'I don't know, I was intoxicated, but I was cool and chilled.' Again he laughed. 'I remember going home and taking my clothes off and going to bed.'

His – clearly grossly distorted – account gave me a clue as to what had probably happened. It looked like he had 'tried out' his attack earlier in the day before meeting Chiara. She presumably walked into this human time bomb totally unaware and with little time to react. On an isolated wooded path, she no doubt rebuffed his advances. What followed must have been her desperate efforts to fend off this attack, which he had been building up to for days, fuelled by his pent-up feelings of rejection and humiliation, with little or no conscience to inhibit him, given his callous lack of empathy.

I had to ask him about the rape and with twisted logic he tried to portray it as a consensual act. 'I don't know how good it was because of what I was on.

'I remember kissing her, we must have fallen,' he said.

With horrifying understatement, he said that he 'probably' put his fingers in her vagina.

What he said, despite its distortion, was broadly consistent with the crime scene, although such minimisation of his brutal behaviour was a telling characteristic.

But what about the clumsy attempt to conceal the body?

'Once what happened had happened, I went to a pub in Bexley. I remember getting some crack.'

He then said he went back to 'where what happened, happened.

'I wanted to see if she was still there so I headed back. I'm pretty sure I did try to blow some air into her lungs. I remember putting a pallet over her. I'm not sure if the foot was mangled. I can't remember, it might have been. I can't remember what I told the police about this.'

He said that he was arrested two days later, on Sunday, in Swanley, and had told the police things, including, 'I was out of my tree.'

In answer to the evidence against him, he said, 'I saw the

pictures of her. I felt sorry for the poor little cow,' and, 'I still can't remember a lot.

'The way I see it, what's happened is atrocious but I can't feel no pain or sorrow, I don't give it a second thought, I've got no emotion.

'I wish I could cry about it.

'More or less I don't give a damn.

'I feel back to normal. I've got no feeling for that girl. My heart bleeds for her. My cellmate is in for murder, he gets back flashes [sic], but I sleep well.'

Sitting there, I thought of the Nazi war criminal Adolf Eichmann, and how the writer Hannah Arendt used the phrase 'the banality of evil' to describe his deportment at his trial. Was this what she meant?

'I remember bits and bobs,' continued Watson as the interview progressed.

'Inside I feel mixed up.

'How can I look my parents in the face?

'What am I doing with the other animals in here?'

But then he commented that he felt the respect of other prison inmates. 'Other lads clock what sort of person I am . . . I don't have to lie any more . . . I don't have to glorify myself.'

There was nothing particularly revealing about the Mental State Exam, except that he reported occasionally hearing internal voices in the second person calling him a 'cunt' or a 'tosser'. They were indistinct and had the quality of pseudo-hallucinations, but there was no evidence of true psychosis.

In psychosis there is a loss of contact with reality, often in the form of delusions – delusions of persecution, for example: a feeling that the body is controlled by an outside force, and that thoughts are broadcast outside the head. These delusions can be accompanied by true hallucinations, which may involve commands.

Psychosis can occur in young adults after a normal development, but in Watson's case there was a clear developmental pattern of disordered conduct in childhood – repeated deception, impulsive behaviour, a failure to learn from experience. This maladaptive pattern of behaviour was consistent with what we conceptualise as an antisocial personality disorder.

How does someone become antisocial? This is the subject of extensive research, but rather than being a product of birth, much antisocial personality disorder (ASPD) can be explained in terms of nurture or childhood experience. The diagnosis requires evidence of disordered conduct before fifteen, and adult behaviours such as unlawful behaviour, impulsivity, recklessness and irresponsibility. ASPD is common, with as many as two thirds of male prisoners fitting the description, according to Nicola Singleton and Jeremy Coid's study.[19] But there is a small subset of those with antisocial personality disorder who have a more severe disturbance and who also meet the criteria for psychopathy (or who have high scores on the psychopathy checklist). It's in this group that there is increasing evidence of a more heritable set of biological traits.

James Blair, an American researcher at the National Institute of Mental Health, has suggested that the neurobiology of the brain explains the reduced 'moral reasoning' in psychopaths.[20] The amygdala, a part of the brain deep in the temporal lobe, has been shown in research to be a key structure in the processing of memory, decision-making and emotional responses, such as disgust, fear, anxiety and aggression. In psychopaths, the amygdala fails to send the correct signals to the decision-making brain structures (in the ventromedial prefrontal cortex). But this does not explain everything, and we need to understand how life experiences may provide a link between brain and behaviour.

If you take someone like Watson, with callous and unemotional traits hard-wired from birth, and throw in all the

61

bullying, maladjustment and low self-esteem, then you have the makings of a psychopath. I remembered a boy at my school who had revelled in distressing younger boys by pulling the legs off crane flies (daddy-long-legs). No surprise then that he liked to taunt boys into fights and was expelled later for threatening an elderly maths teacher with a tennis racket. I don't know what happened to him after that, but his later experience would no doubt be critical to the outcome. Let's hope he didn't end up in Borstal. Watson's antics with pigeons and rats were a hint that, although his adult self was possibly shaped by his experiences, he was not the product of his prolonged bullying alone.

One issue linking Hardy and Watson was probably impotence. I only had Watson's account and the post-mortem findings to support this hypothesis, but in Hardy's case it was certainly caused by diabetes, and in Watson's case probably by substance abuse. These were both sexually motivated homicides but committed without 'rape' as rape was then defined in law.

Years later, I would assess a middle-class family man whose sexual deviance had escalated through various, initially harmless, fetishes like cigarette 'objectophilia' (pornography or sexual activity with cigarettes as a feature) all the way through to extreme bondage and sadomasochism, troilism (preference for threesomes) and Candaules Syndrome (taking masochistic pleasure in being cuckolded), to many months of intrusive murder fantasies partly inspired by the horror film *Hostel*. One day he woke up and, instead of driving to his office in a government department, arranged to meet a prostitute and almost beheaded her with a Stanley knife, without any apparent sexual activity taking place. In this case, the murder had become a paraphilia in its own right and can be referred to as 'homicidophilia': an arousal or gratification from killing itself, the end of the road of sexual deviance.

Verdict: murder. Life imprisonment; twenty-six-year minimum term.

As I went away to digest my interview with Watson and start to draft my report, I sought the input of colleagues. First, I suggested that the defence team instruct a clinical psychologist. Clinical psychologists are not medically qualified, but they also have a lengthy and rigorous training over six years, often incorporating research up to doctoral level. We work closely with them, as they provide another perspective, taking a 'dimensional' or sliding-scale approach to psychological and behavioural disturbance, rather than the 'categorical' or 'medical model' diagnostic approach of psychiatrists. Clinical psychologists make greater use of structured interviews, standardised tests and rating scales, and they have specific training and expertise in various non-drug 'talking therapies' essential in forensic settings.

My colleague Ian Hunter, who was on my team supervising the Camden patients, was instructed by the solicitors and performed a battery of tests on Watson over two interviews. Though the first interview was terminated when Watson became aggressive, he had calmed down for the second, and was able to perform some basic cognitive testing to look at IQ and memory. Watson's IQ was in the upper seventies. Given that the average is one hundred, this meant he was not bright, but certainly not formally learning disabled.

Ian also carried out the Millon Clinical Multiaxial Inventory, a detailed questionnaire of 195 items designed to draw out personality traits and clinical syndromes. And finally there was the PCL-R, or 'psychopath test' to quantify the traits I had identified in my clinical interview.

The PCL-R consists of twenty 'scoring items'. These include abnormal personality traits and deviant behaviour patterns such as glib/superficial charm, need for stimulation, pathological lying, lack of remorse or guilt, parasitic lifestyle, callous lack of empathy, failure to accept responsibility, impulsiveness, irresponsibility, poor behaviour controls, juvenile delinquency and criminal versatility.

These scoring items are all carefully defined with a two-day training course to improve 'inter-rater reliability'.

Ian scored up his tests and I wasn't surprised to hear that the Millon test confirmed antisocial personality disorder. Meanwhile, the psychopathy score was high, at twenty-eight out of a possible forty.

These rating scales bolstered our clinical impressions and gave us another angle to aid our understanding of these extremes of human behaviour.

I also sounded out my medical colleagues. I've always considered informal peer review to be an essential part of my practice, and nowadays it is a formal part of every doctor's professional revalidation. After hours, when the corridor traffic had died down, I sifted through the papers and crime-scene photos and presented the case to a trusted colleague and contemporary in the next-door office. It is crucial, in my view, to bounce ideas off others in the field. Forensic psychiatrists who try to practise in isolation miss out, not just on testing their hypotheses about diagnosis, but also on the opportunity to share and defuse the emotional impact of these challenging cases. Bill Hickok and I were developing our forensic skills alongside each other, and as we each took on gradually more high-profile and complex cases, we exchanged ideas and tested our opinions before committing ourselves on paper. I composed my report on Watson over a couple of weekends, and Ian and I presented the case to our Friday seminar or 'journal club', where interesting and complex cases or research papers would be presented for discussion by colleagues in order to further triangulate our views, before a final edit of the crucial 'opinion' section.

All of this preparation is an essential way of checking for weaknesses. I was learning from bruising encounters in the witness box that whatever I wrote now would be pored over by nit-picking barristers, and could come back to bite me months later, under the withering glare of a QC's cross-examination in an Old Bailey murder trial.

Set out over twenty pages or so, my Watson report covered our interviews and all of the testing that had been carried out. I noted his account – confirmed by others – of how repeated lies were used to bolster his self-esteem and magnify his achievements, and to create a 'false self'. After all, he had said quite openly that he told these lies in order to describe things he wished were true, a form of lying behaviour known as *pseudologia fantastica*', 'pathological lying', or 'Walter Mitty Syndrome', after the classic James Thurber short story.

Pathological lying involves the creation of a tissue of fantastic lies, which may begin as instrumental in the sense of bringing an advantage or prestige. In its more extreme form, *pseudologia fantastica* can become a fantasy run riot, which involves self-deception as much as it does deceiving others.

Watson was a loner, with a childhood dominated by anger, bullying and humiliation at school, and an adult life which continued in much the same vein. He had developed chronic low self-esteem and paranoia and created a false-self to cope in social situations. He probably had callous, unemotional traits, as characterised by his hobbies of collecting skulls and weapons, and his torturing of animals. The loss of his job and girlfriend, escalating drug abuse and the attempts by his family and counsellor to confront him about his deceptions seemed to have tipped him over the edge.

With the exhibitionism incident and his sister's report of the photographs of prostitutes in sexual poses in his room, it seemed likely that there had been some escalation in his sexual fantasies and behaviour. But evidence to confirm this would not emerge until years later.

Taking into account Watson's callous unconcern for the feelings of others, gross and persistent attitude of irresponsibility, incapacity to maintain enduring relationships, and low tolerance for frustration, he clearly fulfilled the criteria for personality disorder with predominantly antisocial features.

His inappropriate and fatuous laughter when describing the offence, coupled with his lack of remorse and callous comments about the victim, were all evidence of the psychopathic traits as measured by the PCL-R. The crime scene and post-mortem findings suggested an opportunistic and disorganised attack involving extreme violence and degradation of the victim.

While Watson's crime scene suggested a spontaneous, disorganised killing, Hardy's disturbing offences were planned and organised. These two cases illustrate quite clearly the two types of 'lust murder' described by Ron Hazelwood and John Douglas of the FBI. They conducted a series of in-depth interviews with thirty-six convicted sexually orientated murderers, including Ted Bundy and Edmund Kemper. Bundy was later executed after being convicted of a sample of his offences, although he was linked to over thirty killings. Kemper, a multiple killer and necrophiliac, had been imprisoned, then released against psychiatric advice and had gone on to kill again.

Organised and disorganised offenders leave different crime scenes. An organised offender, like Hardy, will use planning and control, which will be reflected in what is found by police. The organised offender is more likely to use a verbal approach with victims and be of above average intelligence. Hardy, an engineer, had clearly lured his victims to his flat. By contrast, a disorganised offender such as Watson will have committed the crime in the heat of the moment, displaying no pre-planning or thought, and using items (that is, the brick) already at the scene. He or she will also be less intelligent and less socially competent.

However, FBI crime classification was not the issue we had to address for the Old Bailey trial. Ian and I agreed that there was enough evidence to suggest that Watson's mental state at the time of the killing met the legal criteria for an 'abnormality of mind', namely antisocial personality disorder with psychopathic traits. Whether the abnormality of mind substantially impaired his responsibility would be a matter for the court and, ultimately, the jury. Subsequently, the law has changed to put more onus on the expert with regard to what we call the 'ultimate issue'. Experts can opine, but these issues have to be decided by a jury.

I submitted my report to the solicitors. This being a criminal rather than a well-funded civil case, there would be no pre-trial conference with barristers, and no trip for coffee and biscuits in plush barristers' chambers at one of the Inns of Court like Middle Temple. Our discussion was limited to an hour of hushed voices around a conference table in the lofty domed-roof hall – painted with images of the London Blitz – outside Old Bailey court number four in the older, 1907 part of the court building.

The Old Bailey, or Central Criminal Court as it is technically known, exudes history and gravitas in equal measure, built as it is on the site of the notorious Newgate prison. Even the modern 1973 extension is made of solid Carrara marble, with inverted brass swords of justice forming the bannister rail, and eighteen courtrooms dealing with over 150 murders and all the high-profile criminal cases in a typical year.

Ian and I were well aware that this psychiatric defence was in all probability doomed to failure. An Old Bailey jury – no doubt also impressed by the surroundings – would be made fully aware of the depravity of the offence. But in my view, where mental disorder is evident, it needs to be presented to the defence team and their client, for them to decide if it should be brought up in the court. I have gone in to bat for a 'weak diminished' plea on a number of occasions, partly because if the psychiatrist tries to act as judge and jury and unfairly shuts the door, the defendant can blame their defence team for failing to offer them the chance to run a psychiatric defence, however slender. If they enter a guilty plea after taking advice, they may subsequently regret this decision as they will have plenty of time to mull it over. They may later decide to apply to the Court of Appeal, arguing that psychiatric expert evidence denied them the opportunity of a fair trial. This has happened to more than one of my colleagues.

In short, it was our job to faithfully report what we found regarding abnormality of mind. Gambling on winning a reduction to manslaughter, with discretionary sentencing, instead of mandatory life for murder, Watson had been warned that he could add years to his minimum tariff before parole by putting the family through a trial. But he wanted his day in court. One of my mentors and another forensic pioneer, Paul Bowden, had said after years of Old Bailey murder cases that defendants were better off if they started crying and entered a guilty plea. Airing psychopathy in court is a sure way to convince the judge that you are a menace to society, warranting a sentence to match that impression.

Murder trials are, to my mind, a form of cathartic social theatre. The defendant in the dock, the victim's family in the gallery; the prosecution case set out once all the admissible evidence has been agreed. Is the theatre of court, with its robes and wigs, society's way of bringing a sense of order and closure to cases like this, which involve such chaos and cruelty? Does this help the family of the victim or add to their distress? I have often wondered.

With a psychiatric case like this, the only defence evidence would be from Ian and myself, as the facts of the prosecution case for murder were all agreed. The question for the jury was not 'who?' but 'why?' The Crown Prosecution Service (CPS) had hired one of their favourite psychiatric experts to rebut our argument on behalf of the prosecution, this being what we call a 'contested diminished'. The CPS expert was very confident in court, but he had the irritating habit of addressing the jury as if he was a barrister rather than an impartial expert.

Ian and I sat through the last morning of the prosecution evidence. Just before the lunchtime recess, I was in the witness box being sworn in before the jury.

First there were the easy questions from the barrister on my side of the argument, called the examination-in-chief. I then had to steel myself for cross-examination by the prosecution team, with my opposing expert feeding the counsel challenging questions on sticky notes. Over the years, I've learned to anticipate likely lines of enquiry when writing the reports, but it is always a tense and challenging task. A bit like a pass/fail viva exam at medical school with your whole summer holiday on the line (failure in the viva meant you'd have to swot throughout the break to prepare for a last-chance re-sit in September).

'Doctor, you say that at the material time the defendant was suffering from an abnormality of the mind.'

'Yes, I do.'

'Doctor, can I ask you to help us? What is the "mind" and what exactly do you mean by "an abnormality of the mind"? Can you explain this to the jury?'

I once cringed as I watched an expert who was unable to answer that it had been defined in 1960 in a previous case, that of R v Byrne. Like Watson, Byrne had killed a young woman and mutilated her corpse, and he had a history of 'violent desires'. The appeal court ruled that the mind should be taken to mean the mind's activities in all its aspects, denoting not just the perception of physical acts but the ability to form a rational judgement as to right or wrong. The mind would also include the ability to exercise willpower to act in the way that such rational judgement would suggest. The appeal court judges also said, with confusing circularity, that an abnormality of mind must be so different from normal that a reasonable person would term it abnormal.

On the other hand, a psychiatric definition of 'the mind' would consider the mind to be located within the physical and chemical structure of the brain. The function of the mind would be taken to include perception – such as seeing, hearing, smelling – the processing of feelings and emotions, consciousness, language, memory and reasoning. The mind allows us to imagine, recognise and appreciate, and it is the mind that stores our beliefs, attitudes and hopes, and enables us to form a rational judgement. These are complex issues, but a psychiatrist who goes into the witness box to give an opinion on the mind of a murderer, without having considered them beforehand, is going to struggle to persuade a judge or jury that they have the necessary expertise. It may seem amazing, but it happens.

Forensic psychiatry in the legal arena involves mapping contemporary psychiatric concepts on to arcane and often outdated legal definitions. A challenging intellectual exercise for any expert, but especially so in an inexact science like psychiatry, once described by Nigel Eastman, professor of forensic psychiatry at St George's, as like playing cricket with a rugby-shaped ball.[21]

My evidence was interrupted by lunch. In the Old Bailey, judges are addressed as My Lord (never M'lud) as, although they are circuit judges, they are given the honorific of a high court judge. His lordship reminded me, somewhat severely, not to discuss my evidence with anyone during the break, as I was in the purdah of sworn testimony. There could be no question of barristers slipping in to coach their expert. So, though tempted by the sushi bars and bistros of Limeburner

Lane next to the court, I opted instead for the iron rations of a brown bread and processed cheese sandwich in the canteen on the third floor. A chance to re-read my report and prep for the questions to come, many of which would attempt to undermine my expertise as well my analysis of the evidence.

Once the defence case is complete, the CPS expert has the last word in 'rebuttal' of the psychiatric defence. In the USA, the prosecutors may employ a 'death penalty mitigation rebuttal expert' to challenge any psychiatric attempt to avoid a lethal injection. Now there's an ethical dilemma I am glad I don't have to face.

The CPS expert used a clever tactic lifted from student debating society technique. He conceded nearly all the points in our reports but, having agreed with the diagnosis, argued that if sexual gratification was deemed to be a part of the offence, then the jury should consider this as purposeful behaviour, and responsibility must be in no way diminished, despite abnormality of mind. This calculated ploy allowed the CPS expert to avoid having to argue against our carefully considered diagnosis. It also dodged the central issue, namely, did the abnormal mental state explain the killing?

The second part of the defence to murder, which asks whether there has been a substantial impairment of criminal responsibility, is a moral issue, not a medical one. I always avoided opining on responsibility unless pushed very hard by a judge for an answer. Even then I would say that the jury must judge that for themselves: 'My Lord, I would argue that the abnormality of mind was capable of substantially impairing responsibility, but whether it did impair responsibility at the material time is a matter not for me, but for the triers of fact – the court, and ultimately you, the members of the jury.'

Watson was convicted of murder on a unanimous verdict. We had been played an interview tape where he broke down in tears. Given what he had said during our interviews, we all agreed that he was crying for himself and not his victim. The sentence: life imprisonment with a minimum twenty-five years before first parole review.

Years later, during a cold case review, Watson would be convicted of two serious sexual assaults and a particularly aggressive rape that took place in the period before this final rape and murder. It made sense to me, as such a sudden escalation to a sexual murder had seemed extreme at the time.

When I asked my final question in my original interview of Watson, I was thinking about his Belmarsh regime. He was kept in maximum security – in other words, in a single cell for his own protection, twenty hours a day behind the door, food on a tray, no natural light, exercise-yard trips without any company, body cavity searches before and after each legal visit, restricted and monitored phone calls, no alcohol or drugs and pretty dreadful food. I asked him how he was coping with all that. He smiled and said, 'I'm fine, Doc. It's warm, and I feel very safe here. I finally feel like I'm in the right place.'

Watson's trial was concluded in 2004, but I had to wait until 2005 for the publication of the Hardy inquiry. The inevitable delay started eating into my enjoyment of the sunnier days as we waited for our verdict.

When it was finally released, I couldn't attend the press conference – that would have been too much. But as I drove through Muswell Hill one clear morning, I heard news of it on the radio, which in the papers the next day was reported as, 'Psychiatrists exonerated in Camden Ripper Inquiry'.

The inquiry found that Hardy could not have been detained longer under the Mental Health Act on the basis of what the mental health professionals knew at the time of his release. The original murder charge from January 2002 had been dropped, so the two psychiatrists who saw him in Penton-ville prison were correct in diverting him to psychiatric hospital from court. He was dealt with on the basis that he had committed criminal damage while drinking heavily and, given his background of bipolar disorder, a period in psychiatric hospital was thought to be a better option than release straight from prison.

Once in hospital, he had cooperated with treatment, including taking medication in the form of lithium for his bipolar disorder, and had agreed to engage with the community drug-and-alcohol service to address his drinking. He had been in hospital for several months and not been disturbed in his behaviour. The grounds for his detention were scrutinised by an independent panel and they had to judge whether further confinement was 'necessary for the health or safety of the patient', and/or whether it was necessary 'for the protection of other persons', as the treatment 'cannot be provided unless he is detained under this section'.

With the burden of proof for these tests falling on the hospital, and as Hardy had agreed to community treatment and follow-up, there was no way to keep him in. Regarding the multi-agency or MAPPA referral, this was a procedure that was very new and it turned out that his criminal damage was too low-level an offence and would not have qualified him for MAPPA (which requires more serious offences).

The considerable unease of staff who worked with Hardy arose from the fact that Rose White's death had happened in circumstances that were unexplained, and from the perception that Hardy was untrustworthy, manipulative and emotionally detached. In other words he made people feel 'creepy' – not enough to detain someone, of course.

The inquiry found no evidence of negligence and said his bipolar disorder had not contributed to the murders. They also found that further detention, under section in psychiatric hospital under the Mental Health Act, would not have reduced the risk of him going on to murder. The inquiry chairman, Robert Robinson, acknowledged that this provided no comfort for people wanting reassurance that such events could not happen again.

Of course, we now know that Hardy was in fact a stone-cold sexual sadist and must have been in between his first and second killing in a series of three when he was admitted to St Luke's. He did not have the 'glib and superficial charm' of a psychopathic killer such as Andrew Cunanan or Ted Bundy, but his untrustworthy and manipulative nature meant that the standard psychiatric interview was never likely to reveal the whole picture. The only way his true diagnosis was going to emerge was on the basis of his behaviour being identified correctly by the criminal justice system. In other words, serial killers don't admit what they have done unless or until they are caught.

At the time, there was also a debate about whether psychopaths were treatable anyway, even if Hardy had been diagnosed. The Mental Health Act was reformed in 2007 to address this, in order to encourage greater hospital treatment of more benign personality disorders. But for the psychopaths at the severe end of the spectrum, the hospital-based units for dangerous severe personality disorder (DSPD) have all been subsequently abandoned, as at least half the psychopaths refused to even engage in the therapy, never mind make any progress. They are also adept at putting up a false front and 'pseudo cooperation', of course. The management of this group has, in recent years, been moved back into the high-security prison system, in places like Whitemoor prison.

It all came down to the inaccurate and negligent post-mortem. If that had been performed correctly, Hardy would have been serving life, with a likely tariff of at least fifteen years, and never have been free to kill his two other victims later that year. So for me, relief, after nearly three years of tension. I could move on from Hardy. But he would leave an indelible mark on my practice for the rest of my career. Every case required a thought given to the worst-case scenario and the need to anticipate every possible outcome meant that 'What would they say in the homicide inquiry?' became a common refrain when considering whether or not to take a particular course of action.

Hardy had most likely channelled his resentment, misogyny and diabetic impotence into sexual sadism, humiliation and murder. The killing and body disposal was part of a perverse and sadistic need to exert control over life and death. The depression and bipolar disorder had been a red herring, and in any event, a suggestion of relevant psychiatric issues at the time of the offence was pre-empted by his guilty plea to the three murders.

But psychiatric diagnoses and crime-scene typologies are still only descriptions of the internal life and murderous actions of our subjects. Despite the advances of neuroscience, forensic psychiatry and criminology, we will always struggle to make sense of terrible crimes such as Hardy's. More recently, an increasing number of men have tried to avoid a murder conviction by claiming that death has resulted from rough sex gone wrong. But you can't consent to your own death. Hardy's implausible claim was that his victims died by being suffocated under his body weight after he had fallen asleep, leaving us to speculate about his true motivation and behaviour. He will, in all likelihood, take the full details of what he has done to his grave.

Psychotic Homicide

Case Study: Daniel Joseph

5

A trickle of carmine venous blood ran across her forearm, to be soaked up by the sterile white gauze. With surgically gloved hands, I dabbed more blood clear and continued to seal the skin with interrupted 3-0 silk sutures on a swaged needle. Cheryl, the patient, had used a razor blade to cut two long wounds lengthways along her left forearm. The cuts were clean-edged and deep, through to the yellow subcutaneous fat underneath.

The year was 1998, and we were in the Crisis Recovery Unit at the Bethlem Royal Hospital. The unit's remit was to manage those who repeatedly self-harm, often having being diagnosed with a borderline personality disorder. Most of the patients in the unit had a history of abuse or adversity in childhood. Developed by Dr Michael Crowe and the consultant nurse Jane Bunclark, the unit used a novel approach: rather than physically trying to prevent repetitive, non-suicidal, self-harm behaviour, the aim of treatment was to bolster self-control.[22] This meant that, unlike in many standard psychiatric units, sharp implements were not hidden away and treated as contraband. Instead, patients were allowed access to sterile razor blades (and even, on one occasion, caustic soda), which, in turn, meant that it was standard procedure for the junior psychiatrist (or 'registrar' as we were called in those days) to stitch up any wounds. As the only psychiatrist or doctor of any kind on night duty, it was our job to deal with out-of-hours medical and psychiatric problems. My recent experience in A & E proved more useful than my fledgling psychiatric skills in this regard.

As for the self-harm, we were asked not to reward the behaviour but also not to punish it. In other words, you couldn't be too consoling, and so provide positive attention, while on the other hand, you couldn't be overly harsh and dismissive. This is because the motives for self-harm are complex: the shedding of blood, the experience of pain, the wish for punishment and the response of others can all be 'reinforcing'. Instead, what was needed was a 'Goldilocks' or 'just right' approach, which meant maintaining a calm, neutral attitude while diligently repairing the damage done.

I drew up another 5 mls of lignocaine and warned Cheryl that there would be a sharp scratch as I infiltrated the local anaesthetic around the second wound. I paused to let it take hold and then, in an atmosphere of calm silence, applied eight stitches to the second wound and dabbed the fresh blood clean. The nurse helped me by spraying some povidone-iodine and applying sterile dressings. Cheryl smiled and thanked me for the suturing. I did my best to keep my features neutral. No sign of exasperation. No attempt to console her.

The procedure complete, I let myself out of the ward – this being an open unit without a locked door – and returned to the on-call doctor's car, a dilapidated Nissan with a faulty gearstick and a full resuscitation kit, including defribillator, in the the boot.

It was a damp and cool night, so I wiped the mist off the inside of the windscreen, pulled out the choke and turned the ignition over. I had another couple of calls to make before turning in, and I followed the hospital site's internal road, sticking to the fifteen-miles-per-hour speed limit. A fox scuttled in front of the car as I took a side road into the car park of the medium-secure unit, my last call of the night. All around me the hospital was quiet.

The Bethlem, also known as the St Mary of Bethlehem. And perhaps even better known as Bedlam. No doubt you're familiar with the name. Once the archetype for the inhumanity of the asylum era, it inspired William Hogarth's *The Madhouse*, the final canvas of the *Rake's Progress* series, which in turn inspired the eponymous 1946 Boris Karloff movie. In 1998, the hospital had just celebated its 750th anniversary. The Bethlem started life in 1247, housed at Bishopsgate outside the walls of the City of London, then moved to Old Street, Moorfields, in the seventeenth century. A further move in the early nineteenth century took it to St George's Fields in Southwark (now the Imperial War Museum). A wing of the Southwark site became the first criminal lunatic asylum, later separated and moved to Broadmoor. Bethlem's most recent transfer to spacious grounds (with open grass areas, an orchard and even a cricket pitch) near Beckenham in Kent was in 1930. It was later linked to the Maudsley Hospital and evolved into a cutting-edge, modern psychiatric hospital with national centres of excellence, the forensic unit being the most recent addition. Not all changes are for the better, however. During an expansion in 1999, bickering and rivalry led to the 752-year-old name Bethlem being dropped in favour of the bland 'South London'. Imagine Johns Hopkins being renamed 'East Baltimore'.

Still, the hospital's notorious past is memorialised in Caius Gibber's statues that depict 'raving' and 'melancholy' madness. Once they adorned the hospital entrance; now they are preserved in the hospital museum.

Call-outs for the duty doctor could be to anywhere on the Bethlem site: to deal with patients such as Cheryl in the Crisis Recovery Unit, for example, or to the National Psychosis Unit, an open ward dealing with treatment-resistant cases of schizophrenia, referred from around the country. Or I might be called to one of the other specialist units: for learning disabilities, phobias, alcohol detox and recovery (long since shut in the wake of slashed budgets for addictions), brain injuries and eating disorders, which had an intensive programme for life-threatening anorexia and bulimia. Most of the patients were free to come and go as they wished as, on the whole, any risk they posed was more likely to be to themselves than to others.

My last call of the night was to the medium-secure forensic unit, the Denis Hill, a new-build from the late 1980s, where I was due to write up some repeat prescriptions. I buzzed and a nurse let me through double-airlocked doors made of heavy glass. Inside the ward, which had twenty-four bedrooms in two corridors, it was eerily quiet. Just a couple of patients were watching late-night TV in the communal lounge area. Forensic patients, once they're established on treatment and with a focus on rehabilitation, are generally settled and doing their best to move on with their lives (until they're not, of course, and then it really is bedlam). And so tonight all was calm. The intensive care or de-escalation area (a separate part of the ward where a disturbed patient could be managed away from the others) and the seclusion room were empty.

I spent a couple of minutes filling out two charts and cross-referencing medical records to check a treatment plan. Patients' case notes were lever-arch files with handwritten notes on paper – red corners for inpatient periods and blue corners for outpatient spells. In forensic units, the files tended to be bulky but well organised, with a detailed background history and an analysis of the most significant criminal offence that had led to their psychiatric admission – which we and our patients refer to as the 'index offence'. It was this rigorous approach to assessment that had attracted me to forensic psychiatry, along with the composed response of the senior nurses, who seemed unruffled in the face of disturbed behaviour. This was in contrast to the chaotic atmosphere of the wards for psychiatric patients in the community on short-term admissions, where occasional patient aggression seemed to cause unnecessary panic.

My duties finished for the night, I returned to the hospital's spartan on-call quarters, a one-bed flat with a small galley kitchen and sitting area. Compared to a busy night in a general medical hospital, it was usually pretty quiet at the Bethlem after midnight. Unless there was disturbed behaviour requiring rapid tranquillisation or an acute medical emergency, there was a reasonable prospect of getting a few hours' sleep.

I cleared up the leftovers of my takeaway curry. Having missed the canteen, I regretted the choice of extra spicy chicken jalfrezi, delivered from the curry house in nearby West Wickham. I knew I'd pay for it with a rumbling stomach the next day.

I struggled to sleep for a bit, still wired by the excess coffee that had got me through the fifteen-hour day, but I must have eventually dozed off.

I awoke with a start. The porter's lodge was fast-bleeping me to go to the forensic unit ASAP. I didn't bother with the car, just threw on some clothes and jogged over.

It had been almost time to hand over the bleep to the doctor coming on duty, but this call was mine to deal with. Buzzed in through the airlock, I saw that everybody seemed very tense and heard shouting from the de-escalation area. It had a low wooden slatted bench held securely with brass screws, soft furnishings and a television behind a heavy-duty Perspex screen. Sylvia, the charge nurse on duty, said that a patient had been transferred a few hours before from the low-secure PICU (psychiatric intensive care unit) up at the main hospital, the Maudsley in Camberwell.

Details of the patient's offence were sparse at that stage, but those terrible events are described in detail in the independent inquiry report and I will summarise them here. At about 7.45 a.m. on the morning of Thursday, 22 January, Daniel Joseph, eighteen, had kicked in the door of his friend

Carla Thompson's flat, burst into the bedroom where she slept and dragged her out of the room by her hair. He began severely beating her, smashing up the flat at the same time, battering her head against a radiator and the door frame, kicking her in the head, stamping on her. During the savagery he tried to set fire to her hair, but that didn't work, so instead he looped a tow-rope around her neck and dragged her out of her blood-splattered flat and into the car park outside.

There he took a length of wood and smashed several car windows before throwing a brick at the kitchen window of a flat belong to fifty-three-year-old Agnes Erume. He then went into Agnes's flat and dragged her outside and down the steps. He laid her down next to Carla and tied the two women together by the neck, continuing to kick and stamp on them both long after they were unconscious.

By this time, several police officers had arrived on the scene and Daniel took up kung fu-type stances in front of the women. The officers used CS gas, but it seemed to have no effect. With reinforcements called, the police officers advanced on Daniel as he climbed on to the bonnet of a car and beat his chest 'like Tarzan', then jumped down and began throwing objects at them. In all, it took them over twenty minutes to subdue him and get him into a police van.

Twenty-one hours later, Carla Thompson died from over fifty different injuries. Agnes Erume, although initially not expected to survive, made a remarkable recovery and merci-fully can remember nothing about the attack.

Normally after a homicide, the arrested person is held overnight by the police, appears before the magistrates in the morning and is remanded in custody to a Category B prison, where a psych assessment can follow. But this was already an unusual scenario. Sylvia said they wanted me to go in with the response team to administer rapid tranquillisation, as the patient was agitated and not responding to reason.

Rapid tranquillisation is only used *in extremis*, when the safety and health of the patient is paramount. This was just such a case. I asked for a standard rapid tranquillisation kit to be drawn up, including a butterfly needle, alcohol swab, two 10ml syringes, and several vials of Diazemuls (a white, milky, injectable form of diazepam which we no longer use in psychiatric settings) and haloperidol, an antipsychotic that can either be given intramuscularly or, in those days, intravenously.

Once we had that ready, we briefed the response team (summoned from other wards) on the plan of action. Restraint has a bad name, and if it is used, it must be rigorously monitored and reviewed, preferably by CCTV. The techniques, called PMVA (prevention and management of violence and aggression), are designed to restrain the patient in a controlled, safe and humane way for just a few minutes, to allow the administering of emergency medication or a transfer to seclusion.

We were ready to go in when the two nurses observing Joseph came piling out, slamming the door behind them. I peered through the glass observation hatch and got my first good look at him. A very heavily built, toned, muscular young man, six foot seven, he was engaged in trying to prise off one of the wooden slats from the bench. Testing the design to destruction, he easily broke through the heavy brass screws and then started smashing the shatterproof cover over the screen of the TV recessed into the wall. There was real concern he might harm himself, but also that he was capable of breaking out of the intensive care area and attacking us.

At this point I heard sirens and we were told that the Territorial Support Group (TSG), or riot police, had arrived. Going out to the car park, I saw three vanloads of riot police putting on their kit, and I spoke to the sergeant in charge, who told me they'd already been called out twice, once at the point of arrest and secondly after Joseph had started to smash up the low-secure ward.

Behind the riot police vans was a police car and van, with a dog handler and two armed officers, each carrying a Glock sidearm and a 9mm Heckler & Koch MP5. 'If he gets past us, he's not going to get past those two,' explained the sergeant, noting my wary glance.

By now this was clearly a serious incident and, sure enough, I saw my boss pulling into the car park. Dr David Mottershaw was experienced, decisive and no-nonsense. A Lancashire man with the accent to match. He'd been briefed about the situation on his way in to work and joined our huddle, telling me that there had already been a discussion at a senior level. Given the disturbance of this patient, he clearly needed to be held in a maximum-security facility, and Broadmoor Hospital in Berkshire had already agreed to accept him without their usual lengthy referral procedure and admissions panel.

As I was discussing the situation with Dr Mottershaw, an ambulance arrived. The TSG sergeant, firearms lead and police gold commander came over to work up a plan. Since Joseph now had wooden slats broken off the bench as weapons, PMVA was too risky, so it was agreed that the TSG would help us restrain the patient with shields. We would try to sedate him and if we could safely achieve that, then we'd think about the practicalities of a transfer to high security.

Meanwhile, Joseph was continuing to smash up the intensive care area and, after some further delay for discussion, Dr Mottershaw was becoming impatient. He told the sergeant they needed to get in quickly because there was a real concern Joseph might attempt suicide. The sergeant asked Dr Mottershaw to brief his team about what to expect, and the TSG assembled in an expectant group, about thirty of them, complete with tactical helmets, visors, leg guards and riot shields.

David Mottershaw looked at them and in typically direct style, said, 'He's six foot seven, a wrestler and a body builder, and he's completely mad. He'll probably think that you've come to kill him and he's deaf anyway, so don't bother trying to reason with him. Just get him on the ground with your shields. We'll sedate him and take it from there.'

I could see the officers' eyes widening beneath their visors. This was no ordinary riot scenario. It was clearly way outside their comfort zone.

A psychiatrist's ability to get butterfly needles, cannulae and intravenous drugs in the right place diminishes rapidly with each year away from 'real' medicine. It was something in the forefront of my mind as I realised, when Dr Mottershaw told the officers 'we'll sedate him', he'd actually meant *me*.

All the other patients had been escorted to other wards, so the TSG went through the airlock, which had been wedged open, shuffling forward like a phalanx of Roman legionnaires until they were outside the door. A nurse was ready with the key and, after a quick countdown as agreed, the door was opened.

The officers charged inside, shields held high, shouting for Joseph to get down, evidently forgetting what Dr Mottershaw had told them. Either way, they must have been a terrifying sight for he was quickly subdued. A few shouts and muffled grunts later and the officers were yelling, *'Medic!'*

That was me. I entered to find Joseph on the floor with his muscled forearms double-cuffed in a rear stack, and I knelt to administer the injection. The technique for intravenous sedation involves swabbing with alcohol to sterilise the skin. With a twenty-three-gauge green butterfly needle, a suitable vein must be found on the forearm. The syringe plunger is then withdrawn to get a backflush of blood to check the needle is in the right place. The Diazemuls can then be slowly injected while the respiratory rate and pulse are monitored.

Diazemuls is a sedative commonly known as Valium in its more familiar oral form, and is from the group of psychoactive drugs known as benzodiazepines. Given intravenously, it can induce sedation and semi-consciousness at a dose of 5–10 mg in the elderly, or higher doses in a fit young adult. Working in Australia, I had once administered over 100 mg to an enormous rugby player who was suffering a bipolar relapse while high on cocaine and who had needed mounted police for his apprehension on Manly Beach and transfer to the East Wing at Manly Hospital. Nowadays, for safety reasons, we inject into the muscle, but in the 1990s it was standard practice to inject intravenously. As was also standard practice, I followed it up with 10mg of haloperidol (again, intravenously), with the aim of providing a longer-lasting calming effect and a reduction in psychotic symptoms like paranoia.

Soon, Joseph was quietly sleeping and, as the nurses monitored his pulse and respiratory rate, I went outside to confer with Dr Mottershaw and the gold commander.

'How long is he going to stay asleep for, doctor?' asked the commander.

'Difficult to say. It'll be forty minutes to an hour until the Diazemuls wears off.'

'So what's the plan after that?'

'Broadmoor have accepted him for high security.'

'Broadmoor ready to take him now?'

'Yes, there's a bed on Luton, the admissions ward. We're cleared to drive him straight in through the gates. We just need to get him there safely.'

'Right,' the DCI said, 'let's blue-light him to Broadmoor, but I want the TSG and the ARV (armed response vehicle) to stay with us in case he wakes up.'

It was agreed that Julie, a senior nurse, and I would ride in the ambulance with Joseph on a stretcher. We would have two riot officers in the ambulance with us, and the other officers would follow in vans.

Joseph was loaded into the ambulance by the paramedics,

attached to a pulse blood oxygen meter, cardiac monitor and blood pressure cuff, peacefully asleep for now and therefore not handcuffed. I took a small bag with extra medication and belted in to the jump seat for the journey. A police car led the convoy, a column of six vehicles including the armed response van, ambulance and TSG vans, and we were going around eighty to ninety miles per hour, top speed for the ambulance. I had recently driven to Broadmoor for a seminar and it took me an hour and a half to get there from the Bethlem, but that day we got there in forty minutes flat.

As we arrived, the gates opened and we swept in to park beside the admissions ward. Paramedics wheeled the still-sleeping Joseph into the custody of reassuringly heavy-set psychiatric nurses, several of whom were tattooed and looked like they might be the front five of the Broadmoor staff rugby team. They in turn carted Joseph into a featureless, safe admission room, complete with moulded bed, moulded toilet and sink, and absolutely no ligature points or sharp objects. There he was laid carefully on the bed, nurses monitoring his physical health.

After a full handover lasting about half an hour, the ambulance crew agreed to give us a lift home and we headed back up the A322 towards the Bagshot junction with the M3, feeling the tension release. I realised that my shirt was soaked with sweat and my feet were hurting. For the first time that day, I started to feel the cold. To make matters worse, the ambulance juddered to a halt and pulled over to the side of the road with its overworked engine steaming. By chance, the three vanloads of riot police had come along the same route and cheerfully offered us a lift. They were eating sandwiches and Cornish pasties and in good spirits after a successful deployment. Thus rescued, we pottered our way back to Beckenham, listening to a car chase in south London on the police radio scanner.

Back at base, I went into the nurses' station for debrief and then to my office to work on a case summary for presentation to colleagues at the weekly peer review on Friday. I was struggling to concentrate, and when the porters rang me to say that the duty doctor wanted the flat key, I retrieved my overnight bag and headed home to Camden. The flat was empty, and I poured myself a large glass of red wine and dropped on to the sofa, relieved that my eventful thirty-six-hour on-call shift had ended without disaster. Even so, I was shaken as I digested the impact of the day's events, thinking about the consequences of abnormal mental states for which I would be taking responsibility.

The adrenaline was only now beginning to ebb away and I found I couldn't concentrate enough to watch the news. Feeling zoned out but not yet ready for sleep, I just stared vacantly out of the window, lost in thought.

Dr Mottershaw had seemed so calm and unruffled by it all. Would I be able to reach his level of confidence and experience? I wouldn't have had a clue what to say to those riot police, but he had been blunt and succinct, told them all they needed to know for the task at hand, and Joseph had been safely transferred to the most secure psychiatric hospital in the country, with no injuries or harm to staff or patient. I still had a lot to learn.

The following morning, the full background of the case began to emerge. Daniel Joseph had been deaf since birth. After disruption to his education, his sign language had never properly developed, so he still had major communication problems. Joseph's troubled life story and history of contact with psychiatric services before and after he killed Carla is outlined in great detail in the inquiry report. Diagnosed with bipolar disorder, he was described by those who knew him as a likeable and friendly boy, albeit of immense physical proportions – a gentle giant who was good to have around. He had grown obsessed with becoming a world-famous wrestler and, through gym and diet, had honed his substantial frame into a physique compatible with professional wrestling at the highest level. Latterly, he had suffered a psychotic breakdown, during which these unrealistic beliefs had reached delusional proportions and he became convinced that he could banish his deafness, live in the hearing world and become a World Wrestling Federation wrestler.

One night he took an overnight bag and his passport to a WWF wrestling bout at the London Arena in the hope that he might be able to travel back to the United States with the wrestlers. When he was escorted home that night by Arena security, he became agitated with his family, claiming they had stopped him going to the US. Matters escalated and Joseph ended up throwing a kerbstone through a front window of the house; police were called and Joseph, having been seen by the psychiatrist Dr Peter Hindley, was admitted to hospital for the first time.

Later, Joseph would be let down by the poor coordination of deaf and mental health services; indeed, a subsequent inquiry set out the various difficulties of coordinating psychiatric care and the limited availability of mental health practitioners with sign language.

Unfortunately, after a further psychotic breakdown, Joseph had moved to a different area of south London, covered by another mental health team, and been placed in a community hostel, which he later chose to leave. He had been befriended by Carla Thompson, a former alcohol and drug abuser (who may have had mental health problems in the past). Carla had found religion and welcomed several young people with drug or mental health problems to share her one-bedroom flat. Unfortunately, she persuaded Joseph to stop his medication and use prayer as a substitute. This, in retrospect, was a catastrophic, and ultimately fatal, mistake.

Joseph had been sleeping on her sofa for a number of weeks when, following concerns about him, mental health workers carried out an assessment (unfortunately hampered by the late arrival of the sign language interpreter, who had been given the wrong address). This assessment described the living conditions as untidy and dirty.

Meanwhile, Joseph stayed briefly at another friend's home and then, a day or so later, returned to Carla's flat at about 9 p.m., when there was a dispute about whether he might have made a young woman pregnant. According to the inquiry, this was the last time the two spoke before the attack.

After the attack, once the TSG officers had eventually subdued Joseph, he was put in handcuffs and ankle restraints. He was taken to Brixton police station and seen by a doctor there, who gave him wet bandages for his wrists. Communicating through an interpreter, Joseph was found to be anxious and excitable.

An experienced chief inspector, Sue Hill, was called in to deal with the situation. She immediately realised that, despite the seriousness of his actions, Joseph was a vulnerable young man who needed help. DCI Hill later described to the inquiry that Joseph seemed extremely frightened. A decision was taken not to interview or charge him, but to arrange transfer to hospital as soon as possible. There were a number of phone calls trying to find a psychiatrist who would come to the police station and, eventually, the duty senior registrar (senior resident, one level below consultant) from the Maudsley was contacted on his mobile. On his way to the Maudsley to deal with another matter, he agreed to go to the police custody area, where he decided to recommend that Joseph be admitted to the Maudsley for further assessment under Section 2 of the Mental Health Act. Joseph was placed in seclusion on a low-secure ward for acutely disturbed psychiatric patients, which we call a psychiatric intensive care unit. Despite the best efforts of this ward, where staff are accustomed to violent and challenging behavious, Joseph became so violent that riot police were called for the second time to transfer him to the medium-secure Denis Hill Unit, which was where I came in.

Joseph was too disturbed to be brought to Camberwell Magistrates' Court and a special sitting was convened at Broadmoor. There, he had responded quickly to the reinstatement of his medication and, after one minor incident, reverted to the engaging and friendly young man he had been before the attack.

There were four local inquiries and a full public inquiry into his care. It was agreed he had suffered a relapse of bipolar disorder, characterised by his grandiose delusions and his agitated and aggressive behaviour. The inquiry set out the lack of mental health professionals able to sign, and problems handing over care between different teams, a common theme in homicide inquiries. A number of recommendations were made about mental health care for deaf people.

As was common in the late 1990s, this was a searching review, which sought to improve services. The reality, some twenty years later, has been the fragmentation of community mental health services, underfunding, and closure of beds for short-term admission. So, despite the work of the confidential inquiry into homicides and suicides by the mentally ill, and against a background of falling homicide rates generally, the homicide rate by those with, for example, schizophrenia has resisted efforts to reduce it. It seems that many of the lessons learned from these inquiries have been ignored or forgotten. With ever greater pressure to reduce the cost of psychiatric services, many of the local psychiatric hospital beds have been closed. These are the type of unlocked units where someone like Joseph could have been helped through a crisis, but this is an option that's frequently unavailable.

6

In psychiatry, we divide major mental illness into two broad categories: bipolar disorder (or manic depression as it used to be known), and schizophrenia, and have done since 1899 when the distinction was first defined by German psychiatrist Emil Kraepelin, the father of modern psychiatry.

As it happens, recent genetic research now suggests that this separation needs to be reconsidered, and in any event, there is a third category, called schizoaffective disorder, which is in between the two. But until the research evidence becomes clearer and is translated into clinical practice, we continue to distinguish between bipolar and schizophrenia.

In mania, you see racing thoughts, reduced sleep, euphoria, infectious good humour and increased sociability. Years later at HMP Holloway I assessed a pub landlady with a long history of bipolar disorder, who was singing cheerfully as I walked into the cell to interview her. During a manic episode, drinking heavily and dancing in her underwear in the front garden, she had left candles burning in her ground-floor flat. A candle fell and the smoky conflagration overwhelmed and killed her elderly upstairs neighbour, whose charred corpse was found by the fire brigade slumped on the toilet, resulting in murder and arson charges for my patient. It emerged that a psychiatrist hired to provide temporary cover (a locum) had recently re-diagnosed her with personality disorder and stopped her lithium – with inevitable consequences. (Did I mention that psychiatrists often disagree?)

Bipolar disorder is not usually associated with violence, and is compatible with a normal working life in between episodes. It has even become a fashionable diagnosis, especially in its milder version, Bipolar 2. However, irritability, disinhibition and features of psychosis, such as delusions, can result in life-endangering reckless behaviour, or violence, as was the case with Daniel Joseph.

But what do we mean by 'psychosis', and how can it lead to murder? 'Psychosis' is a catch-all term that covers any severe mental disorder where thought, perceptions and emotions are so impaired that contact is lost with external reality. Psychosis is seen in schizophrenia, but there are other disorders which feature 'psychosis' or 'loss of contact with reality', such as delusional disorder, brief psychotic episodes and drug-induced psychosis. Yet it is bipolar disorder and schizophrenia which concern us most of the time. Of the two, schizophrenia is the condition that is evident most frequently among forensic patients, and in fact a diagnosis of schizophrenia is found in around three-quarters of our secure unit inpatients.

As with bipolar disorder, most of those suffering with schizophrenia are not violent. It's a relatively common condition with a prevalence approaching around 0.7 per cent of the adult population. The majority of people with the condition are more likely to be victims than perpetrators of violence, as well as being at a greatly increased risk of suicide. However, a survey of twenty studies by Seena Fazel found that those with psychosis are nineteen times more likely to commit a homicide than the general population.[23]

In the past we couldn't agree how to diagnose schizophrenia consistently. Until the early 1980s, a few days of hearing voices could earn you a diagnosis. These days it is much better defined. For example, a brief episode of psychosis doesn't count as schizophrenia until there have been at least six months' alteration in mental state. But schizophrenia can appear with a wide range of features in different people. First episodes are usually in the late teens and early twenties, which is why it used to be called 'precocious dementia', before the confusing label of schizophrenia was introduced. (Confusing, because schizophrenia doesn't involve a split mind, except in the sense that a person's mind can operate in a very different way during an acute episode than when mentally stable.) The illness can start either suddenly or with an insidious onset and often has repeated episodes, with a gradual decline in social functioning over the years, although some have a good outcome after a psychotic episode and go on to recover.

Schizophrenia is defined by abnormal experiences and behaviour such as hallucinations, delusions, disorganised thinking and speech, behavioural disturbance and negative symptoms. Hallucinations appear real to the individual and voices may comment on the individual's actions. In some cases, the voices may give commands, which the subject may decide to obey. This can have alarming consequences, for example when the hallucinatory commands are to kill. Delusions are fixed beliefs that resist challenge and will often involve themes of persecution, grandiosity and religiosity.

'Delusional perception' is a delusional interpretation of a normal perception (for example, a car flashing a light may be interpreted as a sign of a surveillance programme). This may be preceded by a 'delusional mood' (a sense of unease or strangeness). Delusions about being under surveillance, or feeling under threat of attack or being killed, can result in withdrawal and fear, or lead to aggressive behaviour in self-defence. There are delusions of love, jealousy (more on this later) and misidentification (loved ones replaced by imposters). Delusions of being targeted for surveillance or mind control are very distressing and often impact on the behaviour of those afflicted – for example, provoking them to lodge complaints against and harass those they believe are persecuting them, or prompting them to wear bizarre protective headgear. These beliefs are sometimes harmless and may also occur as a variant of the psychosis we call a 'delusional disorder'. But delusions of being targeted have also been found in perpetrators of mass shooting incidents in the USA, such as Aaron Alexis, who shot thirteen people at the Washington Navy Yard, believing he had been targeted by ultra-low frequency radio waves.

Some delusions may be horrific, like being experimented on or having internal organs removed. In a bizarre example of life imitating art, some believe they are being driven mad by 'gaslighting' (a term adopted from film adaptations of the Patrick Hamilton play *Gaslight*). Equally deluded family members can fuel or reinforce delusions in a *'folie à deux'* (a shared psychosis), while online communities may validate the beliefs of people sharing 'group' delusions in a *'folie à plusieurs'*. At the National Psychosis Unit, we admitted a young woman whose psychotic mother had convinced her that her insides were rotting. Separated from her mother, the beliefs quickly subsided and it became clear which of them really needed treatment.

The bizarre delusions and diverse hallucinatory phenomena of psychosis often occur in combination, pitching the person into an alien and frightening world. This distressing experience provokes an intense emotional response. Their mind is disturbed so pervasively that their ability to reason is impaired.

To help understand it, think of *The Truman Show* flipped on its head. Imagine that there was no show, but that Truman's deluded imagination was causing him to interpret radio interference or the odd behaviour of others as evidence that he was surrounded by actors and his life was being controlled as part of a reality TV show. That is what delusions must be like – for the sufferer, they can be as frightening as living in a horror movie made real.

Behaviour changes may include agitation, aggression and catatonia. Negative symptoms, such as flattened emotions, poverty of speech, and reduced drive or apathy, tend to occur later on, after acute psychosis has subsided with treatment.

These descriptions of the strange internal experience of psychosis are hard to imagine until you have heard them firsthand. When I started at the Maudsley on the National Psychosis Unit, I saw a patient who described microchips in their carburettor listening to their thoughts; a young man with cat delusions who got himself mauled by Arfur the lion at London Zoo; a young student who had run down the M1 to escape persecutors; and, on one particularly memorable day, a patient who arrived handcuffed, escorted by three British Transport Police officers, with heavy black grease marks all over his face and clothes. It turned out he had jumped on to the underground rail tracks at Lambeth North tube station in a suicide attempt that he'd miraculously survived. When an appointment letter to see me at the outpatient clinic at the Maudsley was found in his pocket, the officers decided to bring him along. Severely depressed and psychotic, he had heard angels calling him to 'the other side'. I was so concerned that I arranged a second opinion to admit him under section, for his own health and safety. I didn't think the tube journey home would be a good idea.

As I started gaining experience and developing some clinical skills, a degree of exhilaration came in being able to manage situations like my underground train jumper (much as I had experienced as a medic when doing my first chest drain or central line into the heart). I quickly started to develop that sense of pattern recognition, all the while keeping in mind that every case is different, of course.

Psychiatrically disturbed behaviour can be dramatic and bewildering for those family members who come across it for the first time and then find themselves visiting a relative at the Bethlem or Maudsley. But for anyone trying to learn psychiatry you couldn't be in a better place. By working in a national referral centre, I got to meet a highly select group of patients, exposing me to the full range of psychotic phenomena, while at the same time I was learning how to manage acute psychiatric crises at the out-of-hours emergency clinic (EC). This clinic performed an important function by providing a safe space for careful assessment, as well as keeping some of the acutely mentally disturbed out of King's College Hospital A & E across the road (although it was closed in 2007 to cut costs).

I encountered many other bizarre but intriguing examples of psychosis during my first six months at the Maudsley, and I quickly realised I had discovered the medical speciality that suited me best. Added to that, I found myself witnessing profound changes at ground level in psychiatric practice and services. Back in the early 1990s, the focus of research activity and grant funding was shifting away from environmental and social factors in psychosis and towards genetic and biological. It was becoming clear that schizophrenia is a disorder of disrupted neural (brain tissue) connections, with genetic and environmental risk factors influencing brain development.

Using brain imaging, we know there are structural changes in the cortex of the brain. But as well as abnormal static images, 'functional' imaging has looked at the brain as it works, scanning subjects while they perform a mental task like a calculation. These functional scans have found changes in memory, decision-making and emotion-processing. But schizophrenia is not all about genes and the physical structure of the brain. Stressful life events, cannabis use or head injury can all tip someone over the edge into psychosis. In other words, it's a combination of nature and nurture, but more skewed towards nature than other mental disorders.

So how do we treat it? The answer is mainly with the use of antipsychotic drugs first developed in the 1950s and improved and refined ever since. These are not without side effects and involuntary treatment remains a thorny issue. I spend a lot of my time with a patient assessing their capacity to understand the treatments on offer, and there are strict safeguards if they don't want to take medication.

Of course, in the not-too-distant past, psychiatric treatment had a really bad name, thanks to the use of insulin coma therapy and psychosurgery as depicted in the Jack Nicholson film *One Flew Over the Cuckoo's Nest*. The problem was that psychosurgery (that is, operating on the brain, such as the lobotomy given to Nicholson's character) had uncertain benefits and could have terrible side effects.

I know this only too well. My maternal aunt, Georgina, suffered a post-partum psychosis in the late 1950s. She was hospitalised and treated with frontal lobotomy. It seems to have arrested her psychosis, but she was left with impaired social inhibitions, one of the milder side effects of deliberate surgical damage to frontal brain white matter, which meant she would often have to be reminded not to tell rude jokes in front of the children at Christmas. She also couldn't stand teddy bears or dolls – something I only came to understand later.

Attitudes to mental illness are improving along with greater public awareness, but stigma still lingers. My aunt's mental illness, and that of other family members, had not been discussed openly amongst us and although I was aware of some parts of the story, it was only after I started psychiatric training that I began probing older family members for more details. On the whole, they seem to have found it cathartic to talk about mental illness in a way that was previously off limits.

But I wasn't at the Maudsley to go on a DIY *Who Do You Think You Are?* quest – at least not then. Although I had a growing sense this was a field that suited me, at this early stage in my career I hadn't yet begun to unpick all the factors which had contributed to my decision to go down this path. I was far too busy treating patients.

At this point I must emphasise that medication is not the only treatment we use. Far from it – we also employ proven psychological treatments, along with a range of other approaches, such as working with families and finding meaningful occupational activities. In fact, research has shown that family interventions can reduce relapse rates in schizophrenia, although funding and provision for this is sadly inadequate despite the research base.

However, antipsychotic drugs are crucial to my day-to-day practice and can have dramatic, life-enhancing beneficial effects – and they can prevent homicides.

They are thought to work by blocking or partially stimulating dopamine receptors, to interfere with the pathways that give rise to abnormal perceptions, like auditory hallucinations, and abnormal thoughts, like delusions. Some patients respond very quickly. Those who have killed while psychotic might recover after a few weeks of treatment. Once they've regained insight, they then have to face the terrible consequences of what they've done.

We're getting better at helping those with serious mental illness like schizophrenia, but this progress can be hampered when patients don't qualify for treatment because of service cuts and ill-considered, financially driven re-organisations.

Society in the late 1980s and 1990s became unwilling to accept that violent psychotic incidents, including homicides, were random events. Increasingly there was a need to find a person or organisation to blame, as well as a drive to unpick systemic failures which might have led to any adverse event. This has been reflected in other areas of health and safety: the Clapham rail disaster, the *Marchioness* tragedy and, later, the Haringey child protection inquiries. The case of Christopher Clunis and the campaign of Jayne Zito, his victim's wife, was instrumental in drawing attention to inadequacies in community care and homicides by the mentally ill, showing that in the early years, after asylum closure, this care had been ill-planned, over-optimistic and poorly coordinated. There were significant improvements in practice and procedures in the late 1990s and early 2000s.

The Zito Trust was closed in 2009, its work apparently complete, only to re-open as the Zito Partnership in 2016, after yet another homicide in the wake of continued cuts to services.

Nevertheless, the impetus to move psychiatric and learning disabled patients into the community, which continues, is commendable and important. Although we try to avoid psychiatric hospital admissions, there are times – especially during a relapse – when a week or two of respite as an inpatient can be crucial. Medication may need to be changed, suicide risk managed safely, and violent behaviour tackled with a graduated return to the community via a period of trial leave. These short-term admissions can then be followed by high-quality community care, ideally from a single catchment area team.

However, even these small numbers of beds have been progressively cut, meaning that rushed admissions of one or two days are common. With fixed, minimal bed numbers on the general adult wards, there are daily meetings with the aim of running through the current patients and discharging the least disturbed in order to make way for the latest crisis, regardless of day-to-day variations in the numbers of patients who would be better off staying a bit longer.

At the same time, the pathway into mental health services has been made more complex, with opaque and bureaucratic referral procedures and separate teams for patients at different stages of their illness. My colleague Simon Wilson recently published a paper[24] about these problems, on which I was a co-author. We pointed out that people suffering a psychotic breakdown in which they have completely lost contact with reality are now expected to deal with letters asking whether they would like to opt in for help with their mental illness. As you can imagine, this creates further barriers, as they may not have a fixed address – because the delusional and persecuted often move around – or the post may lie unopened on the doormat of someone experiencing a profound mental breakdown.

Meanwhile, geographically based teams that used to accept referrals of all types have been replaced by smaller teams, such as crisis-resolution teams, early intervention teams and prodromal psychosis teams, who only deal with cases showing the very early symptoms and signs that precede the characteristic manifestations of the acute, fully developed psychosis.

So it's harder to get into treatment than it used to be, while at the same time the pathway out of psychiatric treatment can be brutally rapid, with discharge to overworked GPs increasingly common. It recently took me five months to persuade a mental health service to assess a patient with high-risk behaviour. This was a case where the patient's mother had also noticed a change and was asking for help. One thing I have learned in my job is that concerned mothers of those with mental illness should always be taken seriously as, tragically, psychotic violence is often directed to those close by: that is, friends and family – especially mothers.

Royal princes and retired football players talk passionately about reducing the stigma and improving treatment access for general 'mental well-being' (as opposed to more serious 'mental illness'), as well as for depression, anxiety, PTSD and addiction. This is clearly a noble aim, but the reality is that although there are now more psychological therapies through the Improving Access to Psychological Therapies programme (IAPT), specific addictions treatments are facing a downward spiral of cuts. And for major mental illness, while the NHS rhetoric is about care in the community, the reality, again, is financial savings. Inpatient beds do cost money, as they require staff around the clock, but we have gone way below the critical mass needed to provide safe care.

So, despite all the platitudes about equivalence between mental health and physical health, the reality is that these crucial crisis beds have been closed and the gulf between the well-funded forensic units and the chaos of general adult care in the community is growing ever wider. Patients are referred for forensic opinions about risk, but sometimes it feels as if the referral is actually a request for the forensic team to interview the patient and write a report, as the general adult teams are so overwhelmed by their outpatient caseload they haven't themselves got time for a more in-depth assessment.

As we've said, schizophrenia can be linked to violence in a number of ways, and general risk factors – being a younger man with a past history of violence, personality disorder, drug use and impulsivity – must all be factored in. Many of our forensic patients have the 'triple whammy' of a neglected and abused childhood adversely affecting their personality, early drug abuse and a psychotic breakdown as a young adult. Throw in a serious violent offence or a homicide committed during that first psychotic breakdown, and you have a fairly typical forensic patient.

But violence in schizophrenia can be driven by psychotic experiences alone, especially command hallucinations, persecutory delusions and delusions of being controlled by outside forces.

Peter Adeyemi, one of the most psychotic patients I have ever interviewed, said, 'I think I was being influenced . . . I suspected that I had enemies . . . they were using chemicals on my brain, put into my ear . . . acids, powders, gunpowder, caustics and hydrochloric acid . . . I suspected someone had a set of spare keys to my flat.'

He believed his thoughts had been intercepted by telepathy and that people he knew had been replaced. 'Someone is not really the one I know, they are clones. There are people who look the same, but I didn't have substantial proof.'

He said voices were 'competing against what I want to do until I become exhausted and then I give in and do what they say', and he suspected a 'miniature limpet speaker' powered by 'body salts' had been placed in his ear.

With a mental state like this, his brutal killing, with multiple stab wounds to the neck, of an elderly neighbour who he thought was involved in his torment is no less shocking but perhaps less surprising.

Managing a case like Peter will always be a challenge. His care was criticised – he was not taking medication, and had been missing appointments – but he had not been seriously violent before. But how good are current mental health services at managing cases known to have a clear risk of violence?

You only have turn to the press reports about Simon Grachev. This was not a case of mine, but a report in the public domain outlined Grachev's long history of mental illness, going back to his university days, when he had become a heavy cannabis smoker. He had been sectioned on multiple occasions and used knives to threaten his parents and a psychiatrist. His condition stabilised with treatment for around a decade after 2000.

Prior to the attack, he had been staying with his mum, but he began to feel mentally unwell as his psychosis started to relapse. Both he and his mother made contact with mental health staff and repeatedly asked for him to be admitted to hospital. Grachev told one mental health worker that he thought he 'might harm his mum'. He was identified as needing a psychiatric admission, but no bed was available.

Two days later, while waiting for a psych hospital bed, he stabbed his mother to death and then set fire to their flat.

The case highlighted not just the missed warning signs but the trust's decision to axe more than one hundred beds in the previous four years.

Quoted in the press reports was the chief executive of a mental health charity, who said: 'It is a scandal that Aileen Grachev lost her life . . . mental health services are in meltdown.'

Grachev pleaded guilty to manslaughter on grounds of diminished responsibility and arson, having previously denied murder. The Crown court judge made a restriction order under the Mental Health Act to keep him in hospital indefinitely.

So the message is clear. If you have a major mental illness and you want high-quality psychiatric hospital care, with a detailed assessment, access to tailored therapies and diligent risk management, then sometimes it seems the best way to get this is to become a forensic patient.

The police are accustomed to dealing with the mentally ill, and often use their powers to transfer them to a place of safety in hospital, only for them to be discharged the same day. A 2018 report by Her Majesty's Inspectorate of Constabulary and Fire & Rescue Services said, 'The police service is stepping in to fill shortfalls in health services . . . transporting someone to hospital because an ambulance isn't available; waiting with someone in hospital until a mental health place is available; checking on someone where there is concern for their safety. Often, as a 24/7 service, police are the only professionals available to respond because the person is in crisis out of hours. We believe there needs to be a rapid investigation into this situation and, if necessary, proposals for fundamental change.'

Tragically, in some cases, where assessment or treatment is delayed or denied despite warning signs, only after an act of serious violence or an arrest for murder will the system ensure care is provided.

Recent research has shown a decline in homicide in the general population. Homicide by the mentally disordered has also fallen, but by less than the fall in the general homicide rate, while homicides by people with schizophrenia have risen.

Is this the result of mental health service cuts? It is too early to say, and homicide is still a low base-rate event, with infrequent occurrence, so trends are hard to interpret. But the way services are organised now, it feels to me more like a roll of the dice than a risk-management programme.

The mentally disordered may kill in an abnormal mental state, but like many murderers, they are also more likely to kill a family member than a stranger, often in the context of a quarrel or an argument. Those who kill in a profoundly psychotic state may have previously led blameless lives or have a history of antisocial behaviour before the killing. But even if they have a background of violence – being a gang member, say – the killing is usually extreme and out of the ordinary compared to their previous offending. As you might imagine, it is the antisocial gang members who kill while psychotic that are the most challenging.

Homicides by those with schizophrenia number around five to eight per cent globally, so in the UK we might expect around three per month, two of which would have been committed by someone who had had previous contact with a psychiatrist.

But what about those cases not known to mental health services? It is probably a fact of life, or an 'epidemiological constant', that a certain proportion of people with undetected mental illness will commit homicidal violence in any one year, during a first psychotic breakdown. The issue of these killings is the same around the world.

After I had been at the Maudsley for two years, I'd grown confident enough in my new-found skills to take up a six-month work exchange in Sydney, New South Wales. While there, I met forensic psychiatrist Olav Nielssen, a researcher at St Vincent's in Sydney. He has pooled studies from around the world and found that one-third of all homicides carried out by mentally ill people were committed by first-onset cases: people who had never been diagnosed or referred to a psychiatrist before they killed. In a further international study across four countries, Olav made another important finding. The killing of a stranger by those with schizophrenia is extremely rare, occurring at a rate of one homicide per fourteen million people per year – that is, around three per year in the UK. The stranger homicide offenders were more likely to be homeless and to have exhibited antisocial behaviour than those who killed family members, and they were less likely to have ever been treated before.

So sometimes a murder may be the first sign that someone has had a mental breakdown, by which I mean a psychosis. The only way to prevent these killings is to improve awareness of what emerging psychosis is like – particularly for relatives of those who are developing it for the first time. Perhaps this book will help.

Case Study: Jonathan Brooks

7

At a forensic service in London where I was working as a consultant, our referrals meeting would be held at 10 a.m. on a Friday. Most of the forensic trainees, and members of the nursing staff and other disciplines, would gather to run through the inpatients and highlight any upcoming discharges or potential flashpoints. After that, the referrals would be reviewed. There could be anything between one and eight per week.

Jonathan Brooks's referral came in as routine. Although clearly psychotic, he was not aggressive and had already started treatment. HMP Wormwood Scrubs, where he was being detained for murder, wanted us to consider his transfer to hospital for an assessment.

In the UK, as in Nordic countries, it is relatively easy to move a prisoner to a secure hospital if they need it. Even a sentenced prisoner can be moved under section, although they remain subject to their sentence and may be returned to prison. The position is very different in the United States. There, the only way a prisoner can go to a secure psychiatric hospital is for them to be found legally insane at the time of their trial, which means a number of severely mentally ill inmates languish among the two million prisoners. In many other parts of the world, secure psychiatric treatment of mentally disordered offenders is a luxury of civilised society which just cannot be funded in the face of other priorities.

I was booked on to the Scrubs official visits list, and had decided to skip referrals that week. It was August 2013, and I drove along the A40 listening to the parliamentary debate about military intervention in Syria, and then switched to a

CD. However, the discordant tones of John Coltrane's *Live at the Half Note: One Down, One Up* made me feel more irritable, so I drive on in silence before taking the exit for White City, left past the Hammersmith Hospital and on to Scrubs, a red-brick Victorian prison that housed over 1,200 inmates in vast galleried wings.

I parked in the potholed gravel visitors' car park and then dodged puddles on my way to the visitors' entrance. Prisons have a way of making even official visitors feel unwelcome, and Scrubs used to be notorious for being unhelpful, even when we'd come at their request. Add to that the smell of sweat, rubbish, prison food and Lysol floor wash, and the overall effect is to leave you feeling like you need a shower by the time you come out again.

I passed through the usual X-ray screening and, to avoid the trudge back to the car, had to throw away a favourite Rotring 0.3mm fibre tip, because it was in excess of the permitted two pens.

My escort walked me down the side of B Wing, taking a wide berth to avoid the detritus of cigarette butts, unwanted food and bags of excrement thrown from the cell windows above. I was reminded to keep my eyes to the left in case of flying projectiles.

Waiting in an interview room, I looked up from my papers as Jonathan Brooks was brought into the room. A master's degree post-graduate in his mid-twenties, dressed in a prison tracksuit, he walked slowly and seemed fearful. When we talked, he seemed subdued and spoke softly, although he warmed up as the interview progressed.

After asking about his current situation – food, exercise and visits – I enquired about his background. He said that his father, Paul, had worked in marine consulting, having been in the Royal Navy. He'd been based in Southampton but also used to travel to Annapolis, Newport and Boston in the USA.

The interview was painfully slow as I coaxed the story out of him.

I cleared my throat and began. 'I want to ask you about your family. Tell me about your father, what did he do for a living?'

'I lost my dad,' he told me.

'When was that?'

'This year.' As I was discovering, he kept his answers short and did not spontaneously elaborate.

'Did you get on all right with him?'

He shook his head. 'I didn't know him well. We didn't get on.'

My questions continued and as he became more at ease I managed to glean that his mother, Veronica, was fifty-one when she died, and that she had been a dinner lady at the local primary school.

'My sister, Ann, is a paralegal,' he told me.

'Was she living with your mum, too?' I asked.

'She was moving into her own place, before this all happened.'

I nodded, pleased that we seemed to be getting somewhere at last. 'Tell me about your education. How did you get on at school?'

'School was okay . . . I didn't have many friends.'

'Tell me, what did you do after you left school?' I asked. 'Study? Training? Work?'

'I went to Hull to study a BSc in economics.'

'How did you get on?'

He shrugged. 'It was okay . . . I got a 2.2.'

We pressed on.

After much effort, Jonathan had enrolled on a master's degree course in finance at Anglia Ruskin, but his father died just before the term ended. During his time in Cambridge, he lived in a student house and again appears to have been somewhat isolated. He completed his master's degree and returned home to live with his mother and sister. There he began to apply for jobs and was hoping to obtain a further training position in computing or finance.

He went for an interview for a trainee accountancy post, but said he became wary when he was asked to take his jacket off, and that after the interview he was introduced to another candidate in the waiting room who he thought was 'suspicious' and was there to try and 'get information' from him. He said that he had a 'general feeling' there was something 'strange' going on in this situation.

'Everything seemed larger than life,' he told me, adding that he remained uneasy for a few days after this interview, but that these thoughts gradually improved – until he went for another interview, on Thursday, 11 July 2013.

This interview was at a software company. 'The office telephoned me to confirm the interview was going ahead.' He caught a train and arrived in good time, but he felt the interview did not go well. He thought that maybe the long journey had affected his performance. He caught the train back and bought a cup of tea on the journey.

He said he did not see the assistant make the tea, but that it was produced from under the counter of the buffet car. He drank it and subsequently fell asleep for about two hours.

'I passed out until someone shook me awake. I felt so tired.'

The next day he began to suspect that his tea had been spiked. He started feeling sick every morning and believed he'd been drugged but had no idea why, or who might be responsible. This worried him and he attached significance to a radio report he'd heard that talked about plastic contamination of water.

He said he'd told his mother about his concerns and that she advised him to see the doctor. He had wanted to see the police rather than his GP, but his mother persuaded him there was insufficient evidence to take to the police. He continued to feel anxious, scared and convinced that something bad was happening throughout the following week, and described going to post letters with his mother on Saturday and how he had been fearful of a white van parked next to the corner shop, which he believed was a surveillance van. He saw a man blowing dead leaves, but thought he was pretending and that he had a rifle hidden under the hedge. In a local park he also believed people were listening in on their conversation.

When he switched on a light early on the morning of Monday, 15 July, a fuse tripped out, and Jonathan began to suspect that someone was in the house. He insisted that his mother set the house alarm before going to bed each night and became so scared of being in his own room that he slept on the floor in his mother's bedroom on Tuesday. He believed there were vehicles circling outside the house. He also started to hear whispering, which seemed to be people describing his movements, although he couldn't see anyone. Were these echoes from listening devices? he began to wonder.

On Wednesday he visited his grandmother's house with his mother, but refused to eat any sandwiches or cake, as he saw a photograph of his grandfather with some male friends in suits and began to think the Freemasons might be involved in some sort of conspiracy to keep him under surveillance; he thought this was all linked to his job interviews.

As he described his experiences, I could see how he had developed a delusional mood, persecutory delusions, auditory hallucinations – all classic symptoms of schizophrenia.

Witness statements and exhibits included in the Crown Prosecution Service bundle provide a further window into his mental state, such as an email from Brooks to human resources at the software company:

I recently attended for interview . . . I was surprised by the peculiar behaviour of the panel. Firstly, I have never been to an interview where the lead interviewer has suggested that I take off my tie . . . secondly, when I briefly hesitated in response to a question the chairman said, 'Are you all right?' He then said, 'Did you say "yes"?' I simply and categorically did not say, 'Yes.'

I was concerned by the behaviour of a member of staff in reception who was clearly bogus. I am also concerned that a member of staff was observing my arrival on camera while I was attending for interview. In view of the above, I wish to withdraw my application for employment at your establishment . . .

Yours sincerely,
Jonathan Brooks

Brooks's preoccupation with surveillance had evidently begun, and it would escalate to reach delusional intensity later. The external recruitment record of that interview from the other side of the desk provides further evidence of his withdrawal into a psychotic state. Remember this is a master's level student quite accustomed to interviews:

Monosyllabic answers with only one or two sentences despite lots of probing . . . No evidence of inter-team interaction except to provide technical knowledge . . . Jonathan's a very withdrawn candidate, who appeared quite reluctant to talk, despite prompting and probing by the board. Communicating with him was very difficult.

Ann Brooks, his sister said,

Jonathan began to talk about something very odd. He said he thought that someone had put something in his tea when he was travelling on the train. He thought that he had passed out for about two hours. He was adamant that he remembered nothing of the journey and believed someone gave him a shove when the train reached Birmingham to let him know he had arrived and wake him.

He said a taxi driver was weird and everything was strange. We tried suggesting that he probably fell asleep. Jonathan was adamant that someone had put something in his tea. Jonathan hadn't mentioned this business on the train before Saturday. I tried to reason with him and asked where he had got the tea. He said that he had got it from the refreshments on the train . . . but I didn't believe this could have happened.

On Monday Jonathan was still being physically sick and couldn't eat anything . . . Jonathan spoke to me about there being a power cut the night before . . . Jonathan was saying that he thought someone was targeting our house. He was going on about Freemasons.

Neither Mum nor I could convince him that it was a power cut that had affected the street. He believed that someone had specifically done something to our house . . .

I was feeling worried about his behaviour so I took my parrot in its cage to my new flat.

I spoke to Mum that Monday and on the Wednesday. I suggested that Jonathan should see the doctor. Mum thought it might be nerves causing an upset stomach. Mum said something like, 'He hasn't been right for a while.'

On Thursday at 8.54 a.m. a witness, William James, called 999, and complained that a neighbour, Mr Brooks, had appeared in his driveway and looked terrified.

Later another witness, Post Office worker Andrew Wong, described Brooks entering the shop and looking agitated, constantly looking over his shoulder. He said Brooks was clearly distressed and exhibiting signs of mental health problems.

Amelia Davenport also reported seeing Brooks outside her partner's building on the same day. She was alone in her car when she saw a man walking towards her, clutching a set of keys. Although he didn't seem agitated, she said that he looked completely zoned out and was staring.

Also that morning, a friend of Brooks's mother called the police. He was concerned, having not seen Mrs Brooks since the previous Friday at around 2 p.m. Police visited the address, quickly gained entry to her home and found her dead from multiple stab wounds.

At 9.54 a.m. the same morning, police received another 999 call from a corner shop approximately five minutes' walk away. Staff had seen a man in the street with blood on his hands. Police attended at 10.05 a.m. and found Brooks hiding in a large bin in the forecourt of the nearby railway station. He had cuts on his right hand and blood on his clothing and arms.

Nearby youths were filming and laughing, and were asked to refrain from doing so as 'the male was clearly unwell'. When attempts were made to persuade him out of the bin, he resisted fiercely, until he was restrained, cuffed and taken to a local police station.

Jonathan told me what had happened. On the morning of the offence he got up at around 8 a.m. and went into the kitchen to get breakfast. He ate cornflakes but shortly afterwards felt nauseous, and attributed this to drinking poisoned tea on the train journey (even though the interview had taken place almost three weeks previously).

Next he became suspicious that someone was interfering with the radio in the house. Every time he changed the station there seemed to be a report referring to environmental pollution and he thought this was linked to him being poisoned deliberately. He believed that somebody was controlling the information coming into the house and when he saw a news headline referring to corrupt politicians, he became sure this was further evidence of a conspiracy.

He said that during the week between his last interview and the day of the offence he had been convinced his life was in danger. Everything he saw, heard and felt seemed to confirm his worst fears. He added that he had begun to feel suspicious about his mother, as there was no one else in the house, so she might be involved. Over several days he then became certain that his mother was a spy who was controlling his life.

She didn't seem herself to him, and was behaving strangely, and he started to think that someone had assumed her identity while his real mother had been abducted. He was frightened there was something outside the house and also believed his mother might have been responsible for his morning nausea – in other words, that she was poisoning him. He continued to hear whispering voices describing his actions and it was as if the voices were conversing among themselves.

He remembered rushing into the kitchen from the hall and hitting his mother with a shoe, then taking a kitchen knife and stabbing her in the neck from behind.

He felt as though he wasn't really in control of what he was doing, and described how his mother ran for the telephone in the hallway and he followed, repeatedly stabbing her. During the attack, he cut his fingers as they slid down the blade and he remembered dropping the knife to the floor. He then realised that the surveillance was continuing and ran outside to try and find somewhere safe to hide. He had vague memories of seeing other people, but by this stage was convinced he was going to be killed.

He denied having any violent thoughts prior to the attack or having planned the attack.

He said, 'I really did feel as though I was being watched . . . I had been poisoned . . . I blamed my mother for it.'

He still couldn't understand how he had done it.

Staring into the distance, clearly perplexed by what had happened and with his symptoms fading on antipsychotic medication, yet still unable to accept his persecutory experiences hadn't been real, he said, 'It's a terrible tragedy . . . I haven't been allowed to go to a service for her.'

Jonathan was charged with the murder of his mother, Veronica Brooks, on Thursday, 18 July 2013.

From this interview, you can identify Brooks's psychotic symptoms. Around the time of his job interviews, he had a 'delusional mood' and delusional interpretation of normal events: the white van, the leaf blower, the family photograph and the way he was given a cup of tea on a train, a sign of it having been poisoned. He became convinced that he was under threat and subject to surveillance and he gradually incorporated his mother, replaced by an imposter, into those persecutory delusions.

This was probably his first episode of major mental illness in the form of schizophrenia, although only time would tell. Incontrovertible was the fact that with such profound psychotic symptoms, this master's-level student had become a killer.

Four psychiatrists, including me, agreed that he was psychotic from a recognised medical condition at the time of the killing, substantially impairing his ability to form a rational judgement. The CPS accepted a guilty plea to manslaughter on grounds of diminished responsibility, so there was no need for a trial by jury. This is a partial defence to murder, thus criminal liability is reduced but isn't absolved completely, while of course the abnormality has to provide an explanation for the killing. In this case there was no alternative rational explanation for him killing his mother (something the police will always seek to rule out). At the sentencing hearing, an order was made for his detention in secure hospital with a restriction on release without limit of time. Now he had to begin the long process of treatment and rehabilitation, and coming to terms with what he had done.

The local press said, 'A schizophrenic who stabbed his mother to death has been detained indefinitely in secure hospital. He has not given a reason for his savage attack at the family home.'

Although of course he *had* explained it, and it was quite rational in his deluded state of mind. After all, who wouldn't take action against an imposter who was involved in a conspiracy to poison you and had you under surveillance? The analogy of the horror film made real applies again here.

In Jonathan's case, I hadn't really needed to interview him to make the diagnosis. The whole story was clear from reading the witness statements. His sister had correctly described his psychosis, but how could she or her mother have been expected to understand what was happening?

I remember reading the case papers. It was one of those late summer afternoons just before the schools go back. I had worked my way through the statements with a growing sense of awful inevitability about where the story was headed.

Of course, if a psychiatrist had interviewed Jonathan in time and made the diagnosis, and offered some treatment, then the killing might have been prevented. Hindsight is always tempting, but this was yet another reminder to me always to extrapolate the possible adverse future outcomes in any given psychiatric case.

Those who kill their own mothers are around six times more likely to be found to have a psychotic illness compared to other homicide perpetrators.[25] Which is why forensic psychiatrists take distressed mothers seriously. We always accept referrals of matricides, as they are invariably 'one for us'. I have seen many cases of those who've killed their mothers while in the grip of delusions about witchcraft or 'juju', or being possessed by evil spirits, or the devil, and often with bizarre crime scenes to match: decapitations, mutilated pet reptiles, forks stuck in the body. To kill your primary caregiver, your birth mother, you must be mentally abnormal, right? The statistics speak for themselves.

Think of the impact of this on Jonathan's sister. She has not only lost her mother but also her brother, to a lengthy spell in secure psychiatric hospital and the inevitable, lifelong distance created between them by what he did to their mother, however disturbed he was.

A death by suicide has a terrible impact on families, far worse than death by natural causes, as relatives can be left with thoughts of what might have been done differently. But the death of a family member at the hands of another often means that two lives are lost; the victim as well as the perpetrator.

8

My own family experienced this double loss of life in a way that would profoundly affect the lives of my grandparents Edward and Katherine. My maternal grandfather, Edward, joined the Royal Navy just after the end of the First World War, and while serving on HMS *Iron Duke* he witnessed the evacuation of Greek refugees during the great fire of Smyrna in 1922. He spent most of the inter-war period on battleships in the Mediterranean Fleet.

His tough exterior masked a softer demeanour as a kind mentor to the younger men under his command, although as I recall from my childhood, you had to scratch quite hard to find it. He was an accomplished boxer and Imperial Services Boxing Association Light-Heavyweight Champion in the early 1930s, when the British Empire's military was still huge. Boxing tournaments would be held on board battleships – in Edward's case HMS *Revenge* vs HMS *Hood*, before it was sunk – or at naval bases like Portsmouth and Malta. The inter-service boxing finals were held at the Stadium Club, High Holborn.

A press cutting from an edition of the *Evening Standard*, around 1931, describes his victory against Kennedy of the army in the light-heavyweight division: 'Kennedy made no attempt to disguise his intention of winning by a knockout, but he had a big shock in the second round when Alberts dropped him on the canvas. It was a thrilling fight in the last round. Alberts put Kennedy down five times and in some wild fighting towards the end, Alberts himself twice visited the boards but he did sufficient to get the verdict with something to spare.'

He qualified as a diver and during the Second World War, when HMS *Queen Elizabeth* was holed by an Italian manned torpedo in Alexandria harbour, he was lowered into the murky water with a traditional diving helmet and lead boots to deal with the damage to the hull. He was mentioned in despatches twice for these exploits and somehow managed to avoid ending up on a sinking ship, unlike some of his comrades.

But the naval life took its toll on my grandmother Katherine. Edward was almost permanently away at sea in the thirties. Their oldest child, my aunt Georgina, didn't meet her father until she was past her third birthday, and when he did come home, she was apparently angry and resentful at the loss of her mother's undivided attention. Katherine was left alone with Georgina and their second child, also called Edward. Like many others, Katherine spent the war as a single parent, eking out wartime rations. There was real fear that Germany would invade, and my grandfather had left a revolver with instructions for Katherine that, in the event the Nazis arrived, she should shoot the children and then turn the gun on herself. Portsmouth was a major target for the Luftwaffe and frequent trips to the air-raid shelter at the bottom of the garden added to the stress.

Despite V-1 rocket doodlebugs in Portsmouth and minisub torpedoes in the Mediterranean, all the family survived the war. Edward returned to Portsmouth and extended his service to become an instructor at the gunnery school, no doubt dining out on his war stories. But as must have been common for many wartime couples, the long-awaited reunion was not so happy. Georgina was a difficult child and always seemed to get between my grandparents, exacerbating tensions. As a teenager, Georgina started to develop a form of paranoia, believing that everyone at the bus stop was looking at her. She also became paranoid towards her own family, accusing her parents and siblings of snooping in her bedroom and – bizarrely – of tampering with the nose-pads on her glasses.

My mother and her younger sister were both born shortly after the war and it seems that with four children, and Georgina's problems escalating, my grandmother's nerves became increasingly frayed. A split developed, with Edward regularly taking the other children out cycling or for long walks along the sea front while Katherine stayed at home to look after Georgina, who couldn't tolerate being out with her siblings.

I have only recently heard the full version of this story and, as you can imagine, it still provokes tears when it's spoken out loud. Although Georgina had her troubles, to external observers, theirs was a normal, respected family. But my mother has early memories of trying to keep the peace indoors, not only between her parents, but also between Georgina and her siblings.

My uncle Edward later left Portsmouth and became a journalist at the *Manchester Guardian*, but Georgina stayed at home and trained as a secretary. She started dating Charlie, who was also serving in the Royal Navy, thus setting herself up for the separations and loneliness of the naval way of life. It is said, in my profession, that children sometimes repeat, in an unthinking and compulsive way, the life choices and mistakes of their parents. Were Georgina's decisions an example of this?

Georgina and Charlie were married and travelled out to Malta to join the Royal Navy community there. Not long after the wedding, Charlie was posted back out to sea and their first child, Louisa, was born in Malta. But she was a colicky baby who cried constantly and, with no support from family (health visitors were non-existent), Georgina was unable to cope. In desperation, she wrote to Charlie saying that she 'wouldn't be around' when he came back. The Royal Navy hierarchy got wind of these troubles and must have realised this would be no good for morale on board, so

Charlie was posted back to a shore establishment near Portsmouth. Charlie and Georgina then went to live in a flat near the family home there, just around the corner from the Queens Hotel in Southsea.

Back in Portsmouth, although she had Charlie with her, Georgina still didn't cope well with motherhood. Louisa was not a settled child and cried frequently. Despite this, my mother recalls cuddling her five-month-old niece, taking her for long walks in the pram and feeling so proud of her sister.

But Georgina's mental state deteriorated, her paranoia worsened, and she developed the delusional conviction that others were observing her with intent to do her harm. Convinced, also, that she had been contaminated, she scrubbed herself with Vim scouring powder in the bath. She gradually descended into a post-partum psychotic state, but there was little understanding of this condition back then and, with the support of others, she continued to parent her baby.

Some time later, my mother, then around fourteen, was at home when Charlie paid a visit. My mother entered the living room, puzzled to see her father sitting with his head in his hands, devastated by what Charlie had just told him.

It must have been hard for Edward to describe to his child what had transpired between her older sister and her niece. He explained that Georgina had killed her baby and that the police had taken Georgina away. Bewildered by this news, my mother remembers being taken to the local police station by her father. But when Edward went into the custody area to visit Georgina, my mum was left outside to wait. She remembers feeling profoundly upset and angry at what her sister had done to her little niece Louisa. Once the visit was over, she walked home arm in arm with my grandfather, who was understandably in tears.

My mother says what hurt the most was seeing her toughened 'war hero' father so reduced by what her sister had done.

The next day, my mum was queueing in the post office for some stamps when she overheard two older women talking. One said to the other, 'Did you see the news about that woman who killed her baby? I hope they hang her.'

At that moment, my mother felt her anger towards her sister shift towards sympathy and compassion, mixed with a deep sense of shame. Because, of course, the abolition of the death penalty was still more than five years away, and Georgina did indeed face the prospect of being hanged for murder unless there was some psychiatric explanation.

Over sixty years later, Georgina described the events to me.

Louisa was constantly crying. There were brief periods of respite, for example walking her in a pram, only for the wailing to start again once the motion stopped. Tormented by her paranoia and still feeling unsupported – it seems that Charlie had resented his ship posting being curtailed – Georgina continued to struggle.

One morning after Charlie had gone to work, Georgina could bear the wailing no longer. She said that she picked up the pillow, put it over Louisa and was 'too frightened' to take it off.

Her memory of what happened next is sketchy, but Georgina said she realised what she had done. The arrival of the doctor and then the police are a blur. She remembers being taken to Holloway prison, having all of her possessions taken away and being placed in a single cell. She was told she couldn't go on to a wing for fear that the other women prisoners might kill her, once they found out she had killed an infant.

Georgina says the single cell was awful and she begged to be moved out of her solitary confinement. But when she was eventually placed in a dormitory, this was worse. She was in a bed next to a woman who had killed two babies, apparently to get back at her husband, who'd left her. Georgina witnessed fights and saw one woman urinate on another's clothes during the night. After about five weeks, she was too mentally disturbed to remain in prison, so she was moved to St James's Hospital, Portsmouth. Her delusions of contamination had become more severe, and she couldn't bear anyone touching her clothes or her bed.

She made a number of suicide attempts. Before long, she was treated with electro-convulsive therapy. Meanwhile, her case had started to make its way through the courts, and so Georgina began the journey of all mothers who kill their infants.

Women Who Kill Children

Case Study: Grace Kalinda

9

It was mid-morning, and Colin was driving his double-decker bus from West Croydon to Perry Hill. There were just a few passengers on the lower deck after the morning school rush, and the bus stops ahead were mostly empty. As he looked along Northcote Road, however, he saw a couple sitting at the next stop. They were an odd sight. While the man clearly hadn't washed in days, the woman looked well turned out, and when Colin brought his double-decker to a halt and opened the door for them, they made no move to board the bus.

It was only then he noticed a young girl, four or five years old, sitting between them. A little girl with a bruised face. Her eyes swollen shut. As he watched, the woman lifted a can of lager towards the young girl's lips. Anger welling up, Colin was about to intervene, but thought better of it. Instead he fumbled for his mobile phone – a Nokia 6300 with a snake game that his own six-year-old daughter liked to play – and dialled 999.

The officers took just seven minutes to arrive and even less time to call for back-up. They whisked the little girl off in the back of the squad car, the 'blues and twos' (blue lights and two-tone siren) blasting as they rushed straight to the nearest A & E at the Mayday Hospital, Thornton Heath.

Arrested at the scene, Grace Kalinda from Uganda and David Johnson from Catford were both taken to South Norwood police station. At 11.31 a.m. they were charged with child neglect and being drunk in charge of a child.

And no doubt Colin gave his own little girl a longer-than-usual hug when he arrived home from work that night.

The Mayday Hospital, notorious for being both extremely busy and under-resourced, served the large catchment area of Croydon, and – now renamed the Croydon University Hospital – still does. I knew it well. When I qualified back in 1990, I had to complete two six-month house jobs in medicine and surgery before full registration as a doctor. We were allowed one academic post at the medical school and had to do the other at the coalface of medicine. Thinking the experience of a busy district general would do me good, I signed up for a post in respiratory and general medicine at Croydon.

My first on-call was a hot weekend in early August. I'd sat in the canteen at the 9 a.m. handover, sipping anaemic canteen coffee with the medical team, which consisted of Rhys Thomas, my fellow houseman; Graham Berlyne, the senior house officer; and Charlie Easmon, the medical registrar. In those days, Charlie was in charge, as we would only see the consultant physician at the post on-call ward round.

'Well, it seems pretty quiet,' I said.

'Just you wait,' said Charlie, 'it won't stay that way for long . . .'

Sure enough, within a few minutes we were bleeped to our first referral, and over that weekend we assessed forty-eight referrals from A & E. I had to learn quickly and work hard. My fifty-six-hour shift, starting on Saturday at 9 a.m., finished at 5 p.m. on Monday. This was before the campaign over junior doctors' hours and worries about safety had started to gain traction.

The transition from student life was a massive shock, not least having little or no time for a social life. One Monday evening, after a shift like this, during which I'd only snatched a couple of hours' sleep, I was due to meet some friends for a drink. It was around 6 p.m., so with an hour to spare, I decided to take a quick nap in my on-call room before going out. I woke up after what seemed like a moment, but looked at my watch to see it was already Tuesday morning. I had slept for thirteen hours straight, was already late for my next shift, and would never get back that longed-for evening out.

Now, years later, it was to the Mayday Hospital they took little Nancy Kalinda. On arrival, she was distressed, but thought to be in general good health and well nourished, with her weight right for her age, her verbal and motor responses indicating a normal Glasgow Coma Scale (the fifteen-point scale used to measure conscious level), a normal neurological examination, and with no evidence of sexual interference or longer-term abuse.

However, as the previous observers had noted, her face was bruised and swollen with both eyelids shut, and she also had a number of other fresh bruises and scratches around her body. In all, the clinical picture was indicative of acute non-accidental injury.

Sedated in order to allow the paediatric ophthalmologist to examine her eyes, Nancy was found to have subconjunctival haemorrhages, the whites of her eyes tinged vermilion from ruptured capillary blood vessels, suggesting blows to the face. Happily, her vision was normal, with no signs of inflammation or raised pressure in the eyes.

Back at South Norwood police station, it was quickly established that the male adult at the bus stop, David Johnson, was a skid-row alcoholic. In a chance encounter, he had offered the woman, Grace Kalinda, a drink from his can of super-strength lager, which she'd accepted, although she wasn't intoxicated when breathalysed. In view of the injuries to her four-year-old daughter, Nancy, Kalinda's charge was upgraded to Assault Occasioning Actual Bodily Harm Contrary to Section 47 of the Offences Against the Person Act.

Meanwhile, Kalinda had been behaving bizarrely in her cell in the police custody suite. By 11 p.m. that night, she was observed chanting, laughing and making strange hand gestures. The custody sergeant asked for the forensic medical examiner (a forensic-trained GP), who noted, 'She was shouting . . . hostile and distressed at the same time, agitated, believing we had come to kill her . . . jumping from subject to subject . . . talking about Jesus, the devil and child sacrifice.' She was deemed not fit for interview and the mental health team were called to assess in more detail.

On the hospital's children's ward, Nancy, no longer sobbing, was being coaxed by a nurse to sip some juice. She asked the nurse about her sister and, when questioned further, seemed to be saying that she had a sister at home, sleeping in her cot.

This was quickly relayed to police officers, who were still trying to establish Kalinda's identity and address. Once they'd worked this out, uniformed officers were dispatched to a terraced house sub-divided into two flats with a communal front door. There, the officers found the communal door slightly open but the flat door locked. When no answer came after they had hammered and rung the bell, they forced the door, using their police powers to enter premises without a warrant in order to save life, and began to search the place.

The flat looked clean, but there were signs of a recent disturbance, with broken crockery on the kitchen floor. PC Brown searched the empty galley kitchen, living room and Nancy's room, the smaller of two bedrooms. The master bedroom was dark, the curtains drawn, with bed linen strewn around the floor. In the corner was a simple white IKEA cot with a very young baby, asleep, neatly tucked under a white crochet blanket.

However, as PC Brown approached, it was clear to her that the child was not breathing. What's more, she was cold and rigid to the touch, with severe bruising all over her arms as well as her torso, and a discharge from her nostrils. This was Nancy's sister, six-week-old Dembe.

Dr Peter Herbert, the police forensic medical examiner, attended the scene and pronounced life extinct at 13.03. The little body was taken to the Mayday hospital mortuary, to await the post-mortem.

After the discovery of baby Dembe's body, Grace was re-arrested and her charge further upgraded from assault to murder. She made no reply to caution, staring vacantly ahead, seemingly preoccupied by some abnormal hallucinatory internal experience. Two psychiatrists were called to examine her. Despite some disagreement as to whether the chanting might be part of a religious cult, perhaps, and better dealt with in prison custody, Kalinda was sectioned for an inpatient psychiatric assessment.

She was transferred to the nearby low-secure psychiatric ward at the Bethlem, where she told the staff that God had 'given me power . . . since last week . . . the devil is around me . . . Jesus Christ was sending me to heal people.' There, her mood changed rapidly from periods of calm to episodes during which she'd jump up and stare at staff in a threatening manner, in one case pointing at a nurse: 'That woman has got a demon.' She was placed on two-to-one observation for her own safety, but was left off antipsychotic drugs so a baseline mental state could be established. In the meantime, she was diagnosed with probable post-partum psychosis, the most severe psychiatric complication of childbirth.

The weeks after childbirth can be joyful, but of course new mothers are vulnerable to a range of possible altered mental states, like the baby blues (well over fifty per cent), post-natal depression (over ten per cent), and much less common, post-partum psychosis (around one to two per 1,000 live births).

Post-partum psychosis can appear within a few days or weeks after birth. If missed by family or health visitors, it can result in seriously disturbed behaviour, or even the baby's death at the hands of their mother.

This had been Dembe's tragic fate, and also that of my cousin, Louisa, smothered to death by my aunt Georgina. Unlike Grace, Georgina didn't go straight to psychiatric hospital and her case had to make its way through the criminal justice system. As we shall see, nothing good comes from cases of infant children killed by their parents, but these terrible events are not always as a result of psychosis. How common is this awful offence and how does it vary around the globe?

10

In the nineteenth century, the economic and social options for unmarried mothers were severely limited, increasing the risk of infanticide as an act of desperation. Indeed, in the twenty-four years between 1863 and 1887, 3,225 children under the age of one were killed by a parent in England and Wales, making an average of around 150 deaths per year.

The law had been recognising these issues for some time, with the potential for acquittals or royal pardon for those found insane. By the middle of the nineteenth century, the insanity defence had been codified in the M'Naghten Rules, following the acquittal of Daniel M'Naghten for a murder committed while suffering from persecutory delusions. The M'Naghten Rules, which remain the law on insanity in the UK and the USA, require that the accused was 'labouring under a defect of reason, from disease of the mind' at the time of the killing.

The emerging view was that any woman who murdered her own child must, by this definition, be insane, and couldn't be held responsible for her actions. After the Royal Commission on Capital Punishment in 1864, women would be sentenced to the mandatory death penalty but never have their sentence carried out.

The 1922 Infanticide Act brought in the new offence of Infanticide, so that the prosecution could start with a reduced charge, but the issue would still be put before a jury, and a murder verdict remained possible. In 1938, the revised Infanticide Act – which remains the current law – increased the age limit to up to twelve months, so that Infanticide is defined by law in the UK as death at the hands of the mother occurring up to one year of age, when the 'balance of her mind was disturbed . . . having not fully recovered from the effect of her having given birth to the child or . . . the effect of lactation consequent on the birth'.

The language of these legal definitions may seem archaic, but despite the advances in psychiatry (for example, lactation is no longer seen as the cause of mental disturbance), we still use these rather outdated legal criteria. Given how far back these legal provisions go, it is clear that the law has long tried to make allowances for mothers who kill, because while murder of all types is overwhelmingly committed by men rather than women – a ratio of 10:1 – a high proportion of female murderers have killed their own children.

Why? The 'desperation' issues of the Victorian era have largely been eradicated. These days the causes are more likely to be psychological and anyone working with psychologically distressed women would recognise that they, more than men, tend to direct their aggression towards their own bodies, or to their own reproductive system, in a general sense, or their child. Estela Welldon wrote that women were not solely the victims of violence, but could also be perpetrators. In her book *Mother, Madonna, Whore*,[26] Welldon argued that women have aggressive impulses, that their aggression can be concealed and that their violence may often be towards their offspring.

This, of course, challenges the notion that mothers couldn't possibly decide to harm their children unless 'the balance of their mind was disturbed'.

Children under one year of age are, in fact, the age group most likely to be the victim of homicide. In 2018 in England and Wales, there were sixty-seven victims of child homicide (below sixteen years), and in the average year around half to three-quarters of child victims are killed by a parent, with only a handful of child victims killed by a stranger (a statistic often obscured by the massive press attention on the, thankfully, rare paedophile abduction homicides).

As we've said, child killing is more commonly committed by mothers rather than fathers. And mental disturbance of one form or another is frequently found in the mother of those killed, for example in the context of delusions or acute psychosis, as with Grace Kalinda, and also, many years before, with my aunt Georgina.

Mental disturbance is not limited to post-partum psychosis, of course, as severe depression, where the mother can see no future for herself or her children (in its most extreme form known as nihilistic delusions), may involve what we call an 'extended suicide', sometimes called a familicide.

An example reported in the press was that of Navjeet Sidhu, twenty-seven, who suffered depression brought on partly because her first-born child was not a boy, and partly because of pressure on her from her extended family. After an arranged marriage seven years earlier, there had been conflict with her husband Manjit during a trip to India. He had only returned on condition that he not do any housework (if you are not a feminist already, you will be by the time you finish this book).

On 31 August 2006, while travellers at Paddington station were boarding a high-speed Heathrow Express train, Navjeet left her home in Greenford, west London. With her twenty-three-month-old son Aman in a pram and her five-year-old daughter Simran walking beside her, the trio's movements were caught on CCTV cameras as she made her way to Southall station. Witnesses later reported seeing Navjeet with her two children, apparently loitering around the platform as early as 11 a.m. A Great Western security contractor became concerned and approached her.

'I asked her what she was doing, and she said, "I'm taking

my children to see the fast trains." I told her she was not allowed down there and she accepted that. She seemed very calm and collected.'

Navjeet had phoned her husband, and said, 'I'm going far, far away and I'm taking the children with me.' Manjit drove around the neighbourhood looking for her and finally spotted her entering Southall station, but there was no free space for him to park. By the time he reached the platform, it was too late.

The next person to see Navjeet was the driver of the Heathrow Express train at 1.20 p.m. He saw her holding Aman to her chest and Simran by the hand as she flung herself and the children off the platform in front of the high-speed train. The train driver told British Transport Police that he'd tried to brake but wasn't able to stop in time. Navjeet and her daughter were killed instantly. Simran's body was so badly damaged that she could only be formally identified by her fingerprints. Aman initially survived his multiple injuries, but died two hours later.

When a killer simultaneously takes their own life, there is no criminal trial. At the inquest, the coroner made a finding of suicide for Navjeet and unlawful killing for her two children.

It seems that Navjeet never had the opportunity to receive psychiatric treatment, but Grace Kalinda, by contrast, had been so obviously mentally disturbed that (like Daniel Joseph) she bypassed prison custody and was sectioned straight to hospital.

However, most women arrested for serious violence, murder or attempted murder of their children, like Georgina, will be remanded into prison custody. In 2001 I had started working in HMP Holloway, then the largest remand prison for women in Europe. I will return later to the events that brought me to Holloway, but it was there that I assessed a series of cases from which I learned most of what I know about infanticide, criminal violence, abuse or neglect committed by mothers towards their infants and children.

Andrea Wood, a middle-class military wife I assessed at Holloway, was severely depressed with nihilistic delusions, and had become convinced there was no possible future for her and her six-year-old daughter other than death and decay. She attempted to drown her daughter in a bath and cut her own wrists (serious, deep cuts incising an artery, not superficial self-harm). The daughter survived, Andrea's incisions were surgically repaired, and then she was charged with attempted murder. Later, her depression improved with treatment at Holloway but, still wracked by guilt, she pleaded guilty to attempted murder, refusing attempts by her lawyers to mitigate the offence, and later still, made a very serious suicide attempt, most likely a continuation of the previous one.

This was a desperately distressing case of failure to transfer to hospital. I had referred Andrea to her local secure psychiatric hospital for treatment of what, in my view, was profound depression. But the assessment of the local psychiatrist was that her self-harm was related to personality, not to mental illness, and therefore she should stay in prison (bad rather than sad or mad, in other words).

It was a few weeks later that I received the early morning call informing me she had been transferred to A & E at the local teaching hospital. She'd been cut down from an improvised noose, already blue and close to death.

I reached the hospital to be told that she was in the intensive care ward. Her brain was permanently damaged after being starved of oxygen. So I referred her to her local forensic psychiatry service for the second time, not for treatment of depression but for long-term care in a permanent brain injury unit. This time she was accepted.

These prison transfer decisions are life and death, but there was no exhaustive inquiry into this case. Andrea was just a prisoner. I had been proved right, but it is hard to imagine a more pyrrhic validation of my clinical opinion.

One of my mentors once said that if you want the right outcome, sometimes you have to let someone else take credit for it. I have found over the years that quiet diplomacy and gentle pressure, such as repeated referrals of the same case, work better than a confrontational approach. If you push too hard or are critical of another opinion, then it's likely that the colleague you are trying to persuade will dig their heels in out of sheer bloody-mindedness.

Occasionally, however, I've had to escalate all the way to the top with a threat of a judicial review, manipulation via a court process or formal complaints. One patient's story illustrates this very well.

Cherelle was in Holloway for fairly low-level offences, but was in our gated cell to allow close observation, having become acutely disturbed in mental state and behaviour. She had set fire to her cell, her hair and her clothes, and was self-harming with a razor blade that she'd concealed in her vagina. Although accepted for transfer, she was on a waiting list for weeks while our prison staff tried to keep her safe in a hopelessly inadequate environment. Giving evidence at Southwark Crown Court about her case for the third time, with the transfer to hospital still unresolved, the judge asked if I had any thoughts. I suggested that he might consider asking the chief executive of the relevant NHS mental health service (NHS Trust) to explain to the court why no bed had been found. He duly issued a witness summons and a bed was found within twenty-four hours. I have only used that nuclear option on three occasions that I remember. It has to be used sparingly, but it is very satisfying when it works. Cherelle improved quickly following her transfer to hospital.

But despite the high rates of self-harm and even suicide post-offence, most women who are remanded in custody after serious violence to a child survive to face the court process – as did Georgina, despite multiple suicide attempts. These days the law creates a singular category of infanticide, which from a forensic psychiatrist's perspective can be classified into six subtypes.[27] The first is 'neonaticide', the killing of a newborn in the first twenty-four hours of life, which seems to be different from other forms of 'infanticide', the killing of those between a day and a year old.

Official statistics suggest this is a very rare event, but the true number of neonaticides is unknown as they may be concealed, and even now there are occasionally news stories of mummified newborn bodies or skeletal remains being found in lofts or buried. In 1861, 150 newborn or very young babies were found dead in the streets of London, and foundling hospitals like the one in Mecklenburgh Square near Great Ormond Street Hospital (now a museum) were set up for those found still alive.

Historically, babies have been killed for ritual purposes or because they're unwanted. The Aztecs, ancient Greeks and Romans all did it. The practice persisted during China's one-child policy and continues to persist in parts of India, where sex-selective infanticide occurs as male babies are favoured for cultural and economic reasons. Neonaticide is also common in historical periods or in contemporary societies where contraception is limited or unavailable. Often in young and immature mothers, still living at home with parents, the reality of the pregnancy may have been denied. This can lead to the babies being born in secret in hotel rooms, then being either drowned in toilets or baths, strangled or suffocated.

The next subtype is the Medea Syndrome, sometimes called a spouse-revenge killing.

In Euripides' ancient Greek tragedy *Medea*, the titular protagonist was a woman scorned. Her social status in the Greek world was threatened when Jason left her in favour of Glauce, a Corinthian princess. He planned to keep Medea as a mistress but, unwilling to accept this loss of status (and perhaps, as has been argued, taking charge of her life in a patriarchal society), Medea takes her revenge by murdering Glauce, as well as Jason's new father-in-law, King Creon, with a trick involving poisoned robes. She then stabs to death her two sons from Jason, thus destroying the symbol of their marriage and exacting on Jason the most extreme revenge imaginable.

Over two thousand years later, we refer to Medea Syndrome when children become fatal victims in the toxic psychological conflict between a parent and significant other. The killer might have a mental disorder, such as severe depression, or be a vengeful, narcissistic parent: 'If I can't have them, nobody can.'

This doesn't always involve straightforward revenge, as Medea Syndrome covers all scenarios where the motivation for the killing comes not from an issue with the child but from a problematic relationship between the child's parent and another person or persons (who may or not be the other parent).

A simple example would be the arrival of a new partner (usually male) who finds the children inconvenient, leading to the mother disposing of a child to avoid losing the new relationship. This may sound incomprehensible, but it has happened. In a more extreme case, Louise Porton, twenty-three, suffocated Lexi Draper, three, and strangled sixteen-month-old Scarlett Vaughan in Rugby, Warwickshire, in 2018, seemingly because the children 'got in the way of her sex life'. She did not seem distressed by Lexi's death and accepted forty-one friend requests on the dating app Badoo a day later. The jury took just six hours to find her guilty of both counts of murder after a four-week trial at Birmingham Crown Court. During the trial, the court heard evidence that Porton would often leave her daughters in the care of others, or alone, while she went out to pursue men for sex and cash. Porton was convicted of murder twice over and sentenced to life imprisonment with a minimum term of thirty-two years.

Cases in this group include a 'family wipe-out', typically caused by a parent involved in a childcare dispute after a failed relationship, who may also take their own life at the same time. In a demonstration of the twisted ambivalence of the parent who kills their own child in this context, the instinct to nurture is maintained despite the murderous act. They often leave the child victim or victims tucked up in bed with their favourite soft toys, showing residual affection towards the child. But the urge to appease or exact revenge on their partner or lover is more powerful.

I have seen crime-scene photographs of such killings and they can be too much to bear: the body of a dead six-year-old boy, for example, killed by his father but neatly laid out on his bed in his favourite Nike Air Max 95s and Superman costume, with his mother also lying dead in the neighbouring bedroom. You may have seen the typical headline in a case like this: 'A family of five have been found dead. Police are not looking for any other suspect'.

Another example appeared in the *Sun* newspaper in July 2019. A 'materialistic' mother drowned her own 23-month-old twins Jake and Chloe in the bath at their coastal home in Kent. She was in conflict with her partner after she lost her lavish lifestyle in Qatar and ended up in a 'shithole' in Margate. Police had been called to a collision on the London-bound A299 on 27 December 2018 after she deliberately smashed into the back of a lorry at speeds of up to 100 mph. She was 'hysterical' and said to the police: 'Just let me die. I've killed my babies.' After rushing back to the house, police discovered two children lying in their beds, dead but fully dressed.

The psychiatric experts disagreed as to the explanation for this offence (narcissistic rage vs profound depression) and this was reflected in the 'hybrid order' sentence of ten years, to be served partly in secure hospital and partly in prison.

The fact that infanticides can be grouped into observable subtypes means that the pattern of child murder year-on-year is disturbingly familiar. As well as the smothering of the newborn, psychotic infanticides and Medea Syndrome, there are also 'mercy' killings of severely disabled children, killings to eliminate an unwanted child and the murder of children as an extension of child abuse or neglect.

A well-publicised case in point of a so-called 'mercy' or 'altruistic' killing was Tania Clarence in 2015. Hers was an affluent middle-class family, but she was a severely depressed mother, apparently overwhelmed by the enormous challenge of caring for her three disabled children. Olivia, four, and three-year-old twins Ben and Max suffered from a rare but devastating and ultimately terminal muscle-weakening condition, which required repeated intrusive treatments and surgeries. Tania smothered them in their sleep and then attempted suicide.

Verdict: manslaughter on grounds of diminished responsibility times three. Hospital order.

11

Mothers who eliminate an unwanted child may have no psychiatric disorder other than an abnormal personality, but there can be a history of family discord and maltreatment. The first murder case of any type that I encountered in psychiatry was Stella North, an isolated woman in her early twenties who had been transferred to secure hospital facing a charge of murder of her newborn baby. When I joined the team, she was halfway through a three-month in-depth psychiatric assessment. A report was being prepared to assist the CPS in their decision as to whether the murder charge (with a mandatory life sentence) would be replaced by one of infanticide (where all sentencing options would be open, including a hospital order under section or even a non-custodial penalty such as probation).

In my inexperience, I thought it obvious that, as this was a case of a mother killing a newborn baby, 'the balance of her mind must have been disturbed' – still the legal criteria for infanticide.

I probably had my aunt's history in mind when I made that simple assumption. But forensic psychiatry is a field where you must assume nothing.

Stella's case had been discussed in our weekly seminar with a forensic psychotherapist. To understand murder, you have to come at it from different directions. A psychotherapist trained in psychoanalytic theory can give us a different perspective.

I went into the fortnightly seminar clutching my notes, ready to present the case to Calista, the psychoanalyst assigned to our team. She told me to put away my notes and instead describe Stella's story to the seminar, as well as what it was like to be in a room with her. I laid out the background, from memory, and noted that Stella seemed to be detached from the killing and from her dead baby. The discussion went on to consider not just her disturbed mental state but also her murderousness to her unwanted baby. Stella had concealed her aggression by seemingly separating herself from her actions. She seemed disconnected from any feelings towards the dead baby, as if it had never existed in the first place.

The debate about Stella forced me to re-think my simplistic 'mental illness' model of infanticide. It gave me an uncomfortable thought, too. My cousin Louisa had been an unplanned arrival. She was also a difficult baby who didn't settle. Although there was no doubt that Georgina had been affected by her grossly disturbed mental state, had she possessed a degree of murderousness towards Louisa? At this point, I'd not heard Georgina's account of the smothering, which I now know had been a response to incessant crying, albeit in a highly disturbed mental state. Stella's was the first case of infanticide I had seen professionally, and that must have been when I began reflecting properly on Georgina's story, which in turn set me on the journey of enquiry that ultimately led me to my work at Holloway.

Further details revealed in Stella's case suggested a level of 'murderousness' that was hard to fully reconcile with infanticide. She had telephoned the police from her fourth-floor council block flat, reporting her baby missing. Police officers were all over it: dozens of uniformed staff searched the area, doing house-to-house enquiries and seizing CCTV evidence. After a twenty-four-hour search, the cold, dead body of her newborn was found in the large communal waste disposal bin at the bottom of a rubbish chute, which originated outside the door of her flat.

You can imagine the outrage of the police officers who'd conducted this search, believing it to be abduction, only to find that the mother had disposed of the baby herself. She was not psychotic, but the pregnancy had been unplanned and unwanted – she was immature and isolated and suffering from post-natal depression.

A few years later, I coincidentally found myself as a newly qualified consultant (in an 'acting up' or locum post) supervising Stella in outpatients. After a year in secure hospital, she had been given a non-custodial penalty and made subject to probation supervision with a condition of psychiatric treatment. But she seemed blithely unconcerned about what she had done (dissociated, in psychiatric terminology), often arrived late and frequently cancelled appointments.

She was in a new relationship and thinking about starting a family, despite what had happened to her first baby. If she did go ahead with her plans for another baby, a child protection team would be keeping a watchful eye on her with a pre-birth case conference. They would have to answer difficult questions. Could Stella be safely allowed to care for another child? Would it be safe to even allow her to hold the baby for a few minutes after birth? These were questions I later faced myself while managing pregnant women with serious mental disorders – what we call perinatal psychiatry.

Children killed by parents or carers as an extension of child abuse was a hot topic in the media while I was at Holloway, with the deaths of Victoria Climbié and Baby P in north London attracting blanket media attention. The publicity around those cases focused almost exclusively on the perceived failures of social services and seemed to ignore the culpability of the parents (another example of our contemporary blame culture).

I have seen so many cases of criminal neglect leading to death and deliberate lethal abuse, but a couple of examples linger in my memory.

In Holloway I was asked to see Amelia Stevenson, who had been remanded there having been charged with murder. She herself was a modern-day foundling, abandoned at birth and found in a plastic bag on the doorstep of a hospital before going on to short-term foster placements and a children's home.

She displayed disturbed behaviour at school, dropped out of education and progressed through recreational illicit drug use to heroin addiction. She had several unplanned pregnancies and her first baby died within a few weeks from pneumonia. Her second had been made subject to a full care order by social services and was in the process of being permanently adopted.

Amelia went back to injecting heroin – 'if you can't beat them, join them', she said – and then became pregnant again by her boyfriend, Seth.

During this third pregnancy, social services agreed – oddly, you might well think – that there would be a trial of her parenting with extensive support. She had consented to stay off heroin during the pregnancy so as not to pass her dependence on to the baby. But she quickly relapsed, and managed to hide this from the midwives and social workers (by using 'street' methadone and later switching back to heroin).

When the baby, James, was born, Amelia could see that he was 'very sick', but only she knew that he had heroin withdrawal, which produces flu-like symptoms: muscle pain, fever and chills. The distressed baby was crying frequently.

'Instead of getting professional help, we thought we could manage it ourselves . . . we thought that if we proved we could look after him, they might let us keep him. Joe got some methadone . . . we gave it to him with his feed and he seemed to get better . . . The midwives and health visitors were coming around daily, but we managed to conceal it.'

One day Amelia woke late, feeling groggy from the warm blanket of heroin oblivion.

'The next morning, he was still in bed . . . I had a feeling; I knew something was wrong . . . my boyfriend cried and said, "Amelia, he's dead." I thought he was still asleep, but he was cold. I tried to feed him, but his body was already stiff.'

Manslaughter – five years' imprisonment.

Despite significant self-harm, Amelia was turned down for a psychiatric hospital bed, her negligent homicide not eliciting much sympathy.

In Amelia's case, her neglect of James was hidden from health professionals. This concealment of negligence or abusive behaviour towards children is not uncommon and can take many forms, as I discovered early in my medical career.

By chance, while working on the chest medicine team at the Mayday Hospital, I encountered some unusual psychiatric cases which have stuck in my mind to this day. During those six months there, it had been hard enough keeping up with the torrent of referrals from A & E, chasing blood results and replacing blocked intravenous drips. At that time, I probably came the closest to throwing in the towel and walking away from medicine altogether. Yes, it was that bad, even after six years of training. Despite our exhaustion, we had to stay alert, as the sickest patients were fighting for their lives – and sometimes losing them. But among those genuine patients, we would detect a few who were faking a medical problem. We presumed they were doing so in order to gain the attention that goes with a hospital admission, or maybe to get a kick out of tricking us and wasting our time. But what motivates someone to fake the painful colic of a kidney stone, even surreptitiously cutting a fingertip to drop blood in a urine sample to further convince us?

This was more than just seeking painkillers, as we'd switched away from drugs with abuse potential. Once discovered, these patients would be summarily admonished and banished from the hospital, without so much as an opinion from the 'trick-cyclist' (semi-affectionate, yet denigratory term for my future profession, used by the physicians and surgeons).

One particular case in this group caught my interest. A young woman, Tamara Atkinson, had been admitted to the medical ward, suffering with poorly controlled epilepsy. She'd been accused of poisoning her own child with her anti-epileptic medication and then presenting the child to the doctor with unexplained symptoms. When the child had been admitted to a paediatric ward for observation, Tamara had tampered with the drip, causing a life-threatening infection by contamination of the infusion, and putting her child in intensive care. Next Tamara suffered an apparent seizure in police custody and was transferred to the Mayday emergency room.

Admitted to the ward, she continued to have uncontrolled fits despite adequate treatment and we hastily ordered brain scans and a brain wave test (electroencephalogram), worried she might have a growing brain tumour. When these tests were all negative, we became suspicious. I observed her having a seizure in her hospital bed. It looked convincing, with rhythmic contractions, her head arching back. She even went to the trouble of wetting the bed, which commonly happens in genuine fits.

While we set about confirming these were fake 'pseudo-seizures', Tamara started to develop multiple large, infected, pus-filled boils on her legs and her left arm. The child abuse investigation receded into the background as we became concerned that there was something wrong with her immune system. We checked her blood for HIV and ran a full panel of standard blood tests and microbiology swabs, looking for an unexplained infection. After a search in the literature for rare and unusual conditions, a possible candidate jumped off the page, namely 'Job's Syndrome'. Named after the biblical figure, this was a dysfunction of the white blood cells that usually fight infection and can lead to uncontrolled pustule formation. It seemed to fit the bill, so we booked Tamara in for a test at a neighbouring specialist hospital.

Meanwhile, our consultant had been called to give evidence in court about Tamara's medical status and whether she was fit to attend the criminal and family court proceedings. While we were trying to unravel all of this, a hospital porter came up to me one day and in a conspiratorial whisper, said, 'Doc, I don't mean to interfere, but I just saw something I thought you might want to know about. You know that lady in bed seven? I just saw her sticking needles in her leg.'

It transpired that Tamara had been contaminating needles with her own faeces and sticking them into her skin to produce the boils. She had both Munchausen syndrome and Munchausen by proxy (the deliberate fabrication in yourself, and inducement in a vulnerable other, of a 'factitious' medical condition). Tamara clearly had a significant personality disturbance, and she would have to go to court and face her accusers after all.

Fascinated by the process of unpicking the mental gymnastics that must have been required in order to think and behave like Tamara, I presented her case, complete with slides of the offending lesions, at our monthly medical grand round. Afterwards I was taken aback when the senior dermatologist said to me, 'All very interesting, but next time bring us a real rash.'

I was realising at this early stage that I'd have to find a branch of medicine which was more than skin-deep. Psychiatry was reeling me in. To me, Tamara's affliction was a very real rash. Other skin rashes may reveal underlying medical conditions like scabies, syphilis or systemic lupus erythematosus (an autoimmune disease with a characteristic facial rash). Hers was an open window into her highly disturbed personality: an example of a woman turning her aggression on her own body and reproductive system, namely her child – the process that has been described by Welldon.

The condition, or pattern of behaviour, known as Munchausen by proxy constitutes a severe form of child abuse, and is usually a criminal offence. It is generally found in women who are the mother, carer or nurse of the child. They present the child to doctors with an apparent illness, which is later discovered to have been induced by the caregiver through false reporting of symptoms, or by inflicting injuries on or poisoning the child.

Controversial medical research involving covert surveillance has even found that some mothers of children with breathing problems were actually smothering their own babies. The videos are striking to watch. Mothers can be seen clearly and repeatedly trying to suffocate their own child, while presenting this as a spontaneous cessation of breathing (an apnoea attack). The babies are wired up to breathing and heart monitors and nurses are watching on camera, ready to come in and prevent the worst. This research suggests that, while the vast majority of cot deaths are genuine and devastating, a very small proportion are likely to represent concealed infanticide if the smothering is not detected soon enough. Despite the evidence, there has been a reluctance to accept that mothers are capable of this twisted combination of deception and harm.

Does the deception allow these mothers to deny their aggressive impulse to the child and also feel exultant as they trick the doctors, thus assuaging their own feelings of helplessness? This is one attempt at a 'psychological formulation' but the mechanisms remain largely unanswered. These mothers often show signs of severe abuse or neglect, self-harm or eating disorders, and may have presented with unexplained symptoms and/or had unnecessary hospital admissions and operations themselves.

They also have difficulty vocalising their distress, something we psychiatrists call 'alexithymia', loosely translated as 'the absence of the words to describe a state of mind'.

The experience I had gained as a junior medic, including cases like Tamara's, helped me later understand some of the child abuse cases I saw as a psychiatrist at Holloway prison.

So I had learned that killings of children as an extension of abuse and neglect come in many guises, and the abuse which precedes the killing can be concealed. But sometimes there are cultural and religious practices towards children that may be condoned or even encouraged in other societies, but which constitute criminal offences in the UK, and which, *in extremis*, can lead to fatalities.

Female genital mutilation (FGM) – which affects 200 million women and girls around the world, according to the Five Foundation – is an example of this. In the UK it is illegal, with the acceptance now (at least by parliament) that misguided cultural sensitivities must be put to one side in order to protect young girls from irreversible harm caused by this culturally sanctioned abuse. In a similar way, other physical and emotional abuse which is practised in some communities – in the context of beliefs about voodoo, the occult and demonic possession – must be called out and made subject to criminal sanctions.

But from my point of view as a forensic psychiatrist, these practices need to be distinguished from delusions. Delusions may respond to psychiatric treatment, whereas culturally normative beliefs about witchcraft will not. Non-psychotic ideas about the malevolent forces of evil spirits or witchcraft are surprisingly common, especially in a culturally diverse city like London. For example, beliefs about 'djinn' (or genies) are common in some Islamic communities and 'evil spirits' or 'demons' are often referred to by those from sub-Saharan African countries.

Studies which have surveyed religious and cultural attitudes in different countries have found that beliefs about the existence of evil spirits are held by fifteen per cent of Ugandans and up to ninety-five per cent of the population of Ivory Coast. Cultural beliefs about demonic possession have resulted in significant violence to children, with accounts describing exorcism procedures involving chilli pepper being put in children's eyes, beatings and even ritual murders, particularly of albino children, whose body parts are said to possess special powers.

In 2008, more than 300 cases of murder and disappearances linked to ritual ceremonies were reported to the police in Uganda. The Ugandan government appointed a special police taskforce on human sacrifice, as there were several high-profile arrests of parents and relatives accused of selling their children to witch doctors for ritual sacrifice, to guarantee wealth and prosperity.

Of course, London is no stranger to the ritual murder of children. In 2001 the case of 'Adam' involved the discovery of an unknown boy's torso in the Thames. Following a complex investigation, he is now thought to have been trafficked from Benin City, Nigeria, via Germany to the UK. He had been poisoned (sand flecked with gold particles was found in his stomach), as well as bled and skilfully dismembered, most likely as part of a 'muti' or 'voodoo' ritual murder.

In Holloway prison, I saw other examples of culturally sanctioned violence towards children. In one particularly distressing case, a young Mauritian woman who was in a relationship with a West African man had been persuaded by her partner that their six-year-old daughter was possessed by evil spirits. The couple had beaten her repeatedly, burned her with hot candles and then stitched her into a sack, planning to throw her into the canal near Kingsland Road.

Luckily, they were disturbed by a neighbour and didn't follow through with their murderous plan. It was only when their daughter appeared to be tearful and dishevelled at school that teachers made a referral to social services and the full story emerged. Although her partner had clearly influenced her, the mother showed no evidence of mental illness – she was dealt the full force of the law and received a substantial prison sentence.

Despite the disturbing details of all this violence towards children, I found that by this stage of my career I was able to focus on unpicking the clinical and forensic evidence of murder cases without being too distracted by the nature of the material. It is said that it takes around five years to settle in as a consultant in most medical specialities, which I think is about right. Over time, I found my forensic anxiety had diminished. I'd also learned to manage my stress levels by not accepting every referral or teaching invitation, trying not to be omnipotent in preventing every psychotic crime in my patch, and protecting my time at weekends with a ban on report-writing on Saturdays.

Perhaps forensic psychiatry had become, for the most part, just another profession for me, inured to violence and its consequences. Some people go to work to look at a trading screen, design buildings, teach a classroom of children or read manuscripts, but a few of us traipse around the prisons to interview murderers and try to make sense of them.

When asked, 'What do you do?' at social occasions, I'd just say, 'I'm an NHS hospital medic,' in order to avoid the inevitable discussion about the meaning of evil: 'Surely all killers must be crazy?' or 'Why can't we just hang them all?'

When I went to interview Grace Kalinda some months after her psychosis had been treated, I had to determine, in retrospect, her mental state at the time of the killing. I was also curious to see how she had responded to treatment and what account she would give me of her earlier life and how it had led to the terrible events in her flat.

Born in Kampala, Uganda, Grace had an unremarkable history. There was no abuse in her childhood and she had completed secondary education. She'd arrived in the UK about three years before the killing, aged twenty-three and planning to learn English. She had left the estranged father of four-year-old Nancy in Kampala but returned there briefly, rekindling the relationship and becoming pregnant with baby Dembe. Once back in London, she lived in a privately rented flat in Thornton Heath and had been there for about six months, working as a nursing assistant and a childminder, while attending weekly English lessons in a group. She was a devout Seventh-day Adventist, well known in her local congregation. She said she had no previous experience of demons, 'until I saw them . . . just before my daughter died'. It was clear, then, that her beliefs about witchcraft were psychotic and not culturally or religiously normative.

I asked her what the demons looked like. 'They're dark with eyes, not like human, they were coming into my children . . . I was scared, I was alone with my children.

'I tried to get the demons out, beating them with my hands . . . I hit them on the head and massaged their bodies . . . the spirit told me to do that . . . the spirit told me to get the demons out of them.'

She had become convinced that the only way to get rid of the devil was by 'exorcism', to turn the whites of Dembe's eyes red. Having beaten her until her eyes changed colour, she thought the 'devil had left Dembe', but had 'jumped back into Nancy . . . I thought they were going to wake up.'

I asked her what the consequences would have been if she hadn't beaten the demons out of her children. 'They would have had a bad life . . . the evil spirits would have damaged them . . . The spirit was in my head, repeating to me what I had to do. I couldn't get him out of my head, I was like a prisoner, I couldn't think properly.'

With my interview complete, I caught the fast train back to London. I was under pressure, as usual, to get the report done. I made a strong coffee when I got home and, taking refuge from my son's violin lesson, sat outside in our small patio garden to read through the statements.

A friend who had helped Grace with child-minding said that he'd noticed a change in her behaviour from a few weeks before the killing. She had been sending bizarre text messages and seemed excitable and 'different compared with before'. Another witness described her 'speaking in her own language – she seemed anxious and worried and I thought she was behaving in a strange way . . . like a mad person.' This was consistent with her having developed delusional beliefs about demonic possession and other psychotic symptoms, such as auditory hallucinations, which worsened a short time before the killings.

The police officers who attended the bus stop scene described her as behaving bizarrely and in a disinhibited way. She had been kissing Johnson, who hadn't washed in quite some time. She smelled of alcohol and when they tried to arrest her, she grabbed Johnson's beard, causing him to fall to the floor. She was described as 'smiling strangely' when taken to the van, clutching a Bible and rocking back and forth.

After ten days of observation in hospital, she was treated with antipsychotic medication and, over the course of the subsequent months, her mental state and behaviour gradually improved.

The final diagnosis: 'post-partum psychosis', characterised by religious delusional beliefs, delusions of spirit possession, and the delusional belief that she could cast out demons using violence.

The criminal justice system has provided multiple options for women like Grace to avoid a mandatory life sentence – or, until 1965, the gallows – for murder. It was my task to consider the issues of infanticide, diminished responsibility and insanity, and I had to be mindful of the fact that the legal threshold for these three options gets higher or more difficult as you progress from infanticide to insanity.

It was straightforward for me to argue that she met the criteria for infanticide (disturbance in the balance of the mind) and diminished responsibility (abnormality of mind). But was her mental state so disturbed that she met the higher threshold for legal insanity? Once again, more up-to-date psychiatric diagnoses have to be mapped on to nineteenth-century legal concepts, in this case the M'Naghten insanity criteria from 1843. In order for an insanity defence to be accepted, Grace needed to have been clearly suffering from a 'disease of the mind' at the time of the killing. It also had to be argued that she hadn't known what she was doing was wrong. Given her state of mind, and the fact that she had expected baby Dembe to wake up once the spirits were exorcised, and had made no attempt to conceal her actions or evade the police, the insanity defence was a live issue.

In any event, child killings like this are so terrible that the psychiatric account provides an explanation, which makes the facts of the case more bearable for all concerned, not least the lawyers and doctors involved.

Nobody wanted a trial in this instance, but 'legal' insanity has to go before a jury, even when all psychiatrists are in agreement. The risk is of a jury ignoring the psychiatrists and returning an unexpected verdict of murder. You may remember that in the trial of Peter Sutcliffe, the Yorkshire Ripper, who killed thirteen women and tried to kill seven others in the early 1980s, the jury ignored the unanimous opinion of psychiatrists that he was mentally ill and this had 'diminished responsibility', and returned a verdict of guilty to multiple counts of murder and attempted murder, ensuring twenty life sentences. On that occasion, the judge, jury and society at large were understandably happier with that outcome.

But Grace's trial was short, with only one psychiatrist giving evidence and the judge summing up: 'Members of the jury, the verdict is for you, but it would be an unwise jury, would it not, that chose to ignore the agreed opinions of no fewer than four eminent psychiatrists.'

Verdict: not guilty by reason of insanity. Hospital order and restriction order without limit of time.

Typically, a patient like Grace will spend many years in secure psychiatric hospital and will, of course, likely never have parental responsibility for children again.

In other jurisdictions, such as the USA, there is no specific infanticide law, so mothers who kill their children while psychotic have no other option than to prove that they were legally 'insane' at the time of the killing – which, as I said, is a high bar to clear, legally speaking. Take the case of Andrea Yates in Texas in 2001. She drowned her five children in a bathtub in response to delusions of Satanic influence. She was facing the death penalty after her insanity defence failed, but she was sentenced to life with a minimum of forty years in prison. It was only after an appeal regarding erroneous psychiatric testimony that an insanity finding was made, resulting in her commitment to a secure psychiatric facility.

Around this same period, I had been put off driving by a rear-end car shunt, and so I decided it was time to ramp up my cycling efforts. I would cycle all the way to the secure unit, about fourteen miles each way. The first month was hard. Getting on the bike, especially when the sky was grey or there was drizzle, felt like a chore, but as my fitness improved the cycle home became a welcome time to clear my mind and get my heart rate up. I started to shed the extra pounds accumulated from all those sedentary hours. I could even cycle from Camden along the river to Belmarsh (although I got some quizzical looks from the prison officers as I snuck in to change in the visitor centre loos). I found that after a prison assessment or clinic, forty minutes or so on the bike really blew out the cobwebs.

But the ride to Holloway only took a few minutes, so after locking up my bike, I would show my Home Office ID to the control room at the main gate and pass through the airlock to pick up my keys.

Often while walking around the connecting corridor between the wings at Holloway – with cases like Grace's on my mind – I would be struck by the sight of mothers wheeling their babies in pushchairs or prams after the other prisoners had been safely locked in cells. These women were often serving time for substantial but non-violent offences, like the drug mules from the Caribbean and Latin America who had been caught at Heathrow having ingested multiple packs of cocaine. Prisoners who had arrived while pregnant could apply to look after their child between birth and nine months, under supervision, in the mother-and-baby unit. Of course, there was rigorous screening to ensure there was no risk of harm to these babies. They weren't prisoners and could be collected at the gate by other relatives, as long as those relatives were on the approved list. A series of reports have suggested that it would be better to try and avoid bringing infants into such a tough environment, although at least this way they can maintain contact with their mums during the first nine months of life – crucial for mother-child attachment.

I would later come to better appreciate the effects of separation during those early months, as I reflected on Georgina's prolonged hospitalisation after the death of my cousin Louisa. It would have a lasting impact on her ability to be a good enough mother in the following years.

13

This section has focused predominantly on women who kill children alone, but of course men who abduct and kill may have a female accomplice.

Paedophile abduction murders by men are rare: in 2018, there were only four victims under the age of sixteen who were killed by a stranger. However, the publicity surrounding such cases is huge – and even more so if the male perpetrator has a female accomplice (like the archetypal example of the Moors Murderers, Ian Brady and Myra Hindley).

In 2002, we took a family holiday and, determined to go off-grid, I shut down my phone for our stay in a converted barn up in the hills of northwest Italy. Holidays with toddlers can feel like a logistical nightmare – why would you transport an already stressful feeding and nappy-changing routine to a hot and unfamiliar location? But despite these misgivings, I enjoyed the break, and for the last two nights of the holiday, we drove to Santa Margherita to spend a couple of days by the coast before flying back.

The following morning, enjoying a breakfast in the dining hall overlooking the bay, I saw that *La Repubblica* newspaper had a front-page story with a colour picture of two girls in football shirts.

These were Holly and Jessica, the two victims of the Soham killings. I'd missed all of the media coverage about the search for the two girls, and was unaware that schoolteacher Maxine Carr had been arrested for 'assisting an offender' after she gave suspect Ian Huntley an alibi.

By the time I got back to work, Maxine had been remanded to Holloway and the other prisoners were chanting day and night: 'Nonce . . . child killer . . . the next Myra Hindley.' Maxine was not referred to our team, although I saw her once, being escorted through the prison. It is a matter of public record that Maxine had to be transferred to the local general hospital after her long-standing anorexia became more severe, requiring intravenous fluids, but no psychiatric issues were raised at her trial.

It was accepted Maxine had not been aware that Huntley had killed Holly and Jessica, even after the event, but she was convicted of the lesser charge of perverting the course of justice for the false alibi, and sentenced to three-and-a-half years' imprisonment.

Even so, the hatred towards women associated with male sexual predators is such that Maxine Carr, after plastic surgery and living under a new identity for her own safety, will always be demonised along with Rosemary West and Myra Hindley. When Hindley died in 2002, the *Daily Mail* headline was: 'Myra gets the funeral her child victims were denied'.

The circumstances of mothers killing their children are unbelievably distressing and I have seen many other cases involving extreme violence, such as evisceration to remove evil spirits. For lawyers and doctors, and for society in general, psychiatric explanations do help us understand some, but not all, of these terrible offences. Child-killing is not always as a result of psychiatric disturbance, and women who kill their children through abuse or neglect will not find themselves exonerated by psychiatric excuses.

But what about the case of my aunt Georgina, who had been remanded in custody to HMP Holloway after smothering my five-month-old cousin Louisa? My mother recalls

Louisa's simple burial at Milton Cemetery, opposite St Mary's Hospital. The tiny white coffin was brought to the graveside cradled in the hands of a single pallbearer before being lowered into the ground.

There was no funeral service. No wake, either. When your life is cut short under one year of age you don't get much of a send-off.

Georgina did not attend the burial, of course, being in custody. Clearly suffering from a disturbance in the balance of the mind, her original murder charge was replaced by one of infanticide. Subject to a court order, Georgina was sent to St James's in Portsmouth, but the treatment didn't go well, and after a suicide attempt (not uncommon amongst baby killers), she was eventually subjected to the extremes of psychosurgery.

Nevertheless, Georgina eventually recovered from her lobotomy. Her husband Charlie stood by her, despite the stormy course of her treatment, and eventually she was released from St James's and returned to live in the flat with him. Life settled back to normality and, after a while, she got pregnant.

Of course, the hope was that life would be better for baby David. With ongoing psychiatric treatment and supervision to keep Georgina mentally stable, this was another chance.

But it was not to be. It was a home birth and all was not well. Georgina had been suffering from abdominal pain as a result of presumed cystitis. But then she had a 'show', which is a sign that labour has started. My mother was sent up the road to call for the doctor, but he refused to attend. Perhaps there was some negative attitude to Georgina given what had happened to the baby last time around – and unlike the current practice, there had been no pre-birth child protection conference involving midwives, the police and social workers. David was born heavily cyanosed (a turquoise blue as my mother recalls). He was rushed away to nearby St Mary's Hospital, but only lived for a few hours. Charlie returned from hospital later in the day and said to Georgina in a matter-of-fact way, 'He's gone.'

For my grandmother, Katherine, I can only imagine her sense of grief and failure, after all those years of single-handedly raising four children, only to see her first two grandchildren lose their lives in such needless ways. As well as the inevitable shame around Georgina's infanticide, my grandmother's mental and physical health took a beating. A dark cloud seemed to hang over the family.

However, despite this double tragedy, Charlie and Georgina stayed together, and in 1962 she gave birth to another girl, my cousin Hannah. Hannah received a better start in life than her two siblings and she was the apple of my grandparents' eyes. A precious grandchild indeed.

Still, the impact of the previous events was nothing short of devastating, and it rippled through the family for many years to come. I was not consciously aware of the effect this family history probably had during my early years in medicine, but it must have influenced my chosen career path. I think this background gave me a sensitivity and curiosity about mental disturbance and human destructiveness: and sensitivity and curiosity are essential for forensic psychiatry – more so, perhaps, than other branches of medicine. And after all the infanticide cases it did, of course, belatedly dawn on me that Holloway was the one place where I might develop some understanding of my family's terrible experience over forty years before. Like I said, you don't choose forensic psychiatry; forensic psychiatry chooses you.

I didn't go straight into psychiatry after that crazily busy medical house job at the Mayday Hospital. There's another saying in psychiatry, that it's our medical colleagues who clock whether we'd make good shrinks before we realise it ourselves. My colleague Graham Berlyne was a case in point – when he suggested that psychiatry would be a good match for me, I made a mental note. But I wasn't ready then and so I decided to spend six months in A & E medicine. Amongst all the major trauma, stabbings and cardiac arrests, it was the psychiatric presentations that have stuck in my mind.

And it was there I also treated domestic abuse victims – inevitably men attacking women. As well as suturing split lips and treating bruises and bite marks, I remember even assessing a young bride assaulted at her own wedding after a drunken fight broke out, as well as a woman with spinal fractures who had been defenestrated during an apparently jealous and violent domestic attack. In 2018, an estimated two million adults experienced domestic abuse – that is, roughly six in 100 adults. With this type of violence so prevalent, it's hardly surprising it can often lead to a fatal outcome.

Men Who Kill Their Partners

Case Study: Jai Reddy

14

Lost near Crawley, I found myself in a cul-de-sac that almost took me into the long-stay car park at Gatwick Airport's North Terminal. The road layout must have changed in the meantime, confusing my satnav. I cursed and turned around. If at first you don't succeed.

It was 2009 and I was on my way to see a prisoner called Jai Reddy. Reddy had been charged with the murder of his wife, Jannat, at her workplace some weeks before. After cutting his own forearm, he'd been moved from High Down prison to a secure hospital for an assessment of his mental state. He was, of course, still subject to a return to prison custody, depending on his progress and the outcome of his future trial.

The defence solicitor had warned me he was a difficult client. Sure enough, when he was shown into the interview room, Reddy began by complaining about my lateness, telling me that he was expecting a phone call from his brother, before launching into a rambling account of his wife's failings – all before I'd even had a chance to speak.

He was dressed in a lurid puce polo shirt, and it soon became unpleasantly clear that he suffered from severe halitosis, no doubt explained by the yellowing plaque around his lower teeth. All told, he elicited a very disagreeable impression.

However, my job was to write an expert report for the defence team. I had to retain my objectivity to help me understand what it might be like to be inside his head – or, worse, under the same roof as him – and so I tried to put my first impressions to one side and give him a fair hearing.

He went on in his free-form, time-hopping diatribe, peppered with a post hoc analysis of his late wife's behaviour. He spoke about how their personalities were different and he didn't get on with her family, but then burst into tears talking about his daughter Sarmila: 'I don't want her to be an orphan.' (Sarmila was then studying for a master's at Newcastle University, but as she was a prosecution witness, Jai had been denied any contact since his arrest.)

I passed him a tissue and paused as he regained his composure. We were sitting on easy chairs in an activity room surrounded by 360-degree glass windows. Across the hall, I could see the staff in the bubble of the nurses' station.

Regaining his composure, Reddy said that because he had some knowledge of health matters, it was always his job to care for Sarmila when she was unwell, and that his wife was particularly ineffectual during these times. Medical matters were clearly an issue in the relationship. He complained that, when he was hospitalised with gallstones, his wife was not 'mentally or physically there for me'.

Next he went off on a tangent about an occasion when Jannat had overstayed on a family visit to Malaysia. So eager had he been to see Sarmila that he'd travelled to Kuala Lumpur himself, trying to imply, I thought, that he was the one who had made efforts to keep the marriage going. But recently, their relationship had 'gone worse, from her side'. Regarding arguments he said, 'I was not controlling her . . . perhaps on one occasion I may have hit her . . . on only one occasion.'

Listening to him gripe, I began to wish that I'd left my car in the long-stay car park and jumped on a flight to somewhere hot, or somewhere cold – anywhere, frankly, other than that windowless greenhouse of an interview room with the charmless Mr Reddy. I tried to steer things back to my usual template of biographical information and antecedents to the offence, starting by asking him about his family history.

He told me that his father, Raimaiah, was an Imperial College-educated engineer who had been a lecturer at the University of Kuala Lumpur, and that his mother had worked at a bank. Born in Penang, Reddy had later started, but didn't complete, a science degree, before moving to a job in the state bank of Malaysia. He was a left-arm spin bowler at his local cricket club and a regular blood donor, hence what he considered to be his superior knowledge of all things medical.

Arriving in the UK in 1999, Reddy had studied accounting and, after a series of menial jobs, moved on to a job book-keeping and invoice-processing with Rentokil.

His marriage to Jannat had been semi-arranged. He said he felt that he'd been trapped by circumstance into the marriage, 'but once the marriage had been agreed, I remained with her for twenty-two years . . . I gave her respect and I did so much to provide for her'.

He was subsequently moved to the position of assistant on the bought ledger, with a reduction of £3,000 in pay, and he and Jannat had argued about money. I asked him whether there had been any domestic violence, knowing from the case papers he had been convicted for it. But, despite having just admitted to me that he'd hit her, he said, 'This was false . . . she was falsely accusing me . . . she deliberately framed all of this . . . she knew that it was a Monday and I was stressed, my blood pressure was always high on a Monday.'

In other words, he hadn't hit her, but if he had, it was because she should not have provoked him on a Monday. Who likes Mondays? This was denial and mitigation in the same fetid breath.

In May 2008, he had beaten Jannat with a belt, threatened both her and Sarmila with a monkey wrench and chased them out of the family home. After pleading guilty to an offence of affray, he was sentenced to a non-custodial penalty in the form of a community order, with a requirement that he attend a domestic-abuse programme run by the probation service. He said, 'The domestic violence was fake, but I did the community service honestly. Every Wednesday I had to suffer the mental torture of talking about, "why did you do this?" . . . But I hadn't done this.'

I was feeling irritated by this blatant minimisation but, as usual, I maintained focus on the job in hand, which meant noting down the discrepancy between his account and collateral sources.

But looking back I know what I would rather have been doing. In the car earlier I had been planning that evening's forthcoming trip to the cricket nets in Regent's Park. My boys were working their way through different sporting interests: tae kwon do had been abandoned for cricket, those expensive martial arts suits replaced by cricket whites, pads, bats, helmets and face-guards. It was a warm evening in early summer, and if I managed to pick my route through the traffic, I might just get back in time to catch the end of the session.

Reddy, meanwhile, kept up his minimisation. Despite the battery and affray convictions, he denied anything more than trivial violence. I steered him back to the chronological narrative. In January, he told me, he had heard that his mother had fallen ill in Penang and he wanted to go to the embassy to get a visa to visit her, but he needed identity documents such as utility bills.

'I was upset, it was too much . . . she [Jannat] was cutting my limbs at the knee . . . she wouldn't give me the documents.' There, however, the interview ended, when a nurse tapped on the window to tell Reddy that his brother was on the phone from Johor Bahru, Malaysia.

I headed back to London via the M25, avoiding the endless traffic lights through Purley and Croydon. In forensic psychiatry, you get to know your local geography as well as any photocopier sales rep. Prisons such as Brixton and

Pentonville and courts like Isleworth and Snaresbrook are at all points of the compass, so I use various forms of transport: driving, cycling, overground train, underground, taxis and my favourite – not often practical but always most enjoyable – the Thames Clipper.

I distracted myself with the flute solo on *Tourist* by St Germain as the drive was well over an hour-and-a-half. But I made it to the nets in time to see the last few overs, those precious moments of parental contact I had missed so much when I was their age. The Royal Navy life meant that my father was away at sea for long periods of my childhood. In fact, he only made it to one single sporting event: my last match for the local Winchester rugby club under-18s side, when we suffered a 25–0 thrashing at the hands of the superior Bristol Colts away.

As well as the absences at sea, there were frequent house moves. Shore postings were all around the country from Plymouth to Chatham and Rosyth. This meant that I went to nine different schools, with seven changes before the age of eleven. We seemed to be constantly packing or unpacking tea chests full of crockery, and I grew weary of being the new boy in the playground and of having to adjust to a new curriculum. Later in life I tried to make a virtue of this rootlessness, and before forensic psychiatry, I took every opportunity I got to study or work overseas. But I didn't want my children to have similar instability in those early years. You can't change your own childhood, but you can try and learn from it and give your children a different experience.

As a forensic psychiatrist, I was hearing accounts of far more damaging experiences than mere separations and house moves. Severe neglect and abuse were the norm in the backstories of most prisoners and patients I was interviewing, and the evidence seemed clear to me that there is an intergenerational transmission of abusive and neglectful parenting.

All parents must guard against replicating their own childhood experience.

During my child psychiatry training I'd learned about the research into what makes a good parent, which I will return to later, but some aspects of parenting, you would hope, should come naturally – you just need to be around. That evening, with theoretical analysis of parenting far from my mind, and content that I'd been able to watch my boys, I walked with them up Primrose Hill to catch the sunset, eating ice creams and gazing south over London Zoo and Regent's Park, the Telecom Tower, the London Eye, Canary Wharf, and down to the Crystal Palace radio mast on the way to Bethlem, and, out of sight to the east, the Thames Barrier and Belmarsh prison.

It was a few days later when I returned to the papers in the Reddy case. Running through the bundle, I found witness statements describing him as jealous and controlling. Sarmila said he would become angry after drinking and that he had slapped her around the head and beaten her mum on frequent occasions – a familiar but nonetheless distressing tale of male violence towards a female intimate partner.

Although I tend to see the fatal outcomes, domestic violence that doesn't result in death is all too common. Domestic violence – or 'intimate partner violence' – can occur in any type of romantic or sexual relationship, regardless of the gender identity or sexual orientation of the partners involved. It can even occur in relatively casual liaisons. As you will remember from chapter one, violent acts can be planned and predatory or sudden and 'affective' (emotional). Intimate partner violence falls mostly into the latter 'affective' category.

Violence against women is, globally, a major public health problem. According to data from the United Nations Office on Drugs and Crime, in 2017 an average of 137 women across the world were killed by a partner or family member every single day, accounting in one year for 19,700 murder victims in Asia, 13,400 in Africa, 6,900 in the Americas and 3,300 in Europe. In Mexico the femicide rate has doubled over five years to 1,000 per year. The issue came to a head after Ingrid Escamilla, twenty-five, was murdered on 9 February 2020 by her husband. He said later in his confession that they'd argued about his drinking. After killing her, he had skinned her corpse and disembowelled her in order to flush her organs into the sewer. *Pasala* newspaper published leaked photographs of her corpse under the headline: 'It was Cupid's fault'. In response to this, Mexico's women collectively shut down the country with mass protests against the murder of women and girls, and the failure of successive governments to intervene.

Factors that increase the risk of men being violent to their partners include, as you would expect, poor education, a history of child abuse or witnessing family violence, alcohol and suspicions of infidelity. The risk is greater in societies which ascribe higher status to men than women and/or place emphasis on family honour and sexual purity, or have culturally sanctioned male sexual entitlement at the expense of women's rights.

The achievements of feminism are under attack around the world, and not just in more traditional societies. In Italy, anti-stalking laws introduced in 2009 to protect (mostly) women from stalking were decriminalised in 2017, so that by payment of a fine, the perpetrator can avoid the case proceeding to trial. In the USA, in seven states, a man who rapes a woman can then claim parental rights, while Alabama, Ohio, Mississippi and Louisiana have passed laws banning abortions at any time, with no exceptions for rape or incest – a provision that had previously been a standard component of all abortion legislation. Despite a change in the law and highly effective campaigning by activist Nimko Ali, female genital mutilation has not been fully eradicated in the UK, as some young girls may be taken overseas by parents to have this devastatingly abusive procedure. A Nigerian husband is permitted to hit his wife under Section 55 of the Penal Code, for the purposes of correcting her. In the more puritanical, Wahhabist parts of the Islamic world, the role of women is subject to the most severe restrictions, such as in Saudi Arabia, where women have only recently been allowed to drive. Most pernicious of all is the extreme violent misogyny seen amongst the Taliban and ISIS, with exclusion from education, stoning and sexual slavery. But it is the problem many women have in leaving an abusive relationship which is so striking. In the tribal areas of Pakistan, it may be almost impossible for a woman to leave an abusive husband, but these difficulties can be psychological, as a result of the abuse, as well as coming from legal and cultural barriers.

Being so common, domestic or intimate partner homicides are termed 'normal' homicides – easily solved by police and usually resulting in substantial terms of imprisonment, not hospitalisation. But as we shall see, these murders are not without disturbances of mental state, with personality disorder, intoxication, jealousy, depression and stalking behaviour all playing a part, along with loss of temper or rage.

A few, but not many, perpetrators make it into our secure units, with most spouse murderers serving their time in prison, the main consideration being whether it's a mandatory life sentence for murder, or manslaughter if there is some psychiatric 'excuse'.

On my next trip to Gatwick, I put these considerations to one side. This time I was indeed using the long-stay airport parking for a much-anticipated weekend trip to Italy. I had been training for the Maratona dles Dolomites, a cycling marathon.

The first mountain pass kicks up after the brief false flat into the village of Corvara, but once I got into the rhythm and found a speed I could handle, it became masochistically enjoyable. The pristine mountain air and the sheer relentless effort somehow cleared my mind of all the prison squalor and violence in a way it is difficult to achieve during time off in London. We celebrated our achievement at the post-race barbecue and later with a glass of the deep purple local red called Lagrein in Stefano's cellar wine bar at Hotel Ciasa Salares.

For me, a short but intense break like this pays dividends for weeks. The trouble with a longer holiday is that the week before going away becomes a frantic effort to close out all my reports, and to get up to date with my inpatient NHS key performance indicators (or KPIs), which consist of endless pages of computerised check boxes, most of which are never read. But on this two-day break I had been able to banish thoughts of my caseload until we were back, circling over Gatwick, waiting for a slot to land. Half-dozing when the wheels hit the tarmac, I snapped back to reality and found myself thinking that, somewhere among the lights around the airport, Reddy was safely locked up. I would have to go back to see him, to get the rest of the story.

Returning to Crawley, I was determined to get control of the second interview, and I pressed Reddy to skip ahead to the last twenty-four hours before the murder. 'I had no intention of harming my wife,' he told me. 'I decided to go to TK Maxx where she worked because I was sure she would have the [identity] documents I needed. I thought that if I got the documents I would reach the embassy before they closed and then I could get to Malaysia very soon.'

I pushed him to tell me what happened next.

'Jannat was by the men's jacket section . . . I apologised. I said I needed documents, I was 100 per cent sure she would have them . . . She looked unsure and she took me to the back of the store and said, "Why are you here?"

'She was silent and then she said, "Follow me." My instinct was not to go but I followed her. It was an L-shaped corridor. When she passed the corner, she tried to run away from me . . . she went into an office, but the door lock was faulty . . . I thought she was going to call the police . . . I ran up to her and she pushed me and that kick-started everything . . . only one wound I remember, around the throat . . . I was lost in thinking . . . I hadn't seen the blood coming out . . . I realised the knife was in my hand only about ten minutes later.

'I lost, totally, control of my mind . . . I don't want to make my daughter an orphan, but for so long I've had the anger in my head . . . she caused me pain . . . I couldn't live the life I wanted to live.'

How do we understand this sequence of events: resentment, anger and rage boiling over?

The concept of 'catathymia' is an attempt at an explanatory model of rage-type murderous violence. Fredric Wertham, a psychiatrist based in New York, first described it in 1937 as an explanation for some types of violent crimes. It goes something like this: catathymia is a psychological experience involving unbearable, extreme emotional tension where thinking becomes more egocentric. Suddenly a crystallisation point is reached, with the idea that violence is the only way to release the pressure brought about by the overwhelming sense of tension. After an inner struggle, the violent act is carried out. This is followed by resolution of the emotional tension, but insight into what has happened may not start to develop until months later. This can be sudden or have a slow incubation period.

Catathymia is merely an explanatory theory, not a medical or psychiatric diagnosis. After all, the law expects us to be able to control our feelings of rage and murderous thoughts. You may feel burning resentment towards an office bully, you may even daydream about them being hit by a bus on the way to work (a relatively common murderous fantasy), but if the build-up of tension leads to a catathymic crisis with extreme violence, you will be held responsible for your actions.

In the witness statements, two of Reddy's work colleagues described him making angry comments about his wife, and on one occasion saying he could kill her. Following the murder, police searching outside TK Maxx found a rucksack containing a bottle of wine (Pinot Grigio) and empty packaging for two stainless-steel chef's knives along with a receipt. Comparison of the barcode on the knife pack and computer records at the store showed the purchases had been made at 9.42 a.m. on the day of the killing. There was matching CCTV footage of Reddy buying the items at a local supermarket. The CCTV evidence from TK Maxx, the murder scene, showed him pretending to browse the T-shirt aisles for around twenty-five minutes before confronting his wife when she appeared. The attack was witnessed by a number of people. Jannat's colleagues had come down the corridor and saw Reddy stab her in the chest, push her over and then sit astride her and cut her throat.

A post-mortem carried out by Dr Jacob Swallow gave the cause of death as incised wounds to the neck, chest and abdomen. There was a deep wound across the neck, which cut the carotid arteries, larynx and voice box. There were four deep stab wounds to the chest, one of which had entered the front right thorax, damaging the right lung. There were defence wounds to the right thumb, right index finger and across all fingers of the left hand. Frenzied overkill, in other words, with more than one wound capable of killing.

15

Where does Reddy's case fit into the spectrum of men who kill their partners?

There are some subtle variations in the mindset and behaviours of this subgroup of murders, and the categories are not mutually exclusive, as many killings will have more than one feature. One subtype is those with severe mental illness, as covered in chapter two, who may kill intimate partners in the context of psychosis.

In Reddy's case the killing seems to have been an extension of long-term abusive violence.

But there are other common scenarios, which I have grouped into a loose, unofficial typology, and I will consider them in turn.

Murder motivated by possessiveness and jealousy (with or without mental disorder)

So many of the intimate partner homicides I have seen, as was the case with Reddy, have involved relationships that were breaking down, not as a result of an extension of pre-existing violence, but rather as a result of either possessiveness (don't leave, you are mine) or jealousy (I'm not going to lose you to someone else).

As an example of possessiveness leading to murder, take the case of Harvard-educated charity worker Suzy. Having met a middle-grade architect, Javier, on the London Underground, she agreed to an impromptu exchange of phone numbers – a fatal, sliding doors moment. Later, tired of his possessive and controlling behaviour, she was trying to end the relationship and started exchanging messages with someone more compatible from her Ivy League social network.

Initially unaware of Suzy's new pen friend, Javier was nonetheless unable to cope with the gradual loss of his love object. After he discovered a text message on her mobile from someone called Paul, he simmered for a week, then confronted her. Suzy said she wanted to end the relationship but not because of Paul.

Javier later described feelings of betrayal, anger, blind rage and red mist. He killed Suzy with multiple stab wounds and dumped her in the bathroom. He waited until the following day to call 999, and when the police arrived he handed them a will. He claimed to have written the note after the event, and later told the jury that the attack had happened on the spur of the moment, after he'd snapped, and as a result of his personality traits.

Some killers seem to be aware they will need to get themselves over the hump of their natural self-control. They do this either by pre-loading with alcohol or cocaine, or by engineering a confrontation – half-knowing how it will end. Expert analysis of the metadata relating to Javier's 'will' by a forensic IT specialist showed that he had been editing it in Microsoft Word for a week. This meant he hadn't written it after killing her, and by inference must have been thinking about the potentially fatal outcome. He had researched online the Oscar Wilde quote: '. . . each man kills the thing he loves . . . the coward does it with a kiss, the brave man with a sword.'

Verdict: murder. Life imprisonment; twenty-year minimum term.

Such is often the case at the end of a relationship. Feelings of betrayal, mistrust, resentment, envy and jealousy can all lead to anger and rage. These emotions are part of everyday life, but all may be amplified to a lethal degree – with or without mental disorder – in what Professor Paul Mullen, a world authority on forensic psychiatry, especially the fields of stalking and threat assessment, has called 'the pathological extensions of love'.[28]

Rivalry, envy and jealousy are often confused, but there are important differences, as Mullen explains.[29] Rivalry involves competitive aggression towards a rival who has affection for the same desired person. The aggression is not directed at the desired person. With envy, the rival is perceived to be in possession of the desired person and the destructive aggression towards the rival arises from the wish to deprive the rival of the envied relationship. Jealousy, on the other hand, relates to a situation where the desired person is already a partner, but where there is a rival competing for attention or affection. Jealousy involves both aggression towards the rival and aggression (mixed wth love and desire) towards the partner.

I once heard the difference being explained to a group of forensic psychiatrists like this: envy is what you might feel when you walk past a café and see a couple holding hands and gazing into each other's eyes. Jealousy is how you feel when, as you approach, you realise one of the couple is your wife/husband/partner/significant other.

In other words, envy involves two people (for example, you may envy someone else's happiness) but jealousy involves three people – the classic love triangle.

Jealousy can provoke erotic possessiveness, but also feelings of humiliation with angry and destructive intent. Mullen suggests that jealous men may torture themselves with vivid images of sexual activity between their partner and the rival, or of themselves being ridiculed as a cuckold.

Of course, the cuckold has always been a figure of ridicule. The word is derived from the supposed habit of the cuckoo bird in frequently changing mates and laying eggs in another bird's nest. In Italian popular culture, a soccer referee who misses a foul is taunted for being a cuckold, since he can't see what's going on behind his back (*cornuto* in Italian – the mythical beast with two horns). In *Othello*, jealousy is the 'green-eyed monster' and the cuckold is someone 'who dotes, yet doubts, suspects, yet strongly loves'. But it is the object of their affections and not the rival who is most at risk.

In forensic psychiatry, we try to distinguish between normal jealousy and 'morbid' jealousy (Othello syndrome) where a judgement that an act of infidelity has occurred is based on a delusional belief, rather than on reasonable evidence. The delusion of infidelity with a presumed rival can lead to intensely unpleasant feelings, extensive cross-questioning or abnormally violent behaviour. The problem with this distinction between normal and delusional jealousy is that the 'actual truth' – as to whether the loved one is being unfaithful – may be hard to verify. A patient's cheating partner may not disclose the truth to a psychiatrist or a social worker, for instance.

Sometimes the difference between normal and morbid jealousy can be straightforward, such as when jealousy is clearly linked to the recent onset of other bizarre delusions, like a belief about being deliberately poisoned by the partner.

In other cases, it is the extent of the associated behaviours which make jealousy abnormal or 'pathological', rather than the presence or absence of delusions.

Jealousy might come from a delusional interpretation of innocuous events, like a missed phone call, and then lead to frantic checking – of text messages, the whereabouts of the loved one, even underwear. Severely controlling behaviour in a desperate effort to reduce the risk of infidelity can be termed pathological even if a rival is not suspected. I have seen cases where one half of an intimate relationship does not necessarily believe that their partner is cheating on them, but is nevertheless consumed by anxiety that their partner might be led astray, on a work night out, for example. So although this is not delusional jealousy, the anxiety, possessiveness and harassing behaviour, such as endless phone calls while their partner is out with friends, are clearly pathological.

Pathological jealousy has long been associated with an increased risk of murder, and although the risk is predominantly to the love object, rather than the rival, I have encountered one cuckolded lover who, while both jealous and psychotic, killed his partner *and* her lover, for good measure. Verdict: manslaughter twice over. Detention under section in secure hospital, without limit of time.

Pathological jealousy has been associated with a wide range of mental disorders, including psychosis, depression and alcohol abuse, but also abnormal personalities, such as the superficially narcissistic and self-assured, who underneath have a deep 'thin-skinned' personal insecurity.

When jealousy is clearly delusional, there is often a call for treatment. However, once I, as a forensic psychiatrist, have become involved, I accept responsibility for keeping everyone safe, which is no easy task. What, for example, does a forensic psychiatrist do when a patient makes death threats while in treatment?

The answer is that we use treatment and containment, but must remain mindful that these measures may fail to manage the risk – for example, if the patient refuses treatment, absconds or is released from psychiatric hospital on appeal. We also usually alert the potential victim with what's called a 'Tarasoff warning'.

Tatiana Tarasoff was a student at the University of California in the late 1960s. She had a brief relationship with Prosenjit Poddar, who was a student from Bengal, India. Tatiana quickly realised they had different ideas about the relationship, whereas Prosenjit assumed they were serious. Tatiana rebuffed him, saying she was dating other men. It was the late 1960s in California, after all, so the cultural differences were likely accentuated by the prevailing relaxed social attitudes of the times. Prosenjit was devastated by Tatiana's rebuff, became depressed and neglected his health and studies.

Prosenjit sought help from Dr Lawrence Moore, but during therapy he confided his anger and resentment and said that he wanted to kill Tatiana. Dr Moore took action, involving the police and recommending commitment, but he did not take any steps to warn Tatiana. Dr Moore's supervisor, Dr Powelson, overruled Moore and declared that Prosenjit should not be detained. (The buck stops with the supervisor, right?)

Tarasoff had gone on a long trip overseas, during which time Prosenjit's psychological state improved. But after she returned, Prosenjit creepily befriended her brother in order to stalk her, and in October 1969, he carried out his threat and stabbed and killed her.

Tatiana had never received a warning. If she had, then maybe she could have avoided him, or at least called police upon sighting him.

Would you want the therapist of your former partner to breach professional confidentiality and warn you that your life was in danger if they'd disclosed thoughts of killing you – that's to say, *posing* a threat without *making* a threat to you directly?

Tarasoff laws were brought in, in Tatiana's memory, and they impose on psychiatrists or therapists a duty to warn those threatened by their patients. As the ruling said, 'The protective privilege ends where the public peril begins.'

Tarasoff laws are formalised in statute in twenty-three US states and are influential in other parts of the world, including the UK, but are not actually enshrined in UK law. By contrast, the police in the UK are required to make 'threat to life' warnings to potential victims when such threats are known to police, and they did so on over 700 occasions in 2017 alone.

These signals were introduced after a murder in 1988 where the police had not passed on the threat to the potential victim.

To illustrate how this works in practice, consider Helmut Schneider, referred to me for a second opinion by a local psychiatric team. Helmut had a stable marriage with three children and a devoted wife, Svenja. But Helmut had repeatedly accused his wife of infidelity, despite her protestations and affirmations of love for him, and her acquiescence to his restrictions on her social life.

After extensive social work enquiries, the local psych team were convinced his jealousy was delusional, as there was no evidence of a genuine rival. Helmut had made threats of violence to his wife, but was also so tormented by jealousy that he was suicidal. He was admitted to a psychiatric ward on a voluntary basis for treatment with antipsychotic medication and psychological therapy. After a while he was no longer suicidal, and his 'delusional' jealousy had responded to medication in that he no longer suspected his wife of infidelity. As he was co-operating with the treatment plan, he could not be detained and he was discharged, agreeing to continue with medication, psychological therapy and outpatient supervision.

Before his discharge from hospital, a meeting was arranged with Svenja where she was given a clear Tarasoff warning about the heightened risk of serious, even homicidal, violence from Helmut, and she was advised that separation may be the only truly safe way to manage the risk. But it must be hard to leave someone you love. *How could he possibly want to hurt me? He loves me too much for that.*

It is tough if you love your partner but are exasperated by the false accusations. Helmut agreed to live apart for a while but, with the treatment successful and the accusations in abeyance, the couple gradually spent more time together.

A while later, Svenja and the children booked a holiday to a rented cottage in Cornwall and Helmut was invited in the hope that the trip would help them repair the rift.

Unfortunately, without telling anyone, Helmut had stopped his antipsychotic medication. During an angry confrontation while on the trip, Helmut once again accused the devoted Svenja of sleeping with another man, and during the row stabbed her to death in front of the children.

Everything possible had been done. The psychiatric team could not order Svenja to separate from Helmut and Helmut could not be detained. How could they know that he had stopped taking his medication?

However, reviewing Helmut's interview notes afterwards for the inquiry sent chills down my spine. When asked about his feelings for Svenja he had said, 'I love her so much, I love her to death.'

Verdict: manslaughter on grounds of diminished responsibility. Secure hospital and restriction order without limit of time

This was the case that ruined my honeymoon. Married a few weeks before, and with the ink barely dry on my certificate of specialist training, the news of the murder broke just as I was about to fly to Umbria to spend two weeks by the pool in a rental apartment near the sleepy town of Umbertide.

I was consumed with worry and wanted to be back at the hospital to join the urgent case review to piece together what we might have done differently. The second week of the trip, there was an obscure conference on 'Madness, Science and Society' at the University of Florence. I hadn't planned on going, but I decided I needed the company of my peers. I left Umbertide before 6 a.m. for the madcap 268-kilometre one-day round-trip into Tuscany and back. The plan for the day had been to visit a nearby medieval town. But I was inconsolable and I needed to feel as though I was doing something to influence events, mindful of the stark reality that I can be held responsible if I fail to section someone who goes on to kill.

I was only one of several professionals involved in the case of Svenja – and what's more, I hadn't even been the treating psychiatrist – but even so, I couldn't help being self-critical. Launching on this day trip seemed to give me some sense of purpose, however futile my efforts would be to retroactively change the course of events. But you can't undo the past. Death can come in an instant, and it had done for Svenja, in a way I couldn't help thinking might just have been prevented.

There was no time for a detour to the Uffizi Gallery and Piazza della Signoria, which meant missing the chance to experience a bit of artistic revenge on violent men via Judith's decapitation of male tyrant King Holofernes, as painted by Artemisia Gentileschi and sculpted in bronze by Donatello.

Instead, I stuck to a full day at the conference venue on the outskirts of the city. I do remember full-on Italian espresso coffee in tiny plastic cups – a far cry from the brown dish-water coffee of UK conference venues – but I don't recall any of the talks I went to that day, except for one on vampirism and lycanthropy. By pure fluke, Bruce, one of the junior psychiatrists from the team who had been treating and supervising Helmut, was there. Talking over the case, Bruce immediately understood my disquiet and was able to share the latest with me, namely that the Tarasoff warning had been given and was well documented, mental health detention had been considered, and so on.

Although it was a relief to know we were probably covered in terms of process, it didn't help me stop ruminating about the dreadful outcome. And the two-week break had already been ruined anyway, despite glorious sun.

Thus, the case of Helmut and Svenja stayed with me. Forensic psychiatrists always take morbid jealousy seriously. To come across it during an interview never fails to be a hair-standing-up-on-the-back-of-the-neck scenario (especially for me, after Helmut's case, which I often use as a cautionary tale with my trainees). The only truly safe treatment is geographical, that is, separating the accuser and the lover, either by physical distance, or by injunction or hospitalisation.

As forensic psychiatrists, we always get to see the cases that go wrong, since patients like Helmut will end up in a forensic unit after the event. But it exasperates us when our general adult, non-specialist psychiatry colleagues fail to take signals seriously beforehand.

Not long after Helmut, I was asked to see Andrew who, when his team hadn't been doing well during the FA Cup Final, had attacked his girlfriend, Sarah, making a superficial cut to her throat. He then ran in front of a bus, which fortunately for him was travelling slowly, after which both he and Sarah were admitted to the local emergency room at a London hospital.

Sarah didn't want to make a criminal complaint, but here's where the local mental health crisis team got it wrong. They persuaded the police not to intervene, making assurances that mental health services could handle the situation. Paradoxically, it is involvement of the criminal justice system that provides the impetus for a case getting more attention from mental health services, because criminal proceedings are part of the criteria for admission to specialist forensic services. So if the charges are dropped, then the case will fall down the priority list, even if the violent behaviour was really concerning. This may seem strange but it is a perennial problem in psychiatry, partly because the police have other, more pressing priorities once someone like Andrew is getting some form of mental health care.

As I said earlier, I have seen access to psychiatric care deteriorate over the last eight or nine years because of the fragmentation of mental health services, with disagreements about which team is responsible even before the patient has been assessed. But when the delusions of psychosis are missed, there can be serious adverse consequences, even homicide. Often, in my experience, the crisis teams who are the gatekeepers for acute (non-forensic) psychiatric care are just so overwhelmed that they don't have time for a thorough assessment of history and mental state. Such is the pressure from NHS management to keep acute bed occupancy down that even a short voluntary period in hospital is not available. But these admissions, even if relatively short, would allow a more in-depth assessment of the risk issues.

This was the case here. Nobody ever took a proper psychiatric history from Andrew, and his partner Sarah was not contacted for a collateral history as to what had been going on.

A few weeks after the incident, the decision was taken that perhaps it would be a good idea to request a forensic risk assessment and yours truly was the one to do it. I interviewed Andrew in a windowless interview room, tucked away in the teaching hospital outpatient department. Here, he played down the incident as simply a case of too much to drink and denied any animus between him and Sarah, but he seemed guarded and evasive.

With his permission, I called Sarah to obtain a collateral history. She revealed, to my immediate concern, that she'd been on the receiving end of a litany of previous abuse: jealous accusations, controlling behaviour and a threat of violence. She assured me there was no basis in reality for Andrew's suspicions about her being unfaithful. She had been wondering how to tackle the problem and was getting fed up with it.

So Andrew had attacked Sarah with a knife, but it had little to do with Freddie Ljungberg's second goal for Arsenal, late in the FA cup final, securing Chelsea's defeat – and everything to do with Andrew's pathological, 'delusional' jealousy towards Sarah.

I swung straight into action with Andrew's case. I hastily finalised and circulated my risk assessment. I insisted that Sarah be given a Tarasoff warning, and once the social worker involved was made more fully aware of the risk, Sarah was also referred to a domestic violence project. Andrew was offered treatment but he failed to accept it. After another threatening incident, he was sectioned, but then escaped from a low-secure psychiatric unit. It wasn't easy, but the last I heard Sarah was safe.

For all of this, I got some flak from a non-forensic colleague, an enthusiast for crisis teams, who complained that my forensic report 'carried a lot of weight'.

I could only respond, 'I bloody well hope so.'

Domestic violence in a relationship can start all too quickly, with the short period of blissful contentment cut brutally short. Anger fuelled by jealousy degenerates into rows, beatings and even rape, and ultimately murder. It is common to see accusations of infidelity, even by those who are themselves being unfaithful. In other words, 'I can have what I want, including you, but you must be loyal to me.' The egocentricity of narcissism is a common theme that we find in many types of killers, from domestic abusers to spree killers and school shooters.

Is this toxic masculinity? Has there been a resurgence of male gender roles that expect boys and men to be the alpha male and control their emotions unless it is to express anger?

The excess of male aggression is not a new problem, but it can't be ignored as men make up ninety-five per cent of the prison population in the UK. Neither is it just down to testosterone-fuelled, biological differences as, of course, social and cultural expectations and poor 'modelling' of paternal behaviour all clearly play a part.

Harassment and stalking-based murders
(and how to end a relationship safely)

Stalking is defined as 'repeated, unwanted communications or approaches, which cause distress or fear and/or fear of violence'. Research by forensic psychiatrists Professor Paul Mullen and Michele Pathé (two leading international experts on stalking) analysed the behaviours, psychopathology and underlying motivation of stalkers referred to a forensic clinic for assessment and treatment, and identified five subtypes of stalker.[30] The first, and most prevalent, group contains people who have been 'rejected' by a lover and whose stalking behaviour is targeted on a former intimate. The other four groups are:

- Those who are seeking intimacy – which may include those with delusions that another person loves them.
- So-called incompetent suitors – for example individuals on the autistic spectrum who might be unable to appreciate that their attentions are unwanted.
- The resentful, who are pursuing a grievance or a complaint in an unusually vexatious way, such as against an employer who sacked them.
- The rarer predatory stalkers, who are planning a sexual offence and stalking their potential victim (see chapter one).

In this section, it is the rejected former intimates we are concerned with.

If you are unceremoniously dumped or politely rejected, you can send a few pleading texts, some flowers, maybe some unwanted phone calls. Definitions vary, but after four weeks and ten communications all with no response, it's time to move on. Moreover, if your behaviour causes distress or, worse, fear of violence, you are entering criminal harassment territory. Think of the female character in *Play Misty for Me* who stalks Clint Eastwood, or the male character in *Sleeping with the Enemy* who preys on Julia Roberts.

Rejected stalkers may feel humiliated; they may be over-dependent or narcissistic and overwhelmed by feelings of entitlement. As Paul Mullen and Michele Pathé have described, the stalking behaviour is motivated by a complex mixture of desire for both reconciliation and revenge, or a fluctuating mixture of the two. For rejected stalkers, a sense of loss can be combined with frustration, anger, jealousy and vindictiveness. The stalking is a substitute for lost intimacy, creating a 'semblance of closeness and a parody of a relationship'.[31]

My colleague Frank Farnham[32] was among those who examined a series of harassment cases over a period of years and made a striking finding, much reported in the press at the time: the highest rate of violence amongst stalkers was by rejected former intimates (as opposed to intimacy seekers and other subtypes). What's more, the risk of violence goes up if the stalker has assaulted, or entered the home of, the former intimate, the object of their stalking.

So if your ex pesters you for longer than two weeks or so, then the research suggests there is a much higher chance the harassment will persist beyond six months. The two-week cut-off has been confirmed by Rosemary Purcell's research study of over 400 stalking cases,[33] which showed that stalkers who persist beyond two weeks were more likely to continue their behaviour for six months or more. They were also more likely to place their victim under surveillance; loiter; repeatedly telephone; or contact via letters, faxes or email. They were also more likely to subject their victim to explicit threats, physical assaults and property damage.

If, after sending you unwanted flowers, your ex physically assaults you or breaks into your flat, then you are at risk of serious violence,[34] and even of becoming a murder victim. It's also important to note that rejected men without criminal histories are capable of escalating to sudden homicidal catathymic rage.

In one particular case of harassment by a rejected partner, I dealt with a Mr Francis Chapman, an Audi enthusiast and director of a small industrial contracting company. He was going through a painful divorce from his wife, Rebecca. During a dispute over the sale of the marital home, he sent texts, left voicemails and repeatedly returned to their former joint home to remonstrate with her. He once smashed the greenhouse glass in anger. On another occasion, finding Rebecca out, he broke into the house, ostensibly looking for his post.

'I paid a lot of money for this house; I did a lot of work on it, and she did nothing, and afterwards she wants fucking everything. How am I supposed to fucking save money and buy a new house? The judge should be jailed.' Court papers confirmed he had shouted at the judge and called him a 'wanker'.

As the divorce progressed, he was feeling 'very angry, I wanted my home back or fifty-fifty proceeds from the divorce . . . bloody hell . . . I paid a lot of money for the garden fence. It was fucking robbery.'

The couple had argued over the rubbish disposal. He explained to me that he was always very tidy and organised, but that 'she put the cornflakes box on top of the recycling bin when it was already full, instead of changing the bin bag. She didn't fold the box. She left the last cornflakes inside the cardboard box . . . I threw the cornflakes box on the floor, and she said, "What the fuck have you done?"'

Many non-violent domestic disputes are about money, or sex, or the division of domestic chores and childcare responsibilities, and many couples have differing views on acceptable levels of tidiness, or the appropriate etiquette for recycling and waste disposal. But please beware if the recycling disputes lead to murderous or homicidal feelings.

On the day the decree nisi was issued, Chapman took a knife, intending to plead with Rebecca to split the proceeds of the house and, if necessary, threaten suicide. He said, 'I thought that if I scared her, maybe if she had a little bit of love she might say yes.'

He met Rebecca as she alighted from her regular bus, begging her to share the house and furniture. 'I'm not going to sell, and that's it . . . It's my house now,' she said, according to him.

But instead of threatening to kill himself, he slaughtered her in a vicious knife attack witnessed by a busload of astonished and terrified witnesses. One of them, Jock Hollis, went to see what he could do for Rebecca, but given the gruesome nature of her injuries, soon realised she was dead and covered her body with a coat. Chapman, meanwhile, ran off to the marital home. He was unaware that his mother-in-law had arrived to visit Rebecca. He killed her too.

Crucially, he had bought the murder weapon on the morning of the killing and although he had narcissistic ('it's my house') and obsessional (the cornflakes) personality traits, there was no psychiatric defence. At trial he sought to persuade the jury there had been a sudden loss of control, provoked by Rebecca's last words as she refused again to sell the house. Still angry about the divorce settlement, he was also trying to appeal it from his prison cell.

Verdict: murder, twice over. Life imprisonment; thirty-year minimum term.

All of this begs the question, how do you end a relationship safely? It depends to some extent on the personality traits of your partner. Better to avoid the narcissistic, egocentric, possessive, controlling, jealous or vengeful types if possible (easier said than done!). It's also a good idea to watch out for extreme 'love bombing'. This term, originally coined by members of the Unification Church in the USA known as the 'Moonies', refers to unusually excessive attention, compliments, displays of affection and declarations of love. Cult groups sometimes use it to encourage new members to join them, but it may also be seen in intimate relationships. This behaviour can just be the harmless (if irritating) behaviour of someone wanting to spoil you or convince you to go out with them, but it can also be a sign of manipulative behaviour, and later flip into control and abuse.

But no matter the level of commitment between you and your lover, be it dating, hooking up, marriage, dowry payments, exchanged eternity rings or pre-paid joint burial plots, it is better to have a clean break with a clear message when it ends, something like, 'I'm sorry this isn't working, it's not you, it's me.' And if the pleading phone calls and unwanted flowers persist beyond, say, two weeks, then a formal 'cease and desist' might be in order, possibly followed in due course by a 'stalking diary' and a report to the police for a formal warning, though the current practice is to move directly to further action with a non-molestation order. Finally, an injunction or a criminal prosecution may be required, which can lead to a restraining order, a non-custodial penalty with a rehabilitation requirement or, ultimately, imprisonment.

Stalking is a serious issue that has been grossly underestimated in the past. However, we're catching up, and law enforcement and psychiatry are increasingly collaborating, with innovative joint projects underway. Even so, the fact remains that life isn't straightforward and clean endings can be difficult to achieve. There may be ambivalence, temporary reconciliation and mixed messages. What you think is one-last-time 'break-up sex' could be misinterpreted as 'make-up' sex.

Based on anecdotal evidence of my experience on many cases over the years, I would strongly advise against deliberately inflaming jealousy by telling your soon-to-be-ex that you've found a new lover when, in fact, there is no new lover, and you have merely fallen out of love. A student friend suggested that this might be better than hurting their feelings by telling them that they're not good enough, not intelligent or attractive enough, and that you don't love them any more. No, not a good idea. Your ex-partner's enforced introspection about personality differences, personal failings or dental hygiene are better than tortured imaginings of your sexual congress with a new lover – especially if there isn't one.

Telling someone, falsely, you are pregnant by a rival lover is also a bad strategy. I have encountered two cases where this has led to murder. Post-mortems in both cases confirmed the absence of a pregnancy. In one case, it turned out the victim had been trying to think of a way to categorically demonstrate the relationship was over, and in the vain hope of getting her former partner to move on, she'd lied to him that she was pregnant by someone else.

Witnesses, including a friend and a sister of the deceased, attested that the victim had told them she planned to lie. Her motives, while well intentioned, had awful unforeseen consequences. The murderer reported after the event, at interview with me, that he had become enraged at his ex-partner telling him there was not only a rival in the picture, but that they had made her pregnant.

Sometimes a relationship break-up has to be done under supervision in a police station, probation office or psychiatric clinic, and *in extremis* you might need a refuge placement already lined up, for reasons explored already.

As you might expect, working with these extreme relationship cases which end in stalking followed by murder makes you reflect on your own experience. All of us are likely to have experienced a relationship break-up at some stage, and it hurts once you realise that your affections are no longer reciprocated. It is quite a common response to such rejection to try and salvage the situation, maybe with a heartfelt letter, flowers, a favourite bottle of wine or one-too-many phone calls over a few days. But there is a cut-off point, beyond which sympathy and mild regret on the part of your ex may morph into irritation or even fear if you persist. Anyway, if someone asks you for space, the worst thing you can do is suffocate them with unwanted affection. In my student days, when I was slow to realise that a request for space was just an attempt to let me down gently, a close friend joked unhelpfully to 'Give her so much space she feels like Neil Armstrong.' Much easier to say than do, of course.

Looking back on that experience, if you extrapolate from the understandable and relatable sense of bruised self-esteem, it is possible to see how, in those with abnormal personality traits, these benign feelings can be amplified into a profound narcissistic decompensation. 'How could they say they don't love me? I am irresistible.'

Neuroscientists at UCL have detected increased activity in the cingulate gyrus in the brains of test subjects who are in love. The cingulate gyrus is a curved fold of brain tissue and a component of the limbic system, in the brain which is involved in processing emotions and regulating behaviour. Does brain functioning help us better understand these human experiences and behaviours? Or is it a mistake for us to try and reduce them to a biological process? After all, we have a vast canon of literature, much of it pre-dating modern science, to help us understand that 'the course of true love never did run smooth'.

I once suggested a supervised break-up for an ex-high-security patient. His murder charge had happened when his previous partner dumped him after confronting him about lewd texts found on his phone, sent by a string of casual sex partners. His response to this combination of humiliation and rejection was to kill his departing partner with stab wounds to the face and neck.

A decade later, close to discharge from secure hospital after extensive treatment, he had been dating a young, well-educated professional he met via online social networking. (Yes, even mentally disordered killers can be attractive to some.)

The forensic team ensured that the new lover was informed of our patient's offending history (namely, killing a partner at the time of a break-up) and, undeterred by this information, the relationship blossomed for a while.

But when, some months later, the new lover got cold feet and wanted to move on from this high-risk liaison, we thought a supervised break-up in a safe environment would be prudent. We also arranged a TACAU (treat all calls as urgent) alert for 999, in case emergency services were called to any subsequent confrontation.

The outcome was an amicable separation and a successful discharge to the community, you will be relieved to hear.

Murders provoked by infidelity
(which overlaps with jealousy, of course)

Men who are unable to control anger, or who are suddenly violent in an expression of rage, are most often held criminally responsible for their actions. But partial defences involving either 'loss of control' or 'abnormality of mind' are frequently raised.

In the recent past, claims of loss of control (or provocation, as it was previously known) resulted in murder charges being reduced to manslaughter when a man had killed a female partner after discovering her infidelity. There was increasing concern about this, as well as the fact that women who killed an abusive partner never succeeded with a similar defence.

In 2009, the UK law was reformed with the aim of better accommodating the scenarios in which women might kill an abusive male partner, while at the same time making it harder for jealous and controlling men to be excused for murdering a female victim, especially where infidelity was an issue.

Under the new law, judges have a statutory duty to direct juries to disregard sexual infidelity when considering loss of control as a defence.

The following case illustrates why infidelity must be ignored, and also shows how easy it often is for the police to solve intimate partner killings.

Yet another irascible, controlling husband, Ray Thompson, discovered his wife had been unfaithful. Christine, exasperated by the misery of life with him, was in the very early stages of a relationship with a new man – though not yet intimate with him – and was trying to find a way to end the marriage safely.

Having been told that his wife had been seen with another man at a time when she was supposed to be elsewhere, Thompson did not immediately confront her, but instead offered to pick her up from work early and take her shopping. Instead of driving to the shopping centre, he took her to a secluded road in a park area next to the ponds, whereupon, unhappy with her response to his challenge, he killed her with several deep thrusts of an old military bayonet he'd kept in the garage.

He returned to the town centre and reported her and his car missing. Before long, her body was discovered by a dog walker, although it took the fire brigade three hours to cut into the deadlocked vehicle, as Thompson said there was no spare key. The original, he claimed, had been stolen along with the car.

One of the detectives later said to me at court that he had 'liked' the husband as the prime suspect, but there was, initially, insufficient evidence for a search warrant.

The Metropolitan Police are able to solve around ninety per cent of murder cases. This is because they allocate significant resources to homicide investigations, and large numbers of uniformed officers are deployed during those golden twenty-four hours of evidence-gathering. I once organised a conference during which a senior detective outlined the three most powerful investigative tools in murder cases: mobile phone cell-site analysis, CCTV and DNA evidence – sometimes in that order.

In the case of Thompson, CCTV showed the car driving not to the shops, but towards the ponds, although Thompson couldn't be identified as the driver in the grainy footage. After several weeks of careful analysis, the mobile phone cell-site data (which can geo-locate wherever a mobile phone connects to the network) was complete, and the records allowed police to place the suspect's mobile phone at the site where the car and Christina's body were found, within the pathologist's estimated time frame for the killing.

What's more, the phone call was from Thompson to his uncle, as confirmed by phone records and his uncle's earlier statement that Thompson had phoned him to say, 'Christine's missing.'

On this evidence, the search warrant was granted. The bloodied bayonet was found stashed in a plastic bag, with his DNA and her blood, behind the U-bend under the kitchen sink. Thus rumbled, Thompson then claimed he had 'lost self-control' when she'd admitted her nascent infidelity. The defence of provocation relating to his discovery of her infidelity was proffered and failed because of the purposeful nature of the killing and the attempts to conceal it. Under the new law – introduced since Thompson's case – loss of control must be specifically excluded from the jury's consideration.

Verdict: murder. Life imprisonment.

Depression and diminished responsibility

Putting provocation to one side, is the alternative partial defence of diminished responsibility ever successful when a man kills a woman at the end of a relationship?

The difficult issues raised by a so-called depressive homicide can be illustrated by a late-1990s case of a doctor's wife who had apparently been driven to distraction by her husband's penny-pinching. She had asked for a new fridge. Instead he offered her a second-hand one, used to store samples in the pathology laboratory. And despite having over £800,000 in building society accounts, he insisted on taking the family to McDonald's for their birthdays, and making the guests pay for their own food! Unable to take any more, she had instructed a solicitor, and a petition had been filed for divorce.

But he couldn't accept the marriage was over and repeatedly pleaded with her to reconsider. He began drinking heavily, prescribed himself tranquillisers and appeared gaunt and unhappy to colleagues. One morning he was at home when his wife returned from the school run. As she drank a coffee on the patio, he walked past holding a hammer – apparently intending to break up a concrete path in the back garden – but then 'snapped' when she made a remark.

A post-mortem examination showed that he'd hit her at least seven times with the hammer, and that many of the blows were delivered when she was already on the ground. Next he wrapped her in a bin liner and sheet, dragged her bleeding body to the first-floor bedroom – knowing full well she was still alive – and then threw her from the window, fracturing her spine and causing her death. This is an example of the 'staging' of a crime scene in an attempt to re-direct the police investigation; it is quite rare, occurring in around one per cent of homicides.[35]

He called the ambulance several hours later, initially telling police he had been in the garage when his wife fell from the bedroom, before finally admitting his part, telling them, 'I could not live with the shame.'

Now, you might conclude that a respected professional who suddenly kills his wife in a moment of murderous rage, without any prior violence, must be mentally disordered, right? Sure enough, without a trial, the Recorder of London confirmed the prosecution had accepted psychiatric reports that the consultant was suffering from severe depression, brought on by learning his wife wanted a divorce and custody of their two children. This depression had substantially impaired his responsibility. His team had successfully used the psychiatric defence to reduce the charge of murder to manslaughter, thus avoiding a life sentence. Upon hearing he could be free in just two-and-a-half years, the victim's mother said, 'Is that all my daughter's life is worth?'

The legal test has now become more restrictive and requires that a recognised medical condition must substantially impair various mental faculties, like rational decision-making, and also provide an explanation for the murder. In other words, although depression might explain why someone has a bleak and pessimistic view of the future which impairs their rational judgement, the depression must also explain why they wielded the hammer. I'm not sure this case would be quite so open-and-shut now. Was this the reaction of a depressed man overwhelmed by the loss of his marriage? Or was this the rigidity that can go with the severe parsimony of a wealthy miser snapping and lashing out when faced with losing control over his family and his assets? The alternative interpretation would have added up to a decade more on the sentence. And if he had been a carpet fitter and former squaddie rather than a respected consultant who was also ex-Territorial Army, would he have been dealt with in the same way? These are my thoughts as I look back on that case.

There was an abnormality of mind, no doubt, as I had agreed at the time, but as for responsibility, diminished or otherwise, the issue was – and remains – moral more than medical. Sometimes morality and value judgements are medicalised to make them more palatable, and the prosecution still have to decide whether to accept a plea to the lesser charge. What would a jury make of that case now, under the current, more restrictive law?

Honour-based intimate partner murders

What of so-called 'honour crimes'? These typically involve abduction and murder in order to prevent a woman from exercising her choice of intimate partner, and are used to stop inter-caste and inter-faith relationships. In this context, a husband may kill his wife for becoming too westernised or for trying to leave.

I encountered such a killing, illustrating how concepts of honour can lead to murderous rage. It involved a family from South East Asia who had been living in the UK for almost thirty years. The hard-drinking, unemployed father of the house, Mr Nimol, was angry because, according to him, his wife was dishonouring and disrespecting him, and insulting his parents.

There were multiple incidents of domestic violence, all related to these issues, and mostly when he had been drinking. One night, drunk, and after police had already told him to stay away, he returned home at 4.30 a.m. His wife reluctantly let him back in, the argument resumed and he killed her with two stab wounds, one through the back and into the aorta, and one through the front and through the liver. Either wound was capable of causing death.

He was arrested and, when interviewed under caution the following day, said, 'I felt I was really humiliated as a husband . . . it's unacceptable for a woman, a wife, to disrespect her husband, for oriental people . . . she insulted my parents . . . she dishonoured me the way that she dressed . . . I stabbed her once in the back and once in the front.'

He said that he had been drinking beer and spirits. 'I was just so humiliated I couldn't control myself, I was so angry and upset.' However, he said he had only intended to 'stab her slightly'.

An open-and-shut case, surely?

In this case, the psychiatric evidence became contested in an unexpected way. Once the prosecution evidence was complete, including post-mortem and witness statements, the defence solicitor instructed a psychiatrist to explore possible defences to the charge of murder. We call this a 'psychiatric fishing expedition' as, based on the basic facts of the case, this sounded like a 'normal' intimate partner murder.

In Mr Nimol's case, a psychiatrist, Dr Icarus, was instructed. He had some experience in the lower courts but not in more serious criminal cases. Dr Icarus had interviewed Nimol, in prison custody, three months after the murder, whereas the police had done so immediately after his arrest. By this stage, perhaps in an attempt to rationalise what he had done, the defendant told Dr Icarus that he had felt 'unreal' as he stabbed his wife and that it was 'as if' he felt the 'presence of his dead brother'.

Dr Icarus therefore advanced the opinion that this derealisation was an abnormality of mind, which explained the killing.

There were two problems: the first and most glaring was that the psychiatrist had neglected to read the police interview transcript, in which the defendant had given a contemporaneous and incriminating account. I highlighted this error in my report, and I also pointed out that derealisation is very common and is not a form of psychosis; it is an altered 'sense' of reality but not a 'loss of contact' with reality. It's that spaced-out feeling you can get when you're tired or very anxious – for example, when you're giving evidence in an Old Bailey murder trial, as Dr Icarus was about to find out.

Now we all, eventually, have our bad day in court and my turn would come. But Dr Icarus was seemingly oblivious to what was in store for him and he still didn't ask to see the interview transcript. Expert evidence is like poker, an equal stakes game. If the other side raises the stakes with an interview transcript, you had better call the bet and read the additional material.

Dr Icarus was gently taken through his evidence by the defence barrister. He explained why he thought that the derealisation amounted to diminished responsibility. The friendly and unchallenged part of his evidence over, he stepped out of the witness box and started heading for the exit. But he was apparently unaware of Crown court proceedings.

As he was halfway across the courtroom, the judge said, 'Er, Dr Icarus, please don't forget your cross-examination . . .'

You can imagine how that went. The prosecution QC's questions went something like this:

'Dr Icarus . . . do you stand by your report as it is written?'

'Yes, I do.'

'Doctor, have you considered all the material relevant to forming your opinion?'

Remembering, now, to swivel and answer towards the judge, he said, 'Yes, I have, My Lord.'

'Dr Icarus, would you agree that what the defendant has said about the night in question is highly pertinent to understanding his state of mind at the time?'

'Yes, of course it is, My Lord.'

'Doctor, have you had the opportunity to consider the police interview?'

'Er, no, I haven't.'

'Doctor, can I ask you to read out, for the benefit of the jury, what the defendant said to the police, twelve hours after he killed his wife? You will find it behind the yellow tab, on page seventy-six of the jury bundle, in front of you . . .'

Dr Icarus read hesitantly, '. . . She dishonoured me the way that she dressed . . . I stabbed her . . . slightly.'

'Doctor, can you please explain to the jury why you prefer the version of events he gave to you some three months after the police interview?

'Dr Icarus, can you tell the court what criteria you have used for *abnormality of mind*?

'Dr Icarus, what is the *mind*, exactly?'

Painful to watch, but the Crown wanted a murder conviction, given the facts of the case, and so the expert evidence had to be put to proof.

In the civil courts, a glaring omission like this would be picked up well before a trial via a joint statement of experts. But in the cash-strapped criminal courts, with an overwhelmed Crown Prosecution Service, and barristers instructed at the last minute, it is common for a car-crash defence like this to end up before a jury.

Verdict: murder. Life imprisonment; eighteen-year minimum term.

16

Some months after my first encounter with Mr Reddy, it was time for his murder trial at the Old Bailey. I had interviewed him as the summer was just beginning but now the first autumn leaves of Michaelmas term were swirling in the breeze around Fountain Court in Middle Temple. It was time for a quick consultation with the defence QC on King's Bench Walk, to refresh my memory of the case before giving medical evidence at Reddy's trial a few days later.

In my report, I had pointed out the 'conflict of evidence' between his description of the marriage compared to the accounts of others, including that of his late wife. But I had to acknowledge that work colleagues had described him as being preoccupied with the separation from his daughter, as well as depressed, emotionally labile, tearful and unable to focus on work. The self-harm post-offence could have been a reaction to what he'd done, or a bungled 'extended suicide' attempt (which are also quite common in these types of murder).

Anyway, the psychiatric diagnostic manuals include some variants of mental and emotional states that are not too far away from everyday experience. And so Mr Reddy fulfilled criteria for an 'adjustment disorder', which is described in the international classification as, '[a state of] subjective distress and emotional disturbance . . . in the period of adaptation to a significant life change . . . manifestations vary, and include depressed mood, anxiety, worry . . . a feeling of inability to cope, plan ahead . . . dramatic behaviour or outbursts of violence . . .'

I suggested that this relatively minor diagnosis, although indeed an 'abnormality of mental functioning' and 'a recognised medical condition', would be unlikely to persuade the jury that he had a 'substantially impaired ability to form a rational judgement or to exercise self-control'. But faced with telling their client to plead guilty to murder, start crying and accept a mandatory life sentence, the barrister said it would be better to let him have his day in court. Otherwise, he could appeal, and then spend years blaming the lawyers, rather than the jury, for his sentence.

So I had to go into the witness box and make a robust case for adjustment disorder as a basis for diminished responsibility, though I was aware that the prosecution barrister and opposing expert would be challenging this vehemently.

But the jury were not so much concerned with the minutiae of the diagnostic criteria for adjustment disorder. They had seen the prosecution case set out over several days, with technical summaries of phone records, CCTV footage and till receipts, and they had heard testimony from live witnesses. On top of all this information, they had been given the chance to form their own impression of the man in the dock.

The defence barrister, bringing me up to speed with the evidence from the preceding days of the trial, told me that, when Reddy's daughter tearfully gave evidence about his domestic violence – from behind a curtain in the witness box, so she didn't have to face her father – he had shouted 'filthy slut' across the courtroom.

Sarmila was truly an orphan now, as Reddy had feared. Her mother was long cremated, and her father facing a life sentence – while verbally abusing her from the dock, nonetheless.

The jury were learning, as I had done, what a disagreeable man he could be.

During the last part of Reddy's cross-examination, when he was asked about the deep slash wounds to his wife's neck, which had severed major arteries and caused her death, his response caused an intake of breath from all those present.

'If it wasn't for the wholly inadequate and slow response of the London Ambulance Service, she might be alive today.'

I conceded that his *abnormality of mental functioning* was a minor one, and that whether it *substantially* impaired his abilities was a matter for the jury. But in his evidence, Reddy had revealed to the jury the demeanour and behaviour his wife and daughter had put up with for all those years, and the adjustment disorder didn't really come into it.

It took the jury just ninety minutes to reach a decision.

Verdict: murder. Life imprisonment; eighteen-year minimum term.

First impressions don't always stick, but in this case, they did, and I was glad to put it behind me.

I have described my reaction to Reddy throughout his case history. It helped me make sense of him and I think the likely reaction of the jury members must have helped them make sense of the killing, too.

My reaction to those I assess or treat can take me through a range of highly instructive responses. Sometimes they make me feel irritated, angry, bored or amused. I have one patient who's so funny I can't stop laughing. But he is bipolar, and has been suicidal in the past, so I have to be careful that I don't allow the mirth he induces to cause me to miss his sadness underneath.

These responses tell me a lot when I'm trying to get inside the head of any patient, especially a murderer, and can help me understand why someone has killed, or tried to. I remember being surprised when a colleague announced, 'I don't have any feelings about my patients at all . . . I prefer to remain completely neutral.' For me, that's not the case, and I'm more likely to find that personal reactions arise during assessment interviews and then become more important during prolonged treatment.

Which is not to say that it always pays to be touchy-feely, because at the same time, it's important to maintain a degree of objectivity. Say, for example, a forensic psychiatrist has experienced the suicide of a parent in childhood: they may react emotionally to a case involving parental loss. The challenge is not necessarily to ignore the feelings evoked by the case, but to be aware of those feelings in order to make use of them in understanding the interviewee's experiences, and to avoid those feelings becoming a blind spot.

Psychoanalysts (who are usually medically qualified in the USA but less so in the UK) are required to have both personal therapy and personal supervision of treatment cases as part of their training. In forensic psychiatry in the UK, there is a bit of a split, with some forensic psychiatrists choosing to undergo personal therapy and others not – it isn't compulsory.

When I started training, I was initially sceptical and probably a bit apprehensive about what it might open up. But I ended up choosing to go through personal therapy after assessing a child psychiatry case that resonated with me personally. In my case, it consisted of a brief course comprising a weekly session over about three years. Psychotherapists and psychoanalysts, on the other hand, may have up to five sessions a week for five to ten years.

Whatever route is taken, I still think my colleague was wrong. Deciding that you will have zero reaction to forensic cases means missing out on the opportunity to use a very powerful diagnostic tool, namely:

What is it like to be in the room with this person?
How do they make you feel?
Does your reaction help you understand how others react to them?
Does your reaction help you understand why they murdered someone?

My reaction to Reddy helped me understand some of what his wife must have endured. She had done her best to leave, but had not been able to escape his abuse – and she had paid for it with her life.

But what happens when a woman who can't seem to escape tries to defend herself from her attacker?

The results can be unpredictable . . .

Women Who Kill Their Partners

Case Study: Charlotte Smith

17

It all started after Charlotte had gone to see a woman about a dog. One of her four children, fifteen-year-old Sharon, wanted a dog, and Charlotte, in turn, wanted Sharon to be happy. After all, they had only just been reunited after Charlotte's eight-month stay in residential alcohol rehab. But at last, things seemed to be improving for them.

Or at least they had been, until Wednesday, 29 August 2001, just after the bank holiday, when Charlotte fatally stabbed her partner, Lennie Jones, through the heart with a twelve-inch kitchen knife.

The day I met Charlotte at HMP Holloway, I'd been carrying out my regular half-day of prison 'in reach' to assess new prisoners and follow-ups, looking for cases in need of transfer to hospital, as well as seeing anyone else who officers might be worried about for a variety of reasons: self-harm, suicide risk, or even just the exhibiting of strange behaviour, suggesting possible mental illness.

The role of a prison psychiatrist is very different from that of a hospital inpatient psychiatrist. We are there to manage mental illness or severe psychological distress among prisoners who have caused concern to prison staff, with the simple imperative that, as well as processing prisoners and preventing escapes, prisons must recognise and manage mental disorder, and keep their prisoners alive to face another day.

Holloway, being then the largest women-only remand prison in western Europe, had a capacity of 591 inmates and several thousand receptions per year. It had suffered a damning inspection report followed by a highly critical review, and so our forensic service was approached with a request to provide regular psychiatric clinics to support their over-stretched prison hospital wing. At the time I was just about to start regular clinics at HMP Pentonville, the nearby men's prison. I'd been through the security induction there and issued with keys, so I had to seek authorisation for the switch to join the new Holloway team, causing a bit of an administrative headache.

What's more, working with women in forensic settings is less popular, and seen as more challenging than working with men. As criminologist Loraine Gelsthorpe explains, most crime is committed by men and not women.[36] This may partly explain the observation that women who end up in custody are often more psychologically damaged in the wake of abusive experiences, have a tendency to internalise their distress as well as having high rates of self-harm. Looking back with the benefit of hindsight, my decision must have been at least partly prompted by the infanticide in my family, piquing my curiosity enough to volunteer for this unpopular detail in 2001.

The chief sanction of prison is loss of liberty, but prison doctors in the recent past had seen it incumbent on themselves to ensure any contact with the doctor was substandard and unpleasant enough to be part of the punishment.

Needless to say, we arrived at Holloway with rather more progressive ideas. During training, we'd been taught that you couldn't do any good for a prisoner who stormed out slamming the door, so it was crucial to establish rapport and deal with immediate issues like sleep, food, family contact and suicidal thoughts. Difficult areas, like the offence and traumatic childhood experiences, could wait until later.

It was with this in mind that I made my way to the interview room in C1, the hospital wing in the basement of the prison, where healthcare officers had asked me to see Charlotte.

In the interview room were two old steel-framed chairs and a chipped Formica-topped table. Graffiti scrawls marked the white-painted walls. The only ventilation was a thin slit in a small window of heavy, unbreakable, but scratched glass. Outside was a sunken courtyard, impossible to climb out of, and beyond that, high perimeter walls topped with anti-climb coving.

Charlotte was tall and lean with long, yellow-blonde highlights, a little grown-out and still matted with some of Lennie's blood. It was just two days after the killing. She had dirty and broken fingernails, bruises on her right forearm and a split lip, healing but swollen and bruised. In silence, she stared at the floor.

She had been arrested after midnight on the 29th and spent the following day in police custody. Cooperating with police interviews, she'd made a brief appearance at the magistrates' court, during which bail was denied, and she had then been remanded in prison custody.

I made my introductions and asked her how she was feeling and if there was any way we could help, being sure to focus on the here and now.

She rubbed her eyes and didn't answer at first, until at last she asked how she could get to see her kids.

I asked about them and she began to open up. Lee, seventeen, was preparing for GCSE re-sits; Sharon, aged fifteen, had found it difficult to settle in at her new school; Kevin, ten, was doing well; as was three-year-old Liam, the only one of the four not to have been fostered during Charlotte's time in rehab.

All, however, were in emergency foster care now, and Charlotte was worried about them – whether they'd be together and have each other for support. I reassured her that the social work team would be on to this straight away.

She said she felt 'unreal' and 'couldn't believe Lennie was dead'. Her sleeping problems of about four to six months ago had improved and she had 'pulled herself together'. However, since being remanded in custody, she'd been feeling 'terrible . . . low . . . numb', and she said that it was 'virtually impossible to sleep' in the prison. She told me she was feeling exhausted and had been contemplating ways of taking her own life: OD, cutting, ligature. It was only thoughts of her children that kept her going.

In 2002, there were ninety-five prison suicides in England and Wales, with women prisoners having a twenty-fold increased risk. By 2011, the annual UK rate of prison suicides had reduced to fifty-seven, in part through better health screening of new prisoners developed by forensic psychiatrists Luke Birmingham and Don Grubin.[37] This reduction was also down to improved psychiatric services in prison, as well as innovative work by Professor Alison Lielbling, a Cambridge criminologist who developed a measure of the 'moral quality' of prison environments in order to reduce bullying and boost legitimate staff behaviour.[38] But the prison suicide figure soared again to 119 in 2017, after austerity and savage cuts to prison staff increased bang-up time and reduced rehabilitation and health programmes – a Chris Grayling special. No doubt he sleeps soundly at night, unperturbed by money wasted on ferry contracts, trains running late and an ill-conceived attempt at probation privatisation (the first privatisation of a public service to be so disastrous as to need full re-nationalisation). But I hope the grieving families of those fifty suicides above the norm might give him some cause for regret.

I didn't ask Charlotte any further detailed questions; the main task at this stage was to keep her alive. I went back to the hospital wing office, where two prison health care officers (who have some basic nursing training) in white shirts and black epaulettes were sharing tea with a pair of fully qualified nurses in blue uniforms. We were joined by the social worker and a psychiatric nurse, and we pulled up chairs and discussed the plan. As the only male person in our team of three psychiatrists and a dozen or so nurses, psychologists and social workers, I had to keep in mind the gender politics, especially as my predecessor, with his chalk-stripe suit and patrician tones, had not exactly left a favourable impression.

It was clear Charlotte needed to stay in the hospital wing, away from 'ordinary location', where there were more hardened, habitual prisoners. This way, she could be observed, and we could get her safely through the next few stressful days.

Although she had returned to drinking, she was not fully alcohol-dependent. After a few reducing doses of diazepam to help with any alcohol withdrawal, it was clear she didn't need the full seven-day detoxification regimen. Drug and alcohol withdrawal were so ubiquitous at Holloway that there was already a nurse-managed detox programme for heroin and alcohol dependence, which involved gradually reducing doses of a replacement drug to manage severe withdrawal symptoms (which, in the case of alcohol, can involve life-threatening delirium tremens or seizures).

Once our meeting had concluded, I finished off my reviews of follow-up cases.

These were some of the more serious self-harmers amongst the Holloway prisoners, often with features of personality disorder and histories of abuse. What they really needed was inpatient treatment, along the lines of the Bethlem Crisis Recovery Unit (as on page 79) where I had sutured self-inflicted incisions. But there was minimal provision for this type of treatment, and anyhow, prisoners were rarely accepted for transfer.

We later conducted a study of our Holloway referrals to psychiatric hospital in 2003.[39] Of the sixty we referred, only half were accepted. A significantly greater proportion of those rejected had a personality disorder diagnosis. So, the bottom line was, we often had to manage self-harmers who had borderline personality disorder with the resources we had available to us in the prison.

Charlotte would spend a few days in the hospital wing for observation, but once she had settled, she'd be fit for ordinary location.

My prison session finished, I walked to the gatehouse, where I dropped my keys down the metal chute and waited for my key tally, which I clipped to my keychain, along with my Home Office ID and standard prison whistle (prison procurement having not yet caught up with the shift to electronic alarms – a symbol of how difficult it is to change prison culture).

Driving down the Camden Road and up through Primrose Hill afterwards, I saw drinkers at pub tables enjoying the late summer weather. How many drunken arguments would result in stabbings and murders? Eventually back at home, I checked on the boys and then turned in myself, thankful that they were safely at home, not scattered like Charlotte's children, without either parent to hand.

It has struck me how this line of work starts to affect one's perception of life. After a while, even a simple kitchen knife becomes a reminder of a murder weapon, after seeing so many photographed, blood-stained, as forensic exhibits, then later packaged in plastic to be passed around by the jury. Exposed to all this crime (I was doing reports on robberies, assaults, rape and arson), I had also noticed that I had become more risk-averse. Needing some cash for an early Monday journey out of town, I would think twice about an after-dark trip to the cashpoint on Camden High Street.

A few weeks later, I saw Charlotte again. She looked more together. Gradually, over the course of several interviews, her full story emerged.

On the night in question, she had got a lift, with her daughter Sharon, in a friend's car to go and see the dog, only to arrive and discover that it was no longer available. The woman who'd just sold the dog had got in a row with her partner, so Charlotte spent about forty minutes calming her down.

Leaving the woman, her expedition fruitless, Charlotte needed to sort out tea for all the children, and so asked Sharon to take Liam home after stopping in at KFC on the way back to get some chicken and chips for tea.

Next, Charlotte went to a pub and sat talking to the bar staff, then finished her drink and was about to return to the kids when Lennie walked in and greeted her by way of punching her hard on the arm.

He was angry, she said, because she'd been talking to an ex-boyfriend. She used the toilet, and when she returned, Lennie was sitting at the bar nursing a fresh pint. She couldn't remember much of what happened next, but it seemed like they had several more drinks.

Charlotte had been with Lennie for about a year, after he moved in next door. He had a son, but had lost parental responsibility to his ex, and he blamed the frequent disputes over child contact for his heavy drinking.

As will be clear from the previous chapter, domestic violence can start quickly. Lennie's hard-drinking and antisocial tendencies, coupled with his short fuse, meant that the new relationship quickly degenerated into frequent verbal disputes. Lennie's exertion of jealous control made for a toxic cocktail, with terrible consequences for Charlotte and a fatal outcome for Lennie. Lennie had accused Charlotte of infidelity, while he himself was being unfaithful: 'I can have what I want.' It's that egocentric narcissism again, seen in many forensic cases.

Before long, Lennie wanted control not just over Charlotte, but over her family, too. He was verbally abusing her friends, calling them parasites or slags. At the same time, he was still seeing an ex-girlfriend in Swindon at weekends, and this girl would text Charlotte, taunting her about being cheated on.

Even so, Lennie's jealousy was at the root of most of the arguments, and if he didn't find her at home when expected, this would cause a row. He drank super-strength lager, such as Tennent's, every night, and in recent months his drinking had worsened. With this came an escalation of the verbal abuse.

According to Charlotte, the arguments escalated to beatings about nine months before the stabbing. She found these beatings both frightening and humiliating, and tried unsuccessfully to end the relationship, but he refused when she asked him to leave the house. There were further arguments and beatings, the final being about a week before she killed him.

The abuse meted out to women who have killed their abusive male intimate partner is not limited to physical beatings. In her book *When Battered Women Kill*,[40] Angela Browne suggests that women in this situation only switch from victim to murderer when there is a drastic escalation in the abuse being meted out. Browne noted significant histories of sexual abuse as well as physical abuse. Forensic psychiatrist Gill Mezey studied a series of seventeen cases of women who had killed their abuser, and found that most had experienced severe physical, psychological, emotional and sexual abuse. The sexual abuse included denigration of the woman's size and looks; taking control over contraception; jealous accusations of infidelity; coercing into prostitution ('pimping out'); non-consensual sex with threats and violence; penetration by objects; and, in one case, enforced sexually degrading acts with a dog.[41]

Running out of time, I finished my other face-to-face reviews on C1, made myself an instant coffee with powdered milk, and went through a 'whiteboard' review with the nurses and prison officers.

Satisfied that there were no obvious looming crises, I popped my head into the small occupational therapy art and crafts room. Here the most vulnerable group were doing a session with the art therapist. The therapy dog, an ageing Labrador called Quiver, was dozing under the table. Next I let myself out with my passkey, walking through the heavy steel security grill and into the central courtyard garden, where a group of prisoners were working on the flowerbeds in the middle.

Holloway was built in 1852, and had housed the suffragettes during their hunger strike and force-feeding, as well as Ruth Ellis, the last female prisoner to be hanged in 1955, Myra Hindley, and my aunt Georgina. Rebuilt in the 1970s, it now stood five storeys high and was wrapped around three sides of an irregular rectangle. I followed the perimeter around, past the segregation unit and through the activities block with its art workshops, a gym and even a swimming pool: a very rare treat indeed, even for settled prisoners. Staffing levels meant that, during staff mealtimes, shift changes and at night, the prison had to be locked down, with just one officer per 'landing section' (a group of cells or four-bed dormitories, housing around thirty inmates). As I made my way out through the series of heavy grilled gates, locking them behind me ('Lock it and prove it,' said a poster on the wall), I caught my left ring finger in the last one as it slammed shut. In excruciating pain, I realised I had smashed the nail bed, creating a throbbing subungual haematoma.

I would carry that blackened fingernail for the next six months until it grew out, during which time Charlotte's case was working its way through the system.

And with that, I left HMP Holloway for the evening.

Most journeys home from prison assessments would take me well over an hour, but Holloway was close by. A quick journey is better on the one hand, but on the other, I would lose that decompression time between the forensic world and the happier one of bathtime and bedtime stories. In the car or on the bike, I like to zone out with music, the radio news or just the road in front of me, while on the train I prefer to read a book (non-fiction light reading, usually – *Gomorrah*, *The Looming Tower*, *Unnatural Causes* or maybe some Scandi-noir – a change of mayhem or murder is as good as a rest). It's not that I don't process the forensic material, and neither do I pretend I don't have a reaction to it. I talk over the more difficult and troubling cases with colleagues, sometimes years later, in the bar at our annual conference. But sometimes I have to be able to put the cases to one side, in a box – unless the material is too intrusive, of course, in which case you can't stop it spilling out.

It's also a good idea to spend time with people who are not in the field. On a night out, I might catch up over a beer with an old friend from student days. Many of them had left London, but one, Brad, had ended up working for the television news network ITN. He was often racing around covering movie premieres or press conferences, but once I came out of the Old Bailey and straight into the media scrum waiting for a high-profile verdict, and there was Brad – our very different careers briefly colliding.

Some weeks later, I was told that another psychiatrist had been asked to write an independent report for the defence team and was expected to be advancing a partial psychiatric defence for Charlotte. The CPS had asked me to give a second opinion.

A fifteen-year minimum term on a life sentence for murder would mean Charlotte missing the entire childhood of even her youngest child, three-year-old Liam. How would that affect the next generation? When you incarcerate the mother, you also punish the children. I knew this all too well from visits to oppressive 'care' homes to drop off my older cousin Hannah.

After my aunt Georgina's two older children had died, Hannah's safety and welfare had to be paramount in everyone's mind, and she wasn't able to stay with her mother. But Georgina insisted on Hannah being at a care home near her, so she could visit regularly. Maybe an adoption would have been better, though. Intermittent contact with an unreliable mum while living in a children's home can't have been easy. Hannah was physically safe, but what was happening to her emotional development? I must admit that this was something I would often think about, especially later, when I found myself treating young women in hospital.

Unusually anxious, it seemed, to progress Charlotte's case, the CPS were pressing for my report before the defence report was filed. There had been a delay with the submission of that report, and the defence expert psychiatrist had been issued a witness summons to attend court and explain the delay to the judge. This was sure to discourage further procrastination. 'The dog ate my homework' doesn't carry much weight in the Crown court, and any excuse given in oral evidence will be given under oath.

Ethically, it is a potential conflict of interest for a treating doctor to give an expert opinion on certain legal issues like criminal responsibility, and in the civil courts it is expressly forbidden. But when I am the treating psychiatrist, I have to report back to the court (mad or bad; hospital or prison), and anyway, the tradition then was for prison psychiatrists to do the CPS work. I had also seen Charlotte and assessed her mental state while she was fresh from the murder scene, not weeks later, so that would add weight to my opinion.

I saw Charlotte again and asked about her plea. She told me she was pleading not guilty to a charge of murder on the grounds of lack of intent, but guilty to manslaughter. The issue with intent to murder is that the CPS only has to prove intent to cause serious harm, not intent to kill, so that was unlikely to be enough.

Charlotte was in tears, but with gentle encouragement, she finally carried on with her account of what had happened.

After leaving the pub with Lennie in a friend's car, they had arrived home. Her son, Kevin, was in front of the television and the empty fried chicken bucket had been pushed into the overfull kitchen swing bin. Charlotte went upstairs to check on Sharon and Liam. But Lennie followed and punched her, grabbing her hair, too, and pulling some of it out.

There was a shouting match and Lennie spat in her face, then punched her in the head. 'He called me "a dirty slag" . . . why was I talking to Jeremy?'

Isn't the entitlement and jealousy of the antisocial man tediously predictable? This sort of scenario – of alcohol, jealousy and violence – is so often involved when men kill women: a fight to the death, with men too often the winner.

Charlotte's memory was 'a bit vague'. She went to the boys' bedroom to change their sheets, but Lennie kept on shouting.

'I told him to fuck off out of the house, but he refused to go . . . he was following me round the house.'

She went downstairs to get away from him, to phone for help or just to get him out of the house. But Lennie blocked the front door and refused to get out of her way, and when she tried the back door, he covered the alleyway, preventing her from leaving by that route as well.

Charlotte said she went back into the kitchen. On the draining board, there was a selection of cutlery and kitchen utensils. She was tearful, sobbing as she told me. I passed her a tissue, but I didn't want to interrupt her.

'I just grabbed the first thing I found . . . a long kitchen knife.

'I thought if I was holding a knife, he wouldn't come near me.

'It's really awkward to remember exactly what happened.'
She made a dash towards the door, but Lennie blocked her.
'All I wanted to do was to get out of the flat.
'Lennie started walking towards me.
'I made a jab . . . it wasn't a stab.
'I thought he might have got a nick with the knife.'
After that, he was still walking about, so she threw the knife in a box and went upstairs.

She felt exhausted and was still a bit drunk, with everything in a blur. When she sat on her bed, her hair came out in handfuls. She then went back downstairs for a cigarette, and found Lennie sitting 'slumped against the wall'.

She said that he normally sat like that when he was drunk, so she didn't immediately realise something was wrong. When at last it dawned on her that he wasn't just drunk, she shouted for her daughter Sharon to call an ambulance.

It 'felt like a joke', she said. 'It didn't seem real.'

'Even now it doesn't seem real . . . I still can't believe he died.'

This was as far as we got that day. Charlotte was distressed and started to hyperventilate, so I called an end to the interview. A prison officer comforted her before escorting her back to the wing. My visit over, I bundled my notes into my shoulder bag so I could dash across to Wood Green Crown Court for a 2 p.m. sentence hearing.

With my regular working week divided into half-day sessions, I usually took lunch on the hoof, crossing London between one site and the next. A crusty tuna roll from the Holloway canteen, staffed by prisoners, would be a gourmet alternative to the dismal vending machine at Wood Green Crown Court. I was giving evidence on whether a restriction order should be imposed at sentence for one of my secure inpatients.

I never had less than four elements to my working week at that time: prison, hospital, clinic, teaching and expert witness.

I would get a mobile phone call: 'Hi, it's Peter.' *Which Peter?* I would think. Was that Peter the charge nurse in the secure unit, or Peter at the CPS homicide team in Ludgate Hill? Could it be Peter from public protection at Holborn police station, or Peter from the management team at Holloway? Maybe it was just Peter the plumber come to fix the boiler.

I'm used to shifting from one case to another in short order. It pays to have read the papers the night before, otherwise I'd have to speed-read my report at the back of the courtroom.

But at least I am mobile and not stuck behind the same desk all week. The patient comes to the doctor in most other specialties, but unfortunately forensic patients are mostly detained and not able to travel – besides which, if they could, they would probably vote with their feet and head in the opposite direction as fast as they could. Why didn't I do microbiology? The petri dishes are all in the same fridge, and as you may recall from the case of the miserly doctor who killed his wife, old laboratory fridges can make a perfect birthday present.

Later, Charlotte's CPS bundle arrived. Starting with the witnesses, a Justin Atkinson confirmed that Lennie and Charlotte had been at the pub and had drunk 'quite a bit'.

Another witness, Charlotte's neighbour, recalled the scene outside the pub: 'At about 11.45 p.m. . . . I became aware of a raised female voice and another voice . . . I heard phrases like, "Don't beat me up again . . . if you do, I'll leave . . . he's gonna beat me up . . . this time I am going to leave."'

Ryan Cooper heard '"fucking this and fucking that". There was a lot of swearing from the male and female . . .'

Donna Edwards, a neighbour: 'At 12.40 a.m. I was woken by a female voice screaming hysterically . . . I couldn't make out what she was screaming and shouting about . . .'

And in the house, the only eye witness, ten-year-old Kevin Smith, Charlotte's son, said: 'I came downstairs and Lennie and my mum were there . . . my mum pulled out a knife and Lennie said to her, "Stab me, go on then," and then I just saw it go in . . . pouring out with blood . . .'

When the police and ambulance arrived, Charlotte was kneeling over Lennie. Paramedics tried to resuscitate him, but it was clear he was dead from catastrophic exsanguination. Painting the floor, the still-fresh blood made the kitchen dangerously slippery. Charlotte was quickly cautioned, arrested on suspicion of murder and taken away.

Her reply to the caution? 'He's all right, isn't he? We were just mucking about . . . I didn't mean to hurt him . . . he started it.'

18

Holloway was a victim of its own design. My aunt had experienced the old Victorian building in the late 1950s, but for the rebuild in the more liberal and hopeful 1970s, it had been planned along hospital lines, envisaging that women would be out and about, either working, attending classes or otherwise engaged in useful activities for most of the day. The wings were designed only for sleeping, and so they were isolated, with dog-leg corridors that must have been intended to break up the standard Jeremy Bentham, radial-hub panopticon design of many Victorian prisons.

But in reality, observations of vulnerable prisoners by a single officer per wing were made more difficult, as long periods of the day were spent behind closed doors. Some concerned prison officers, all too keenly aware of these problems, had already developed a number of projects on their own initiative, without any government directives. These aimed to soften the blow or shock of imprisonment, and included wings for general drug detox, heroin recovery, a pregnant women's unit, a mother and baby unit and a mental health assessment unit on C wing. Meanwhile, on the lifers' wing, officers helped those facing long stretches come to terms with their sentences and find a way to make constructive use of their time through education and training. There was extensive provision of forensic psychotherapy – much of which would have been beyond the reach of these troubled women 'on the out' – as well as an impressive range of partner organisations such as the Samaritans, who trained prisoners to be 'listeners' for distressed fellow inmates.

The first-night-in-custody unit had carpeted floors and soft furnishings, in order to ease the transition from the outside world to the harsh realities of 'bang up' for first timers. There, I let myself in to find soft-spoken staff making cups of tea and cocoa.

For this visit, I had been asked to see Amber, an eighteen-year-old schoolgirl remanded the night before on a 'joint enterprise' murder charge. This case sounded like the planned revenge killing of a sexual abuser, but the extent of Amber's involvement was in dispute. Remember, the law has provisions for heat-of-the-moment killings, provocation and self-defence, but once you have had the time to reflect, no matter what the provocation, revenge is always dealt with as murder.

Naive, vulnerable and not at all streetwise, Amber had been lured to a flat by Gregory, a slick and charming thirty-year-old who had a stylish BMW. He had plied her with Malibu cocktails, made her watch pornography and then raped her.

She was so ashamed, blaming herself for going along with him, that she told no one for a week, until she finally blurted out the story to her boyfriend, Shawn. Enraged, Shawn persuaded her to lure the rapist to a meeting near a phone box on the edge of Finsbury Park, where she assumed that Shawn was going to 'box him with his fists' to 'teach him a lesson'. However, as Gregory arrived, Shawn and a friend approached, armed with baseball bats.

'I never expected him to be attacked with baseball bats. I had no idea . . .'

Beaten to death by one metal and one wooden baseball bat, Gregory became a murder victim and Amber an accomplice. With her passage to the wings eased by the first-night unit, she was then to spend her A-level year in a dormitory at Holloway as the case progressed.

Did she have an acute stress reaction to the rape, a pre-cursor to PTSD (intrusive memories/flashbacks, hypervigilance and avoidance)? Possibly, but in setting Gregory up for a beating, she risked a finding that she had intended 'serious harm'. If the prosecution could prove that she had been 'a party to the killing', there was a possibility of a murder conviction, even though she hadn't struck a blow. In the end, psychiatric evidence wasn't called. The CPS must have accepted a plea.

Brent Gibson: murder. Life imprisonment; twelve-year minimum term.

Shawn Elliot: murder. Life imprisonment; thirteen-year minimum term.

Amber Dawson: conspiracy to cause actual bodily harm. Two and a half years' imprisonment.

At this time, my oldest boy had started nursery, so I would pick him up at 6 p.m., a bit earlier if I could, and we would sit on the floorboards, play with his wooden train set, read stories or watch children's TV.

At home I often preferred to avoid talking shop every night, even though it can be a great support to have a partner who works in a similar field. Sometimes, rather than debriefing, I prefer to sift out some of my morbid ruminations about my caseload. When there is a complaint to deal with, or worse a potential homicide inquiry, then compartmentalising just isn't possible. Often, though, the issues that tend to be brought home, as I am sure is the case in most lines of work, are irritations with the bureaucracy of increasing managerialism or petty disagreements with a troublesome colleague. So it's much better, from my point of view, to work my way through my old CD and vinyl collection (as a child of the late 1970s and early 1980s, this ranges from Gil Scott-Heron, Bowie and The Clash to The Jam and Siouxie and the Banshees). I want to keep my home and family separate from the human misery I deal with every day – but sometimes the two worlds collide, despite my efforts.

One evening after Holloway, my mind sufficiently far away from C wing and the lifers' unit, I was changing my son's nappy when a couple of coins fell out of my pocket and landed next to him on the changing mat. A ten-pence coin and one of the tiny five-pence coins.

He was happily giggling and reaching out for the coins when suddenly I realised that I couldn't see the five-pence coin. Only just resisting the urge to panic, I peered into his mouth but saw nothing. Was it lodged in his larynx? I convinced myself he was drooling a little.

Over-cautious as always, especially after my experience of paediatrics as a junior doctor, I was terrified he might choke on the coin. I rushed him to Whittington A & E, where the triage nurse was sympathetic. She asked me to wait for the house doctor to see him and agree to the lateral neck X-ray, which was all I needed to either reassure me or confirm the worst – that he might need a laryngoscopy.

I tried to control my panic, convinced that a respiratory arrest could happen any second. I had worked in that very casualty department as a medical student. Finally, like a true nightmare doctor-patient, I sheepishly approached one of the casualty officers, pulled rank, flashed my NHS Consultant ID, and explained my predicament. She gladly signed the X-ray request form, saving me a longer nerve-shredding wait, and we went to sit outside the X-ray department.

Waiting for the radiographer, I looked down a side corridor and a gurney caught my eye. A young female patient was handcuffed to it. I walked closer and realised that she was a Holloway prisoner, being escorted by a male prison officer. The young woman seemed unperturbed, but I was troubled to see her shackled to the hospital trolley in full public view, with a single male escort to boot.

No doubt they hadn't wanted to send two staff, and prisoners have to be prevented from escaping, but what I observed seemed to be excessive and unnecessarily stigmatising. A few years before, the case of a female prisoner who had given birth while handcuffed to her bed had sparked a fierce debate. 'Don't treat shackled patients' ran the editorial in the *British Medical Journal*.[42] A heated correspondence ensued as doctors working with prisoners pointed out that medical treatment must be available even to those prisoners who are in mechanical restraints because they pose a high risk of escape or violent behaviour. The key issue is that good medical care must not be impeded, and adaptations have to be made where enhanced security arrangements are unavoidable, while at the same time respecting the patient's privacy and dignity as much as possible.

Distracted for a moment from my parental anxiety by thoughts of these ethical dilemmas, I almost challenged the officer, but then thought better of it. *Sometimes you just have to leave the job behind,* I thought, although it still nagged at me.

Of course, there was no coin on the lateral X-ray, and I took a happy, chuckling boy home, with him probably thinking that this whistle-stop hospital trip had been laid on purely for his amusement.

Funny, though, how even in the midst of a family crisis, I'd been wrenched back into the prison world by that unfortunate coincidence.

Later that week, more CPS material on Charlotte's case arrived, and I tore open the envelope at my desk in our spare bedroom-cum-study.

Mindful of my two boys sleeping in their bunk beds next door, and with *The Miseducation of Lauryn Hill* turned down low on the CD player, I took another sip of coffee and shuffled through the crime-scene and post-mortem photographs.

The first pictures showed the exterior of the house, the side alleyway and front door. Inside, shots of the kitchen showed a mess of hastily ripped-open sterile packs and gauze swabs. On the floor were swirls of red, where the paramedics had slipped on Lennie's blood.

Lennie turned out to be muscled but wiry, probably about a super-lightweight boxer physique. He had tattooed arms, and was wearing trousers with braces and no shirt. There was a neat horizontal wound less than an inch across between two ribs, about two inches above and just medial to the left nipple. The wound was gaping slightly in the middle, with darkened clotted blood on the edges and blood-stained yellow adipose tissue visible.

In a separate photograph, the heart had been removed and a blunt dissecting rod was inserted to demonstrate the neat horizontal wound, slightly shorter than the external chest wound, right through the thick muscular wall of the left ventricle, the main pumping chamber of the heart.

It was almost perfect. If you had set out to kill someone with a single stab wound, you could not have placed the knife in a more lethal spot.

The post-mortem report was compiled by a Dr Fox, and read: 'There was a single stab wound to the front of the left chest . . . the wound track penetrated the left chest in a direction front to back, sharply backwards and slightly inwards . . . the collapse may not have been immediate . . . the victim would have been capable of a degree of physical activity following the infliction of the fatal wound' – confirming Charlotte's description – '. . . in the face-to-face confrontation, the direction of the track suggests the knife was held in the perpetrator's right hand, so that the blade emerged from the fist between the thumb and index finger . . . there was no evidence of defence-type wounds to the deceased's hands or arms.'

Lennie's fate – being killed by a female partner – is relatively rare. UK statistics from 2019 showed that only eight per cent of male victims were killed by their partner or ex-partner – compared to forty-eight per cent of female victims. Most men are killed by a stranger or an acquaintance in fights or robberies, or in drug- or gang-related violence.

It is a common finding that women who kill intimate partners have been abused by their victim. In such cases, it is the abused woman who has prevailed in what could have been a fight to the death with their abuser. ('It was either him or me.') But all too often, female abuse victims don't have a chance; the fatal blow coming so swiftly, as it did for Jannat Reddy, in a sudden moment of murderous rage.

So how did Charlotte end up in an abusive relationship like this? Why couldn't she get out? And how did she end up killing her abuser?

However abhorrent Lennie's behaviour had been, killing for revenge is murder by law. With a claim of self-defence looking like a remote possibility, could Charlotte avoid life imprisonment?

In interview, she told me that her natural father had abandoned the family when she was very young. Her mother, Patricia, married her stepfather Curtis (aka 'Geordie') and she remembered regular physical abuse by him from an early age.

Geordie was very violent towards her mother too, and, as so often happens, Patricia tended to placate her abusive new partner at the expense of protecting Charlotte.

School didn't go well for Charlotte. Drinking frequently by the age of fourteen, she was excluded at fifteen and never returned to education.

She self-harmed from her teenage years, cut her wrists and took overdoses. When seen by a psychiatrist after one such incident, she was admitted to hospital for short-term management of suicide risk.

Her first proper relationship was with Russell. She met him while still in her late teens, but the couple had separated by the time she was in her early twenties. Russell was frequently violent after drinking.

After leaving Russell, she met Nathaniel, who was also violent. He left her with a black eye on more than one occasion. Then she met Billy, another hard drinker. Social services prevented him from having any involvement with the children because of his severe alcohol problems.

Meanwhile, Charlotte's own alcohol dependence escalated. Drinking in the morning to stop the withdrawal shakes, she was offered residential rehab and allowed to keep her youngest child, under supervision, while the older children were taken into temporary foster care.

She managed to get dry and stayed that way for eighteen months . . . until she met Lennie.

Charlotte had been given a diagnosis of borderline personality disorder (BPD) – a common diagnosis in Holloway. It involves unstable and intense relationships; unstable self-image; impulsivity; recurrent suicidal behaviour, threats, or self-mutilating behaviour; affective (mood) instability. BPD almost aways arises after serious childhood abuse of one form or another.

Borderline patients have often been turned away by psychiatric services or deemed 'untreatable' (although treatment is much more widely available now). Trying to help can be a challenge, as they have an unfortunate knack of provoking an inconsistent reaction, and sometimes even rejection, from therapists, which the patient's disturbed development has taught them to expect from others.

Put another way, the patient who has been neglected (the mother failing to protect her child from abuse) and sexually abused (by the perverse stepfather) becomes convinced, in later life, that everyone will always let them down or take advantage of them, and so may act in a way that provokes the worst reaction in others, ironically fulfilling their pessimistic expectation.

As a forensic psychiatrist, it is immensely important to be aware of these impulses. In fact, as I have said, it is essential that I monitor my reaction or 'counter-transference' to patients. If a patient makes me irritated, exasperated or angry, I have to make use of what this tells me rather than react to it blindly.

These dynamics are often played out in treatment settings. If a therapist treating a patient with BPD lets them down by being late, cancelling a session or going on holiday, this can precipitate severe denigration of the therapist, catastrophic thinking, vociferous complaints and recurrence of self-harm. If you want to treat this group, you have to be consistent and reliable, as they often struggle to cope with unexpected events.

Therapists in forensic settings need to use an eclectic approach to psychological treatments, tailored to fit each individual patient. Research by gold-standard randomised controlled trials has shown the beneficial effects of several therapies, and the common theme is that these treatments provide a shared language for a therapist and patient to talk about and reflect on the problematic emotions and behaviours.

In cognitive behavioural therapy (CBT), a shared formulation or understanding of a problem (anger, self-harm, illicit drug use, et cetera) is developed between the therapist and the patient. CBT is highly structured and makes use of homework. The focus is on achieving a change in mental state or behaviour.

By contrast, for those who engage in repeated self-harm, Marsha Linehan has developed an effective therapy that emphasises a dialectic – or reconciliation of extreme opposites – combining a Zen-like acceptance of problem behaviours 'just as they are' with efforts to change those behaviours through problem-solving and skills training.

An alternative and effective therapy for borderline personality disorder is mentalisation-based therapy, a sort of psychoanalysis-lite developed by Anthony Bateman and Peter Fonagy.[43] Symptoms such as aggression and emotional crises are seen as conveying symbolic and dynamic meaning, which are being used by the patient in a counter-productive way to drown out painful states of mind. Mentalisation-based therapy is underpinned by an integration of evolutionary science, psychology, neuroscience and psychotherapy, via attachment theory.

It is suggested that insecure attachment to parents impairs a person's capacity to self-reflect, and also damages their ability to understand the desires, intents or beliefs of others. Proponents of this theory argue that it has a neuroscientific basis, as poor early attachments are thought to trigger a switch from the use of the prefrontal cortex (in evolutionary terms, the social brain, responsible for planning, working, memory and anticipation) to excessive use of the posterior cortex (a more primitive part of the brain, associated with vigilance, fight-or-flight and selective attention). Any subsequent trauma has the potential to destabilise the ability to mentalise or reflect, and instead brings about feelings of being overwhelmed and losing control. This can lead to disturbed emotional states, violence or 'acting out' with impulsive behaviour.

In treatment, contact with the therapist aims to cautiously activate the attachment system, to stimulate curiosity, and to 'titrate' any emotional closeness, so as not to push the patient back into 'posterior cortex' mode, or a state of overwhelming emotions.

Now, I know this all sounds like gobbledegook. It even does to me a bit, despite having done the training course, but these therapies are all attempts to provide a replicable therapy for borderline personality disorder that uses a consistent and measurable technique.

A discussion of psychological therapy in forensic settings would be incomplete without mention of psychoanalytic therapy – often called psychodynamic therapy, as this is a less loaded term.

One question you might ask any psychiatrist or psychologist is whether they believe in the unconscious. As it happens, I do. British psychiatry is, to a degree, divided between those who do believe – and who are therefore open to psychodynamic ideas – and those who do not. The dispute is around the evidence base, or perceived lack of one. However, research evidence has been found to support both the neuroscientific basis of some psychoanalytic concepts, such as the role of the forebrain in dreaming, as well as the benefits of treatments, with an effect size comparable to antidepressants in some trials.

Psychodynamic psychotherapy explores those aspects of the self that are not fully known, especially as they come to light in the therapy relationship (see the book *The Examined Life* by Stephen Grosz[44]). Psychoanalytic psychotherapy focuses on a patient's emotions; recurring self-defeating patterns; past experience, such as early experiences of attachment figures; and on how the relationship with the therapist can help the patient to gain better understanding of how they relate to others in real-life relationships.[45]

Full-on psychodynamic psychotherapy, using the interpretation of what is going on in the treating relationship, can be too challenging for many forensic patients. But the insights from a psychodynamic approach can be incredibly useful to the treating team, even if a less 'in your face' therapy is selected for treatment.

In the UK, prescribing psychiatrists don't do the talking therapy. We tend to keep it separate, and we rely on psychology or psychotherapy colleagues to deliver it in parallel with all the other interventions. In the USA, although psychoanalytic psychotherapy is no longer the preserve of those with medical training, a few outpatient psychiatrists still offer a one-stop shop, in that they both prescribe and also offer longer sessions to allow time for psychotherapy. Dr Jennifer Melfi in *The Sopranos*, for example, who prescribes the antidepressant Prozac for mafia boss Tony Soprano, also offers therapy sessions to help him better understand his panic attacks.

A tolerance for and a curiosity about personality disorder, and self-harming behaviour in general, is a key prerequisite for forensic psychiatry, in my view. But it doesn't always follow that all psychiatric or medical staff will feel the same way.

Before psychiatry, when I worked in the emergency room, I had noticed the punitive attitude of some of the A & E staff. For instance, there are two main initial treatments for an overdose: stomach washout (Elton John has one in the film *Rocketman*), which is the most effective, but quite messy and labour-intensive for nursing staff, or administering ipecacu-anha, a less effective remedy, and one that induces severe, painful and involuntary vomiting.

During the day, while senior staff were around, the stomach washout was the preferred option. But while working the night shift, I noticed there was a small group of more hardened nurses who seemed to act on their negative reaction to patients who self harm, and would routinely administer the convulsive vomiting treatment to OD cases. While it avoided the unpleasantness for the nurses of the stomach washout procedure – which I could understand – I also believed it was an unthinking or maybe even a conscious punishment of the patient for blocking up the unit with their self-inflicted misery.

With people like Charlotte, who are suffering from borderline personality disorder and prone to recurrent self-harm and suicidal thoughts, how can we tell when to take them seriously?

Well, one of the crucial factors to weigh in this decision is the lethality of the chosen suicide method. There is often considerable ambivalence about suicide, with frequent morning-after regret or a 'change of heart' being a factor. If the patient has taken an overdose, then depending on the drug of choice, there is a greater possibility of survival, thanks to the stomach washout, activated charcoal or infusion of an antidote. Clearly this is a method of suicide more commonly found in the cry-for-help category.

However, if they choose a method with rapid lethality, then it will be too late for second thoughts. When coal gas (rapidly lethal through carbon monoxide poisoning) was replaced with natural gas (much less harmful) the suicide rate plummeted. All too often in prison settings, the most easily available method is a ligature around the neck, only requiring a strip of cloth, laces or a belt. This can cause rapid unconsciousness and heart slowing through vagal nerve stimulation, as well as asphyxia through strangulation. So common were ligatures that Holloway had distributed Fish cutters to all officers – a plastic device with a recessed blade for rapidly cutting down suspended prisoners.

Sadly, I was all too familiar with the ambivalence around suicide. Too young to remember, I had nevertheless been told that, in the aftermath of the family infanticide, as well as the stillbirth of baby David, my grandmother, Katherine, had become depressed. The social stigma and burden of Georgina's ongoing mental illness took their toll on the relationship between my grandparents and, to add injury to insult, my grandmother developed breast cancer. Katherine started to say that it was all too much, and when things were really bad, she spoke of putting her head in the (coal-gas) oven.

Having exposure to a family history like this can help if you become a psychiatrist. If you haven't had a suicide in the family, or not dealt with one as a doctor, then the prospect can seem remote, even for young psychiatrists – despite the fact that roughly five psychiatric patients take their own lives every day in England and Wales. There is also the 'cry wolf' syndrome. All junior doctors see so much non-fatal self-harm in the cutters and minor overdoses of A & E that, when suicide finally happens, it comes as a slap in the face.

When psychiatrists in training came to Holloway – to get prison psychiatry experience under my supervision – I encouraged them to make referrals to psychiatric services for suicidal prisoners who might benefit from treatment.

I had one enthusiastic but rather over-confident senior trainee who had assessed Arianna, a young woman with borderline personality disorder referred by the prison GP because of significant self-harm. Awaiting her court case for a public order offence, she was in prison for just a few weeks. Arianna clocked her psychiatrist's inexperience. 'You're obviously quite new at this . . . you're very young – and don't deny it.'

He noted that she appeared slightly ambivalent about suicide, but had also said she might try to end her life again.

'When?'

'I don't know . . . It beats jail. Part of me wants to die and a part of me doesn't . . . if I could get my kid back I wouldn't be doing stupid things like arguing with police, slicing myself, trying to hang myself . . .'

He made some suggestions about which medication might theoretically be of benefit, but he didn't prescribe anything. He decided not to refer her to her local psychiatric service in Bristol, thinking she wasn't likely to be transferred to hospital and would soon be out of prison anyway, and thus free to seek help if she wanted it.

Not long after her release, she jumped off the Clifton Suspension Bridge into Avon Gorge, an unequivocal suicide method with no second chances.

As the last psychiatrist to have interviewed her, my senior trainee came to see me for supervision, white as a sheet at the realisation that he would have to explain his decision-making to the tearful family from the witness box of the coroner's court. It is experiences like these that shape you as a forensic psychiatrist.

19

The plight of women abused by their partners has been the subject of much debate. Women are often seen as the victims of men who control and dominate their partners. It may be difficult for some women to leave for reasons of financial dependence, fear of later retribution, worries about losing contact with their children or even fear of an 'honour' killing.

The model of learned helplessness has been suggested to explain this – a state first observed in laboratory rats that showed symptoms of apathy, passivity and loss of motivation when repeatedly exposed to painful stimuli with no means of escape.

Do battered women who see no means of escape from the abusive relationship respond in the same way? Does this explain the feelings of helplessness, hopelessness, lowered self-esteem and passivity?

'Battered woman syndrome' (BWS) is said to consist of a 'constellation' of features seen in women exposed to violence in intimate relationships. Depression and feelings of powerlessness impair their ability to escape from the abusive situation. But is even this too simplistic? Donald Downs, an American professor of political science who wrote a book about BWS, suggests that the syndrome's logic 'denies women their reason . . . reinforcing their victimization'. He argues that women often adopt 'heroic means of survival, retaining accurate, reasoned perceptions [about their abusers]. To portray battered women as irrational and lacking will undermines otherwise valid self-defence claims and hurts women more generally.'[46]

Others have argued that women get caught up in and contribute to the violent relationship, despite repeated experiences of abuse.

Women who fight back against abusive or tyrannical men have been depicted in art and literature with both sympathy and condemnation alike. The mythical tale of Judith's beheading of the tyrant Assyrian general Holofernes, originally described in the Apocrypha, became an allegory for the victory of the weak over the strong; the power of women in overcoming an oppressor; and the pluck of the Florentine republic in facing the threat of foreign powers.[47] The iconic image of Judith is depicted in the two examples mentioned earlier, on p.188, and in Caravaggio's version, a gory chiaroscuro image showing blood gushing from Holofernes' half-severed neck (Caravaggio himself no stranger to homicidal violence, of course). But other murderous female characters have received a different response. Take Thomas Hardy's *Tess of the D'Urbervilles*. A victim of rape by an older man, the cynical and manipulative Alec, Tess's life is sent along a tragic path to unrequited love, an unwanted pregnancy and an infant death.

At the end of the story, Tess realises that Alec has ruined her life and she kills him. The actual moment of the killing is not described, but the workman who finds Alec's body notes that, 'the wound was small, but the point of the blade had touched the heart of the victim', much like the wound inflicted by Charlotte on Lennie. It has been suggested that the killing represents a 'tragic moment of energy and heroism', but it also exposes the extent of Tess's degradation by Alec.[48] One implication of this Victorian narrative is clear: for a woman, happiness is achieved through a stable and happy marriage. Hardy suggests, however, that a man of the cloth cannot be relied on to put love above Victorian social convention. Hardy clearly wants the reader to feel sympathy for Tess, even to view her homicide as justified, but he doesn't let her escape the consequences of trying to break free from the constraints of her subjugated role. The verdict is murder, and she is hanged.

Now, in the twenty-first century, what would Charlotte's experience be? How would her case be resolved at court? Would she be condemned or celebrated, or something in between?

Charlotte's diagnosis? Depression, alcohol abuse, borderline personality disorder, battered woman syndrome.

In other countries, such as the US, alternative charges like third-degree manslaughter may be available. In other words, the District Attorney (prosecutor) has discretion. But in the UK, Charlotte was facing murder, with its mandatory life sentence, unless she could mount a defence. In many jurisdictions, a history of abuse alone is insufficient, but may form part, or a 'limb', of another legal defence.

A survey of battered-women murder-law revealed a range of provisions around the globe. For example, in Victoria, Australia, 'social framework evidence' may be used to contextualise self-defence; in the USA, domestic violence may be taken into consideration when assessing 'reasonableness' in relation to self-defence, and it may affect the issue of 'honest belief' of whether a defendant felt they were in 'danger of death or injury'.

It's easy to see how this could have applied to Charlotte, as she must have had an 'honest belief' that Lennie would beat her again. But was the use of the knife 'reasonable force'? In Hong Kong, provocation has been used as a defence, while in the Indian courts 'slow-burn' provocation is recognised. In Poland, a history of abuse may support a defence of provocation, insanity or 'extraordinary mitigation', while in Brazil, sentencing is more discretionary, and case law allows 'reasons of relevant social and moral value', like domestic abuse, to reduce the sentence. In Japan and Spain, sentence mitigation is the norm, and in New South Wales, non-custodial penalties have been applied.

In the UK, battered women who kill abusive partners have found it difficult to claim self-defence, which, if successful, results in acquittal. And in any event, the only witness, Kevin, had suggested that Charlotte poked the knife at Lennie after he had taunted her, not while he was actually hitting her, so reasonable force might be difficult to get past a jury. But the case law on provocation in cases of battered women is complex and changeable. In 2001, the partial defence (murder reduced to manslaughter) of provocation required not only that there were 'things said or done by the deceased' that constituted provocation, but also that Charlotte must have been subject to a sudden and temporary 'loss of self-control'.

In the late 1990s, attempts were made in various criminal cases to argue that, for an abused woman, there may be a form of slow-burn provocation, which doesn't fit neatly into the legal definition of 'sudden' loss of self-control. The argument is that men kill on the spur of the moment in a domestic dispute because they can, because they're stronger. A serially abused woman, however, may not overpower her abuser unless – as in Charlotte's case – they make a lucky strike straight into the heart. So they might lose control cumulatively, but have to pick their moment. Not revenge, but slow-burn loss of self-control nonetheless.

Luckily, I had some experience of a case like this during my first registrar job in forensic psychiatry. The old medical adage, 'See one, do one, teach one' applies. In 1996, I had been eagerly awaiting my chance to do my first forensic attachment. I had just spent six months on a work exchange in Sydney, at a psychiatric unit called the East Wing at Manly Hospital. So I was adjusting back to London life and already missing the white sands of Shelly Beach and post-work swims in the seawater pools of the Northern Beaches.

My boss was Dr Jim MacKeith, a pioneer of forensic psychiatry, who had developed the Bethlem forensic service at the Denis Hill Unit.

As well as being a thoughtful and compassionate psychiatrist and mentor to many of my colleagues over the years, Dr MacKeith had become an expert in retracted confessions and miscarriage of justice, along with forensic psychologist, magistrate and former Icelandic detective Gísli Guðjónsson. In the 1970s, it had still been possible to be convicted of murder by a confession alone. In some high-profile IRA cases, notably the Guildford Four and the Birmingham Six, 'confessions' to police had been extracted under extreme psychological pressure and, although the confessions were later retracted, the convictions and life sentences followed.[49] Jim and Gísli, working with human rights lawyer Gareth Peirce, had been able, through painstaking work, to persuade the court that there had been miscarriages of justice, at a time when the Old Bailey was highly sceptical about psychiatric expert evidence.

This work on retracted confessions was highly influential, and in 1984 the law was changed to make it mandatory to audio record all suspect interviews. There were provisions to improve legal representation for suspects and to introduce limits on detention before charge. In 1996, I tagged along at Oxford Crown Court to observe the retrial of Sara Thornton, who had originally been convicted of the murder of her husband Malcolm.

Malcolm Thornton was a hard drinker and had subjected Sara to repeated assaults and threats. Police had been called more than once and Malcolm had been charged with assault. On 14 June 1989, he was drunk, and when Sara came home, he called her a whore and threatened to kill both her and her daughter, Fiona, saying he would do this while she was asleep.

In fear of her life, she picked up a knife. She tried to get him to go to bed to sleep off the booze, but when the threats continued, she stabbed him once and called an ambulance.

Meeting at Paddington station that day, I boarded the train with Jim, Gareth, a pupil barrister and the razor-sharp but intimidating Mike Mansfield QC. I had made the mistake of wearing a somewhat lurid tie – a blue one with red tulips. I detected an irritated glance from Mansfield, but his tie definitely won the competition: a florid pattern of blood oranges, an obvious expression of 'radical bar' independence of mind, which would be tucked away once he donned the black silk and white bands of a criminal QC.

The prosecution case was that Thornton was a pathological liar and that the killing was financially motivated, thus psychiatric defences didn't apply. There were the customary four senior psychiatrists at that trial, with some differences of opinion. With Mansfield's incisive advocacy, Thornton got the verdict her defence team had been fighting for through various appeals. On Friday, 29 May 1996, Sara Thornton was found not guilty of murder by the jury. They found her guilty of manslaughter instead, but did not specify whether it was on grounds of provocation, diminished responsibility or a combination of both (the abnormality of mind, in this case, being borderline personality disorder).

She had already served five years, and so the judge went through the formality of sentencing her to time already served, and she was released from the dock at court.

A bit of a fudge, you might think, but the courts were still not allowing slow-burn provocation – no doubt it was seen as too close to revenge, which could not be allowed as a precedent.

The archetypal example of this and a case that was something of a template for the Thornton appeal was the case of

Kiranjit Ahluwalia, who came to international attention after burning her husband to death.

Kiranjit suffered from domestic abuse for ten years, including physical violence, food deprivation and rape. One evening in the spring of 1989, her husband tried to break her ankles to stop her running away and burned her face with a hot iron. Later that night, while he slept, she poured petrol over the bed and set him alight.

Kiranjit was convicted of murder in December 1989. At the trial, the fact that she waited until her husband had gone to sleep was evidence she had had time to 'cool off' and weigh up her actions. In other words, her actions could be seen as revenge rather than sudden and temporary loss of control.

Kiranjit's conviction for murder was overturned on appeal in 1992 on grounds of diminished responsibility, although her submission of slow-burn provocation also failed.

The status of abuse victims is not without controversy. As we've said, it has been argued that casting the woman solely as the victim, rather than acknowledging her own, albeit unconscious, aggressive participation in such relationships, denies women a sense of agency for their actions.

Erin Pizzey, a feminist all her life and founder of the modern women's shelter movement, cautions against accepting a neat division between female victims and male oppressors, reminding us that in many abusive couples both partners are guilty of verbal and physical assault, and that women may choose other alternatives to killing their partners in these violent relationships. Others have suggested that there are dynamics between the couple that contain dependent, aggressive and sadomasochistic elements in both partners.

Women who kill their partners are not all abuse victims, as illustrated by one case that received widespread coverage around the time I was finishing my training. Giselle Anderson, a part-time model, stabbed her boyfriend, Oscar, a bus driver, over forty-two times after they had stopped in his car during an argument in the early hours of 1 December 1996.

It has never been suggested that Oscar was abusive; far from it – he was described as a happy young man. At a press conference three days later, Anderson claimed that a 'fat passenger' with staring eyes had got out of a Ford Sierra and killed Oscar in a road rage attack. Police tried unsuccessfully to track down the murderer, but no one had seen a Ford Sierra. Officers later found the murder weapon hidden in the petrol tank of the car the couple had been travelling in. Anderson was found guilty of murder and served fourteen years of a life sentence, later admitting that she did stab Oscar to death.

Denied the protection of lifelong anonymity, Anderson is said to have completed anger management in prison and, having been released under supervision on life licence, is reported to be living a peaceful life working in a hair salon in a quiet coastal town.

20

In those days, I would dictate my first draft of reports on to analogue tapes, sometimes driving over to my typist's house in the evenings when deadlines were tight. I found that my brain composed faster than my fingers could type and, with interview material and a summary of evidence, a murder report could run to twenty or more closely typed pages. Looking at my report on Charlotte now, it is a little bit loose, and the evidence summaries are quite brief.

I'd also used the Arial font, which is a dull sans serif, popular for NHS letters, but hard on the eye in a long report. As I got more experienced, I tried switching to Garamond, before settling on Book Antiqua, which is a typeface based on pen-drawn letters of the Italian Renaissance and is distinctive and easy to read in a small font size.

A minor detail, you'd think, but impressions count, especially with judges and prosecution QCs. Presenting thorough and detailed work means that your opinion is more likely to be given weight, as a report has to present a persuasive narrative.

Charlotte's defence expert's report was sparse (although padded out with an oversized font, and double spaced) and featured a number of glaring typos. What's more, the opinion was dotted throughout the body of the report, rather than presented tidily at the end, and the language was heavy with hyperbole that undermined the case the expert was trying to make. The style of the report created the impression (false or otherwise) that the author had made up his mind before considering all the evidence, and so he made himself sound as if he were partial to the defence case.

I sat in the spare bedroom-cum-study at home and consulted my copy of *Blackstone's Criminal Practice*, a substantial investment at over £200. We are not lawyers, but we get very familiar with narrow sections of the law. I saw Sara Thornton's case immortalised in black-and-white in the manual and, consulting the legal authorities, I composed my opinion.

Borderline personality disorder was straightforward: instability of affect, impulsivity, self-harm and suicide attempts. Alcohol dependency syndrome with acute intoxication was also certain. We will come back to the effect of drunkenness later, but it was not a 'live issue' in Charlotte's case. But battered woman syndrome was not, and still isn't, a medical diagnosis. 'Feelings of powerlessness' and 'impaired ability to escape from the abusive situation' seemed to describe Charlotte very well, but could they 'substantially impair' responsibility? What about provocation? Were things 'said or done' that were sufficient to cause a 'reasonable person' to lose self-control? What would you have done in Charlotte's situation?

How could you have 'abnormality of mind' and yet be judged as a 'reasonable person'? And, if provoked, can your abnormality of mind be allowed to affect your threshold for sudden loss of control? These are complex issues, which have subsequently been redefined in case law and statute, but in 2001 there was often an elision or fudge of these two mutually exclusive propositions.

There was clearly irritation at the CPS with the poor-quality defence report, and I was asked to attend a conference at chambers in Bedford Row at 5.30 p.m. one evening. I walked along Theobalds Road, past Jockey's Fields, to arrive there and be ushered into an imposing conference room, lined with Morocco-leather-bound law reports and a polished boardroom table. There seemed to be a lot of people: a female QC, a junior barrister, a pupil, a barrister's clerk, a solicitor and a solicitor's clerk. On the table: two pen pots of

Bedford Row logo rollerballs, a stack of new lined pads and trays of tea and biscuits.

Looking back now, the issues are crystal clear, but then, still inexperienced, I had been a little reticent in my opinion. Yes, there was abnormality of mind. I commented on borderline personality disorder and on battered woman syndrome. But as for substantial impairment of responsibility, I thought I should leave that for the jury to decide. Criminal responsibility is ultimately moral, not medical.

I was feeling a bit uncomfortable that everyone in the room seemed to be hanging on my every word. As my murder case experience grew, I would get increasingly used to this. Usually in a murder case, as I have said, all the evidence about who wielded the knife is uncontested – it all comes down to the state of mind of the defendant at the material time, and in order to understand that, the court needed my opinion. At that very moment in time, however, I felt ill at ease, as though it were me in the dock. I distinctly remember the QC clearing her throat to address me. Even though she was a 'friendly', I felt a droplet of sweat tickle my hairline. I swallowed, and hoped that my nerves didn't show.

'Doctor, thank you,' she began. 'We're very grateful for your work on this case. We just need to go through a few points . . . The Crown needs to take a view on the defendant's offer of a plea to manslaughter, as I'm sure you understand.'

Keeping my voice level, I replied, 'Yes, of course. How can I help?'

'Now, you've seen Ms Smith at Holloway on a number of occasions, doctor, am I right?'

'Yes, I have. I first saw her very soon after she was remanded.'

'And you are satisfied that she meets criteria for borderline personality disorder?'

I wondered where she was going with her line of questioning, answering carefully, 'Yes.'

'And you have made a diagnosis of alcohol dependency syndrome, albeit she is abstinent but in a protected environment?'

'Yes.'

She continued, 'And you are agreed that on the back calculation of blood alcohol in police custody she must have been intoxicated at the material time?'

'Yes indeed.'

'But such intoxication must have been voluntary, and therefore is not a live issue, as it is not relevant to abnormality of mind . . .'

'Yes,' I said. 'She has a strong compulsion to drink, but she retains capacity to choose whether to drink or not.'

The QC nodded, looking down at her notes. 'Right, thank you. Now, can you help us with the effects of borderline personality disorder on abnormality of mind?'

'Well, I think the American criteria are more useful. They're more detailed . . . If I can just have a look at my report, I would say the relevant features are emotional instability, impulsive behaviour, affective instability, by which I mean very short-term mood changes, inappropriate anger or difficulty controlling anger . . . frequent displays of temper.'

She pounced. 'But doctor, impulsivity and inappropriate anger could be taken as more of a defect of character than an abnormality of mind?'

'Yes,' I managed, 'but no, but yes . . .'

She stopped me. 'All right, let's suppose that abnormality of mind is accepted, on the criteria you have identified . . . difficulty controlling anger and so on. Do you think the abnormality of mind would be sufficient to have *substantially* impaired her responsibility?'

'Well, let me consider that . . .'

'By substantial, of course you are aware, Dr Taylor, that the threshold in law is more than trivial impairment but less than total.'

'Well,' I said, 'I think substantial impairment is a matter for the court.'

She smiled wanly. 'Yes, Dr Taylor. It is, as you rightly say, the ultimate issue. But you must realise, doctor, that if this case goes to trial, the court will reasonably *expect* you to assist the jury in their deliberations, as to whether, in your professional opinion, there was substantial impairment of responsibility. Let's move on to battered woman syndrome. You are somewhat equivocal on this point. I assume you are familiar with the work of Professor Downs on the subject?'

'Yes, I am,' I replied, trying to think on my feet, still feeling intimidated, 'but there are no clearly agreed psychiatric diagnostic criteria for battered woman syndrome. And Professor Downs refers to the American versions of self-defence and insanity.'

'Doctor, I am sure you are aware that battered woman syndrome has been accepted as abnormality of mind in cases of this type, where a woman has killed an abusive man . . . learned helplessness, impaired ability to leave an abusive relationship, impaired perception of threat, and so on.'

'Yes.'

I detected a tone of exasperation.

'Doctor, I am sure you appreciate that the judge, who has considered all the evidence, including your report, is very concerned about this case. He is mindful that we have four children separated from their mother . . .'

The penny dropped. The CPS knew what outcome they wanted, but they needed an expert opinion to hang it on, and with a poor-quality defence report, the onus was on me.

After further discussion, the QC told me that, in any event, she was advising the CPS that they would need to instruct another psychiatrist for a second opinion.

In tricky cases, it is common to have four opinions, two for each side. When I later found out the identity of the expert the CPS had settled on, I recognised them as an experienced colleague who I knew to have an interest in, and sympathy for, the concept of battered woman syndrome. This was another unsubtle hint, and a learning point for me. If you need an expert opinion, choose your expert carefully.

I must explain that I am not talking about expert opinion for hire or 'hired guns', as they are known. The issue is that, working on the interface of two disciplines with different languages, namely law and psychiatry, there is usually a range of reasonable or acceptable expert opinion. If you fall outside that range, then you risk criticism from judges or colleagues. But some experts are known to tend towards a particular position on finely balanced issues, like whether battered woman syndrome is a useful concept, or whether hallucinations are frequently malingered by defendants after they have heard about them in the prison yard, to give two examples.

I was learning that the law has a way, not of slavishly applying criteria and precedent to their final conclusion, but rather of working backwards in a consequentialist manner. What is the just and appropriate outcome in this case? And how can we work the existing law to achieve this? Does society feel sympathetic to this defendant, or do we need to throw away the key? Does this defendant need treatment in hospital or containment in prison?

Requested to do an addendum report, I was handed the QC's copies of three VHS interview tapes. I had read the transcript, but they wanted me to look at Charlotte's demeanour just after arrest, and to listen to her first-hand account of the circumstances of the offence, rather than just reading the transcript. The jumpy video with time-code bleeps showed Charlotte, her hands shaking, sipping Nescafé and smoking cigarettes as she was led through the timeline, the solicitor having advised her to cooperate with the interview rather than giving the standard 'no comment' responses.

Unsubtle hint number two: if we want to shift your opinion, we will show you some new evidence to give you some wiggle room. I was politely shown out by the clerk as these dynamics were crystallising in my mind.

By now it was almost spring 2002, although there was still a nip in the air. I decided to clear my head and walked along New Oxford Street and into Soho. My destination: Lina stores on Brewer Street, with its sweet smell of Italian cheese and coils of fresh tagliatelle. The pleasing smells and colourful displays of Italian tins and packets were a welcome olfactory and visual antidote to the stagnant air and graffiti-covered walls of Holloway.

I needed an easy supper option, as I had a tribunal report on one of my inpatients to finish before bedtime. The work had become more manageable, through experience and pattern recognition, unless there was a crisis that threw a spanner in the works of a carefully scheduled week. A patient in seclusion, or a recall warrant to be executed with a vanload of police could easily take out half a day.

It's said that it takes about five years to settle in as a consultant doctor in any speciality. The problem is that our training is superb at giving us confidence in managing individual cases, but as a consultant, you also have to show leadership, prioritise and delegate tasks, and anticipate disasters. I was also suffering from FOMO. If I didn't take on this case, no matter how inconvenient, would it mean that they wouldn't send me another? I would feel vibrations in my pocket, only to discover that my phone wasn't there. We call this a haptic or bodily hallucination if a patient reports it.

As in many walks of life, knowing when to say no is a skill that only comes with experience. Life events all come at once. Having done all of my psychiatric training on the south side of the River Thames, I had moved north to become a consultant, and hence I was working with an entirely new network of colleagues. My peer group had mostly all trained together, and they were familiar with the foibles and personalities of all those other psychiatrists who referred us cases – invaluable background knowledge – whereas I had to pick all this up on the hoof. As a parting shot, the senior psychiatrist I replaced said to me, tongue in cheek, 'Dr X is very anxious and will ask for a forensic opinion about everyone. If Dr Y ever refers you a case, you had better send them straight to Broadmoor.'

Yes, it was Dr Y who later referred Anthony Hardy.

The same year I'd taken up the promotion to consultant, we had moved house just four weeks before our first boy was born, barely having enough time to put together the flat-packed IKEA cot.

With both of us working, he had to join a nursery after his first birthday. One autumnal day in 2001, I was giving a lecture to psychiatrists in training at University College when a member of the audience shouted out that a plane had hit the World Trade Center. The teaching session was cancelled and I rushed home, took my son out of the nursery and sat with him, watching the rolling news, convinced, like many people, that Canary Wharf was on the target list. I didn't know it yet, but 9/11 would soon affect the cases I was asked to assess. But once the shock and immediate aftermath of 9/11 was over, normal life resumed. My second son was born that December, and I was back to my routine work.

By the time Charlotte's case was approaching trial, my second boy was coming up to his first birthday and almost ready to join his older brother at the nursery across the road. I set aside a Sunday afternoon to work on my addendum report for Charlotte's case. I had to stick to my guns: that battered woman syndrome, or BWS, is not a psychiatric diagnosis, but I acknowledged it could help explain what Charlotte had done.

'If the court were to accept BWS as an abnormality of mind . . . then the features relevant to substantial impairment would be . . .' and so on.

Using the BWS model, the repetition of the 'violent cycle' over time could have undermined Charlotte's self-belief and created a state of learned helplessness. She was trapped in a 'deadly situation' with Lennie, in which she had 'fought back' with lethal consequences.

For battered woman syndrome to apply, a woman must have been through this cycle at least once, and a cluster of symptoms must have developed: low self-esteem, self-blame, fear, suspicion and 'loss of belief in the possibility of change'.

In the USA, murder is dealt with by the varying criminal codes of individual state jurisdictions, but usually there is a distinction drawn between different levels of seriousness in murder cases: first-degree murder, intentional murder that is wilful and premeditated; second-degree murder, intentional murder not premeditated or planned; third-degree murder, any unlawful killing committed during a non-violent felony; involuntary manslaughter, a lack of intention or negligent act; justifiable homicide, not a crime, often used by police (controversially, at times). But when an abuser is killed – no offence to Lennie – should there be another category: 'praiseworthy homicide'?

A date had been set for trial, and Charlotte's case faded from my consciousness as I carried on with the merry-go-round of my various jobs.

Then came a chance for a break. I was off with a group of colleagues to the American Academy of Psychiatry and the Law conference at Newport Beach, California.

The conference programme that year looked interesting. There were sessions covering: 'The role of defence psychiatrists in death penalty cases'; 'Parricide, a description of forty cases'; and 'Update on the chemical castration of sex offenders'.

As my Virgin transatlantic flight reached cruising altitude, I realised I had seven or eight hours' respite, where no one could reach me. But once we were halfway through the flight and I was feeling rested, I didn't fancy a second movie. I changed seats to sit with a colleague so we could run through a draft report on another Holloway case.

The case was Kathleen McCluskey, later dubbed the 'Cambridge Black Widow', accused of poisoning four fellow heroin addicts with massive doses of methadone concealed in home-made cocktails. One killing began with a Friday night 'sex and drugs' party. Police found photographs of this sex party on some undeveloped film late in the investigation. Suffice it to say that a heroin-fuelled and ultimately fatal sex party was not a pretty sight.

Verdict: manslaughter twice over. Six years' imprisonment.

Forensic psychiatrists work hard, but when we get together once or twice a year for conferences, we play hard, too. We are the surgeons of psychiatry, remember – sometimes a bit larger than life and, for the most part, with a sense of humour to match. We are fond of diagnosing each other. 'He or she's a psychopath, a narcissist, schizoid . . . or on the spectrum (mildly autistic).' 'His reports are interminable. He can't see the wood for the trees.' (By which we mean someone so obsessional that their perfectionism interferes with task completion.)

But we have usually referred cases to each other during the preceding year, or crossed swords in court. So despite vehement disagreements, a late night in the conference hotel bar is a chance to employ a bit of gallows humour as we swap war stories. In my view, this is another form of longer-term decompression, essential for forensic survival. I have seen colleagues come a cropper – and even leave the field – when they try to deal with forensic work by isolating themselves from the opinions of colleagues. Peer support doesn't necessarily involve peer agreement, but as I have said, you do need to make use of the sounding board of colleagues.

After I had returned to the UK, I received a one-line letter from the CPS on Charlotte's case, thanking me for my help. They had accepted a plea.

The sentence was five years' imprisonment (determinate, with release on licence possible after two-and-a-half years). Later, the Court of Appeal cut the sentence by three years, leaving Charlotte to walk free.

Twenty-five years for Lee Watson for killing Chiara Leonetti, and two years for Charlotte: a big difference for taking a life in very different circumstances. Who says the law is an ass?

In 2009, the law would change and battered woman syndrome was no longer accepted as an abnormality of mind, not being a 'recognised medical condition'. In the meantime came a new condition, 'coercive control' – the case of Sally Challen being an excellent example.

Sally killed her husband, Richard, in 2010, having met him when she was sixteen and he was twenty-two. He was charming initially, but gradually the abuse began. He bullied her physically and verbally and restricted her access to her friends, while he had affairs and visited brothels.

She tried to leave him, but was so emotionally dependent that she returned. Not long after this, he sent Sally out in the rain to fetch his lunch as he set up a date with another woman by phone.

She challenged him on her return, and an argument broke out. In the course of this confrontation, she hit him repeatedly with a hammer. Sally was convicted of murder and sentenced to life imprisonment with a minimum tariff of twenty-two years, reduced to eighteen on appeal.

Coercive control subsequently became recognised as a form of domestic violence, its characteristics being psychological abuse, degradation, mind games and control of activities and access to friends, so that the abused becomes isolated and dependent on their abuser. (Sound familiar?)

In 2017, Justice for Women submitted new grounds of appeal with a psychiatric expert report about coercive control and its impact on provocation. Sally's conviction was over-turned and, with a planned retrial abandoned, she was freed in 2019 after diminished responsibility was agreed.

Murder is such an emotive subject that sometimes, it seems, it is necessary to reinvent the wheel.

By 2006, my time at Holloway was coming to an end. In the world of the NHS 'internal market' and competing NHS Trusts, the decision had been taken to allocate the mental health contract to a neighbouring trust with no direct access to forensic hospital beds. Our team at Holloway was to be replaced by a service with a different emphasis, trying to treat more women in prison, and focusing less on referring them out to local services.

Some years later, Holloway prison was further criticised following the sad case of the suicide of a woman with psych-osis who had been waiting for transfer to hospital. Under the stewardship of Michael Gove, then UK Secretary of State for Justice, there was a surprise announcement that Hollo-way would close. Despite its problems, there was much lamenting by the staff of those various programmes which had been built up over the years, like the visiting psycho-therapy team, the lifers' unit and the first-night-in custody wing. Many of Holloway's prisoners came from London, and the replacement private sector prisons in Peterborough and out near Heathrow are much harder to reach, making contact with families and children far more difficult. For this reason, experts on the prison inspection teams had often referred to geography as being one of Holloway's major advantages.

At first there were real concerns that many innovations from Holloway would be lost. The replacement prison, HMP Bronzefield, was a new-build, but bricks and mortar are rarely a solution. 'Let's knock it down and start again' risks losing so much accumulated expertise, especially from somewhere as complex and troubled as Holloway.

But in recent years, thankfully, there has been a major uplift in funding for mental health services at HMP Bronzefield, with an extensive therapeutic programme for those who are in custody for the first time, as well as those on very short remands or sentences, and for lifers. HMP Bronzefield has taken on the mantle of the largest women's remand prison in Europe, and with it the challenge of managing high rates of self-harm, along with all the issues around mothers in prison custody and their babies.

In 2006, when I left Holloway, psychiatric services in women's prisons were being reformed. The unit at Broadmoor high-secure hospital was closed, with the patients moved into lower levels of security. I wrote up some of what I had learned at Holloway in a chapter for *Psychiatry in Prisons: A Comprehensive Handbook*,[50] and doing this proved invaluable, as I was to spend the next thirteen years working with such women in secure hospital.

On my last visit to Holloway, I comically but painfully banged my head on a *No Parking* sign under which I had parked my car. The nurses on C1 patched me up with skin glue when they saw me using a paper towel to mop the blood trickling down my forehead during our team meeting. After all the challenging cases and dramatic events at Holloway, a sore and bleeding head seemed a fitting farewell.

As I left, I reflected on how much I had experienced. If you go into psychiatry, you must have more than a passing interest in the outer extremes of the human condition. And there was no better place to study this than at Holloway. I often drive past now and see the walls and gatehouse, mothballed and awaiting the wrecking ball. I can honestly say that I learned more within those walls than in any of my other placements, from Broadmoor hospital to Brixton prison.

The Murderer Who Forgets

Case Study: Dennis Costas

21

After waiting for almost an hour on a hard plastic chair in Belmarsh's 'legal visits', I finally made it to the interview room, with only forty minutes left before bang up. It wasn't enough time – I knew I'd have to return another day.

In July 2011, my subject, Dennis Costas, a retail manager, had been charged with the murder of his girlfriend, Sophia, and remanded in custody. He'd told police and his solicitors that he couldn't remember what had happened on the night of the murder. It was now November and, as often happens with criminal cases involving amnesia, Costas's memory had been contaminated by what he'd learned from reading witness statements.

In my truncated interview, I focused on the 'here and now'. In other words, his current 'mental state', and his account of the offence, leaving his biography for the next time we met.

The day before the murder, Costas had been drinking heavily all afternoon after having phoned in sick, using his sciatica as an excuse. From where had he made the call? Had it been from the two-bedroom house he'd shared with his wife of ten years, or from his girlfriend Sophia's flat?

'I can't remember,' he told me. 'My recollection is very distorted.' He said he'd taken a nap, but couldn't remember what time he awoke. 'After that, I really don't know what happened. All I can remember is putting out the fire. My vision was blurred. I heard a voice and I came out of the flat door. I went back in again and then out to the lobby. There was a fire in the living room, and I put water on it.'

'What happened next?' I asked.

'I don't know how I got home. My recollection is terrible. It was only when I was told by the police that I heard what happened ... I was horrified ... I remember a fire in the living room, and I heard a voice calling for help ... I think I must have tried to dial 999, but maybe I didn't dial correctly, or maybe I got an engaged tone.'

This was obviously an attempt to deal with the fact that no 999 calls had been made, according to the emergency call logs in the prosecution evidence. Costas would have seen this by now, following 'discovery', which is when the prosecution share their evidence with the defence.

'There was water all over the floor ... I couldn't see where Sophia was, so I went downstairs and out of the building ... I'm not sure how I got home, I think I caught a bus ... My sister-in-law was there [at home], watching TV ... I went into the bedroom and fell asleep. The next thing I knew, the police were at the door and I was arrested.'

And that was the best he could do to recall the events of Tuesday afternoon and Wednesday morning, 22 June 2011.

Costas's fragmentary account was not the first claim of amnesia I have encountered from a murder defendant. Research studies over seventy years have found a consistent figure of around thirty per cent of murderers, other violent offenders and prisoners reporting memory loss for the offence. Given those figures, Costas was no exception.

But what was it that he couldn't remember doing?

On Wednesday, 22 June, at 03.50 hours, police were called to a four-storey low-rise apartment block in Upton Park by a resident saying that someone was banging on their door, trying to force entry. When officers arrived, concerned residents were standing in the car park. Running up to the top floor, the police were met by someone walking towards them. The figure, whose gender couldn't be determined, looked like a monster from a horror movie, flesh melting from horrendous burns to the face and upper body. In a statement, PC Harvey Stewart said that he had never seen anything like it before. 'For a split second, a feeling of unreality overcame me.'

The officers tried to give first aid, but weren't sure what to do. The female gave her name as Sophia. She said she had come home at around 3 a.m. and her former boyfriend, Dennis Costas, was waiting inside, as he still had his own key. She said he had confronted her and, following an argument, doused her in petrol from a can and set her on fire.

By now she was struggling to breathe from smoke inhalation, and the arriving ambulance crew had to cut a new airway through her trachea. In a critical condition, she was transferred to a specialist burns unit.

Inside the flat, the curtains and part of the furniture and carpet were carbonised black, but as the walls were solid concrete, the fire had burned itself out. A plastic petrol can, still containing around three litres of petrol, was found in the kitchen area, which had been untouched by the flames.

Police quickly traced Costas and he was arrested later that morning at the home he shared with his wife, Lina. He was asleep and clearly still drunk. He was so intoxicated, in fact, that he was unfit for interview and had to be left in his cell to sober up.

Closed-circuit television camera images were secured from the area around the crime scene, including a nearby petrol station. The footage showed a man who matched Costas's description walking in a purposeful way, albeit unsteadily. At the petrol station, he selected a five-litre plastic petrol canister, and appeared to have trouble filling it from the pump. After paying with cash, he disappeared in the direction of Sophia's flat. The CCTV time code suggested that he must have been waiting in the flat with the petrol, ready for Sophia's return.

Later, a message came through to the detectives in the custody suite waiting to interview Costas: Sophia had not made it through the night. Cause of death was a cardiac arrest, brought about by respiratory failure from burns to the airways and smoke inhalation.

Having sobered up enough for interview, Costas was brought to the custody sergeant's desk and formally charged with Sophia's murder. At interview, the officers confronted him with the CCTV evidence. After a short break to allow him to consult his solicitor, Costas agreed that it must have been him on the footage, but said he couldn't remember being there. He thought he might have bought the petrol to harm himself, but insisted that he couldn't possibly have set fire to Sophia. 'It may have been an accident as she tried to stop me from harming myself.'

So one of the questions that I had to answer was: was this memory loss genuine?

And if it was genuine, what could have caused it?

As with any murder case, I needed to know the backstory, the relationship between murderer and victim, and the mental state before, during and after the offence, so as to explore any psychiatric issues. But while looking for any abnormality of mind, I also had to consider possible motive, in case there was a more mundane explanation for the killing. All of this information had to be gleaned from evidence such as witness statements, phone cell-site analysis and CCTV, as the killer couldn't remember what had happened.

Costas could just have been lying, of course. Murderers may mistakenly believe that saying they can't remember provides some excuse for the killing, but they soon find out it doesn't. Alternatively, they may think that loss of memory will mean they lack the competency to stand trial. Again, amnesia will not help the murderer avoid trial, as established in English law by the 1959 case of Guenther Podola, who shot a policeman but said he couldn't remember doing it. Although expert psychiatrists disagreed over whether he was genuine, his amnesia claim was not accepted at the trial. Later, he did indeed admit his crime, before being hanged at HMP Wandsworth and buried in the prison graveyard.

Rudolf Hess also tried this at the Nuremberg trials. His claim of amnesia for his activities under the Third Reich was accepted as genuine. But when he realised this meant that he couldn't reasonably defend himself against the allegations, he quickly admitted he had faked his memory loss, and engaged with the trial process.

There is no simple psychiatric test for lying or deceptive claims of memory loss. This is ultimately an issue for the court and not the experts. We don't use lie detector tests in the UK, as they are notoriously unreliable. Psychopaths, with their lack of emotional reaction, may be able to fake a pass, for example. There have been tragic outcomes for participants in tabloid talk shows (such as *The Jeremy Kyle Show* and *Jerry Springer*), who can be falsely accused – on the basis of an unreliable lie detector test – of lying about infidelity, when in fact they're telling the truth. Lawyers rely on cross-examination to expose inconsistent versions of events by murderers, as lies are harder to remember than the truth. They may also persuade a jury to rely on 'demeanour' – that is, does the killer seem shifty in the witness box? This is, in fact, a rather unreliable method, but it is commonly used.

There are some tests, used by specialist neuropsychologists, which may help detect feigned amnesia. These can be trick questions embedded in questionnaires, or they can be easy memory tasks, like recalling simple line drawings of common objects over a very short time, something that would be easy to pass for those with genuine brain damage or advanced dementia. The malingerer may deliberately fail this test by performing worse than someone with brain damage, in a misguided attempt to persuade the psychologist they have a poor memory. Maybe murderers just have a problem accepting responsibility for things they've done 'out of character', during extreme anger or in the 'red mist' of overwhelming rage.

While I was waiting to be allocated an interview room, I observed Costas in the holding cell with other prisoners who were also waiting to see a nurse or doctor. He didn't give much away. Not a habitual criminal, he was keeping his head down. I would have to keep an open mind. In the interview room he seemed subdued. Was this a state of shock, or was he just keeping his guard up? There was no evidence of distraction by hallucinations, and none of the unconcerned or incongruent humour of the psychopath.

One of the major causes of memory loss I had to consider was what we call dissociative, or stress-related amnesia. During highly charged and emotional events (such as when immolating an intimate partner) the events are so traumatic that the brain effectively shuts them out. The memories, loaded into brain circuits at a time of stress, might then be difficult to recall later on, when in a normal and calm mental state again. We call this state-dependent memory. Or it might be an 'unconscious' way of repressing painful events. To quote the philosopher Nietzsche: '"I have done that," says my memory. "I cannot have done that," says my pride and remains unshakeable. Finally, memory yields.' The memory loss may be patchy, with improvement over time, whereas liars will typically report sudden onset and complete memory loss of the offence, with no 'islands' of memory.

Dissociative amnesia is a 'diagnosis of exclusion', namely it may be the only option left once all other causes have been excluded.[51]

So first I had to consider all the other possible causes. In Costas's case, it was most important that I considered whether a brain dysfunction had interfered with the recording, storage or recall of the crime. We call this 'organic' amnesia, which means it's caused by a physical illness affecting the brain. Organic brain disease is fairly uncommon in murder cases (only a handful per year in most studies), but it has to be considered. To exclude a physical cause, I explored whether there was a history or clinical signs of a brain tumour, head injury, dementia or some other physical illness affecting the brain or behaviour.

I'll give you an example from my time at the Mayday Hospital during that first medical 'house officer' post. We had admitted a sixty-two-year-old civil servant. Apparently, he was previously a placid and stable man, with two children and three grandchildren. He arrived at hospital, having become very short of breath over a few days. After X-rays and other tests, we had diagnosed advanced and invasive lung cancer, which had spread to the brain. His family had been by his bedside when we explained there was no more that radio- or chemotherapy could do. A few days later, as I was doing my rounds of the ward in the late evening, I approached his bed to check his prescription chart, which was on a clipboard dangling from the foot of the bed. I must have nudged the bed into his table and knocked over a cup of water.

In the blink of an eye, he leapt out of the bed, lunged aggressively at me, then chased me down the ward. As I passed the last bed, I realised I had nowhere left to run. Luckily there was a large oxygen cylinder on wheels and, by keeping the cylinder between him and me, I managed to hold him off long enough for the trusty porters to arrive.

It turned out that his brain tumour had spread to the frontal lobe of his brain, and the rapidly growing tumour was pressing on the part of the brain which normally regulates behaviour. So his aggression and disinhibition had a 'physical' cause. Had he caught up with me and throttled me to death, his subsequent amnesia for the hypothetical murder would have been genuine, and he could have legitimately claimed diminished responsibility. In my exhausted state towards the end of another thirty-hour shift, this was all I needed. But I was learning valuable lessons for later.

As Professor Rob Anankast told us when we started at the Maudsley: 'In your multidisciplinary teams there will be social workers, nurses and all kinds of therapist in spades. Don't forget your medicine. Your medical knowledge is one skillset you bring to the table.' Multidisciplinary work with a range of other professionals/therapists is essential to the rehabilitation of forensic patients – I have worked with some excellent colleagues. But I have seen one or two forensic psychiatry colleagues who, having lost sight of their role as the only doctor on the team, fail to show the leadership needed to take the tough decisions around physical health, risks to the public and compulsory treatment.

But Costas had no pressing family and social issues – not yet, at least. He had no children to worry about, just a shocked and bewildered wife at home.

Costas showed no symptoms of lung cancer, or any other cancer known to spread to the brain. So what about one of the more obscure physical causes, like an infection or other brain disease?

I have seen a handful of instances in which 'physical' brain disease caused aggressive behaviour leading to murder. One such case was Antonio Rossi. Rossi, a prison service manager, had begun hearing voices and seeing strange apparitions, which, it seems, he thought had been sent by his wife. Believing she was going to kill him, he stabbed her, leaving sixty-eight wounds, according to the post-mortem. He rolled her body up in a carpet and left their flat.

Having severely injured his hand in the process, he walked into the emergency department. However, he had no recollection of what he had done and seemed genuinely perplexed as to what had happened. At first, he claimed to have cut himself on a can of tomatoes, and then he said he'd broken a bottle. These were examples of confabulation, which is an attempt by the brain to fill gaps in the memory that we only see in cases of true brain-damage-related memory loss.

The injuries had, in fact, been sustained as his hand slipped down the blade of the murder weapon whenever the blade encountered bony resistance during the repeated vigorous stabbing. It's an injury commonly suffered by murderers who use the nearest knife to hand, rather than a dagger or combat knife with a crosspiece designed for the purpose. Victims often sustain defence injuries to the hands in a similar way as they try to grab the blade during the struggle.

The severed tendons in Rossi's hand were surgically repaired, and he was transferred to a secure psychiatric hospital. Following transfer, his hallucinations miraculously resolved during the observation period before we started medication.

But Rossi was also losing coordination: he was unable to stand up in the shower, for example. Consulting with neurologists, and after electronic tests of his muscle fibres, we were able to make a diagnosis. The brain degeneration we discovered explained both the transient psychotic episode during which he had killed his wife and his subsequent amnesia regarding the murder. Within a few months of arriving at our secure unit, he was confined to a wheelchair. His condition deteriorated rapidly and he was soon bed-bound. He finally died around two years later.

It emerged that Rossi had developed a rare degenerative brain disease that combines early onset dementia and motor neurone disease. But unlike in Stephen Hawking's case, this type of motor neurone disease is rapidly fatal. The disease starts with a fleeting episode of psychosis. This 'time-limited' psychosis is accompanied by other symptoms of brain impairment, such as disinhibition and aggressiveness. A few months later, muscle twitching appears, along with a progressive loss of the ability to move. The prognosis is poor, and the duration from the onset to death is two to five years.

Rossi is one of only a handful of organic or 'neuropsychiatric' murder cases I have seen. A tragic case, of course, but like stamp collectors, doctors and psychiatrists seek out those that are as rare as Penny Blacks. My detailed report on this 'most complex and unusual case' won me further referrals from both prosecution and defence, as the Old Bailey found this rarity equally fascinating, and I saved them the bother of a time-consuming jury trial.

I reviewed Costas's medical records to rule out any rare conditions in this case. He had a history of backache, chest infection and heavy drinking, but nothing suggesting brain disease. At interview, he had shown no problems with 'screening' tests of brain function, or with normal biographical memory and normal short-term memory, although he still couldn't remember what had happened that night. On further tests of the frontal part of the brain, responsible for regulating behaviour, he was also intact.

Had I found anything suspicious, I would have recommended an MRI brain scan and further tests. But this wasn't necessary, and even if it had been, it would probably not have been funded by legal aid. In a disputed insurance claim with a minor head injury, he would have had the full battery of detailed testing, but this was just a life-and-death case with a potential life sentence – far less important than an insurance company's money.

During our second interview, Costas told me his version of the backstory. He had worked as a retail assistant but progressed to sales adviser and then a sales manager. He had an active social life and liked a drink. He got married in 1999, but his wife lost a child after an abruption of the placenta. They had argued about pursuing the alternative of adoption.

His drinking became heavier. He went from the occasional Guinness to strong lager every weekend, settling on spirits, mainly vodka. He was more of a binge drinker than a regular, dependent drinker, and on a heavy night could get through one-and-a-half bottles of Stolichnaya. He suffered terrible hangovers, but would cope at work by drinking pints of water.

The arguments with his wife continued. However, around 2003 he met the victim, Sophia, at work. Before long, they started an affair. He settled into a dual relationship, spending some nights with Sophia and other nights back with his wife, Lina. Sophia knew he was married, but Lina was unaware of the affair. He told Sophia that he was going to leave Lina, but never did. When Sophia started pushing him to, he said that he wouldn't leave, 'not under her pressure, nor under pressure from anybody else'. His double life continued.

I asked myself, could Costas's pattern of drinking provide an explanation, both for the murder and the subsequent amnesia? After all, it won't surprise you to learn that murder cases are awash with alcohol and other illicit drugs. Stats from 2018 showed that thirty-two per cent of murder suspects and thirty-six per cent of murder victims had been drinking alcohol and/or using drugs at the time of the homicide. When drunk, some people are friendly or amorous, while others become irritable and angry. Alcohol is one factor that can tip the balance from a serious assault to a murder. However, alcohol consumption is a part of everyday life, most drinkers don't kill, and in my experience, alcohol intoxication is never the sole cause of a murder.

Recent government statistics found that around sixty per cent of the UK population consume alcohol and, of that sixty per cent, around a quarter, or eight million drinkers, binge on alcohol on their heaviest drinking day in the week. In short, we're a drinking culture – and I'm no different. But while most of us can relate to a hazy memory after a few too many drinks, alcohol dependency is another matter. While drinking may be integral to a social situation, or happen as a result of peer pressure, it is also used for its anti-anxiety and (short-term) stress-relief effects, or for relaxation at the weekend. It's when this weekend habit expands, starting on a Thursday night and ending on the following Tuesday, that stress-relief drinking can escalate. Habitual consumption becomes daily, with a gradual increase in units leading to dependency – the state where every day requires an 'eye opener' or 'hair of the dog' to relieve not just psychological cravings, but full-blown physical withdrawal.

But Costas had more of a binge pattern than daily dependent drinking, and his alcohol binges were a notch up, even by student standards. I had to consider the potential long-term effects of his heavy drinking and how these might have led to murderous behaviour.

Severe alcohol dependency or very heavy binge-drinking can lead to various acute syndromes or long-term brain damage, which amount to 'organic' or physical causes of disturbed brain and behaviour. Delirium tremens (the DTs) is often misunderstood. DTs can happen when withdrawing from a very high level of alcohol intoxication, leading to anxiety, tremors and sweating, followed by delirium, with clouding of consciousness and hallucinations. The hallucinations can be visual, sometimes small animals or insects, which we call Lilliputian hallucinations – the only occasion in forensic psychiatry when reports of 'little green men' might actually be genuine.

I assessed a man suffering from the DTs who lashed out with a Stanley knife at what he thought were a crowd of people chasing him. He seriously injured a pedestrian who happened to be passing, but luckily the wound wasn't fatal. Delirium tremens usually occurs two to four days after stopping alcohol, and is a medical emergency that may result in hospital admission. It can be lethal if left untreated.

But Costas's murder of Sophia had happened *during* an alcohol binge, not two to four days *after* a binge. Plus, he hadn't reported little green men and wasn't delirious in the police cells.

There is also a severe form of brain damage related to end-stage alcoholism and vitamin B deficiency (in those who have neglected food intake in favour of booze). This starts as a medical emergency with symptoms including confusion, incoordination and abnormal eye movements. If intravenous vitamins are not given urgently, it can lead to a permanent state of memory loss, with an inability to learn new information *going forwards*.

This is the type of amnesia accurately depicted in the film *Memento,* in which the protagonist has to use tattoos and Polaroid photos to collect and record new information as he hunts his wife's killer. In real life, I know of a senior doctor with severe alcoholism who ended up hospitalised with this syndrome. Every morning he would ask nursing staff where his wife was, and every day he would burst into tears on being told that she had divorced him years ago. A sort of *Groundhog Day*, where every day starts off fresh, frozen at the same point in time just before the brain damage happened.

Once again, however, this didn't fit the bill with Costas. There had been no episode of confusion with abnormal eye movements, and he had normal memory testing with no 'going forwards' inability to remember new facts.

Normal intoxication may have a distorting effect on memory, but alcohol memory blackouts, on the other hand, are pretty common, and not just among partying students. These tend to happen following heavy binges that boast a very high peak-alcohol level. The blackouts can be partial, with islands of preserved memory within the memory gap that shrink over time. Or they can be 'en-bloc' blackouts with a very definite onset and recovery. The subject might wake up sensing a lost night or even a 'lost weekend', as depicted in the 1945 Billy Wilder film of the same name.

I described this phenomenon to a judge from the witness box in a murder case involving a thirty-eight-year-old man, Pierre Carter. Carter had throttled to death an older man called Raymond Sanders at Carter's bungalow in Basingstoke, Hampshire. Sanders had taken sexual advantage of Carter, repeatedly, after heavy joint drinking sessions, and was suspected of spiking Carter's drink. Carter later claimed amnesia due to an alcohol memory blackout.

The judge asked, 'Doctor, tell me if I have understood this correctly. Suppose we imagine a river estuary awash with alcohol, are you saying that as the tide of alcohol recedes, we are left with islands of memory in the mud?'

'Exactly, your honour.'

Verdict: amnesia accepted; manslaughter on grounds of provocation. Four years' imprisonment.

Alcohol memory blackouts looked like a plausible explanation for Costas's amnesia. His usual binge of a bottle and a half of vodka was roughly equivalent to fifteen pints of beer, around fifty units. This was supported by the back-calculation of his blood alcohol level based on measurements taken at the police station after his arrest. After all, he had experienced blackouts before. For example, a work friend once told him Costas had phoned him while drunk the night before, but Costas had no memory of making the call. Don't drink and dial (especially if you've been dumped – see chapter fifteen).

I was allocated to the alcohol rehab unit at the Maudsley during my psychiatric training in 1995, and there I was confronted with the terrible consequences of long-term drinking careers. Alcohol dependency often comes to light 'in the fifth decade' (so too late), when it has been escalating for years, is extremely hard to reverse, and has already done so much damage. In those days we offered a six-week detoxification and rehab admission – long since abandoned by the NHS as too expensive. Patients on the waiting list would be told to keep drinking until the day of admission, so as to avoid life-threatening withdrawal seizures. I remember one patient who had clearly followed this advice assiduously, literally falling out of his taxi on the front steps of the Maudsley, with vomit all over his beard. He had to be helped on to the ward by nurses and porters to begin the drying out, safely under medical and nursing supervision. We would give the patients a detox, which was a five-to-seven-day reducing course of 'benzos', which are minor tranquillisers like Valium or Librium. This was to limit the risk of seizures and help manage the often severe withdrawal such as sweating, shaking and vomiting.

Once sober, the patients were put into individual and group therapy twice a week. We'd sort out their mental and physical health problems, replacing vitamins, testing liver function, et cetera. This was my first exposure to group therapy as a co-therapist with one of the experienced nurses, and I quickly realised that it was other members of the group who were most effective in challenging alcoholics about their denial. We had a man who'd run his business into the ground and was close to losing his house. He kept talking about how the solution to his problems was merely to switch the whisky in his glass for apple juice, while doing his neglected paperwork. A young woman who had been street-drinking from three-litre bottles of strong white cider – 8.4 per cent White Lightning – challenged him by saying, 'You're full of shit; you just haven't sunk low enough yet.' She went on, putting it better than I could have: 'You can't start coming back to the surface until your nose has hit the bottom, you prick . . . Wait till you're in a drinking school on Camberwell Green, then you'll understand.' (A drinking school being a collective of severely dependent alcoholics who pool their benefit money to make sure everyone has something to drink.) Patients on the alcohol ward had mostly lived working lives before the alcohol had caught up with them, and most had stories to tell. We had all sorts, including doctors, senior police officers and a trade union stalwart. He reminded me of my grandfather; he had the same frame and huge boxer's hands. His family were old East End, mostly Fleet Street print union members or Smithfield market porters. His drinking seemed to be, in part, mourning for the lost lifestyle, but he admitted that 'the print' had a drinking culture much like the Royal Navy. Sometimes, after a shift, he would end up with a bottle of rum on top of the printing presses as they ran off the early editions. For some, sobriety was just too miserable, and I remember one patient, called Theodore, who had left the ward to go on a final bender. He ended up at King's College Hospital A & E with a catastrophic and fatal haemorrhage from ruptured swollen vessels around the stomach.

Alcohol dependence is a syndrome that was first recognised and defined as a medical condition with a physiological basis by Maudsley Hospital professor, Griffith Edwards. Dependence involves features such as repeated drinking to relieve withdrawal symptoms, narrowing down to one type of booze, and increased tolerance so you need to drink more to have the same effect. Costas hadn't become dependent, but he was evidently an unhappy man, and he seemed to have needed regular alcoholic obliteration for reasons that were unclear.

But are they ever clear? Alcohol has a way of taking control of people's lives and decision-making faculties. When you work with end-stage alcoholics, it forces you to re-evaluate your own alcohol consumption. Working on the alcohol unit in 1995, I was troubled by the lives of my patients, and lost my taste for cold beers and red wine. My strategy that summer was to appoint myself as designated driver on nights out. This period of reflective sobriety was clearly a reaction to my six-month exposure to ward AL3.

22

So I'd found a possible cause for Costas's memory loss, but I still didn't have an explanation for the killing. I had been sent the usual thick bundle of statements and exhibits, and planned to work through them on a train journey to Derby, where I was due for a court hearing. Deciding to cycle and leave my bike at the station, I put a shirt, jacket, tie and lightweight shoes in my bag, along with the two heavy stacks of papers.

As I freewheeled down Regent's Park Road towards Euston, I thought about the case. It must, surely, have been a deliberate and calculated act by Costas to have thrown and ignited the volatile petrol? And how had he, in his drunken state, managed to escape the explosion? I wondered what it must have been like for poor Sophia. Horrific images of the pitiless lashing flames played on a loop in my head. I felt for the police officers who had found her, zombie-like, as she staggered towards them. Sophia must have been an awful sight – no wonder the officers had had no idea how to help her.

It's the smoke inhalation that kills in eighty per cent of fire-related deaths. Inhalation of toxic gases, especially carbon monoxide and hydrogen cyanide, as well as thermal burns to the airways, destroy the ability to breathe even on a mechanical ventilator in intensive care. I knew this all too well from a night shift I spent in A & E as a medical student on the night of the Kings Cross fire in 1987, when thirty-one people lost their lives. I have often wondered what those last moments must have been like for any victim of murder, but death by immolation is unimaginable in terms of suffering.

Turning back to Costas, how had the situation with the two women in his life ended up with his ultimately lethal actions towards Sophia?

His manager described a good record at work with no disciplinary problems. His police national computer record confirmed no prior contact or offending.

But Sophia's sister described Costas as controlling, jealous and a bit of a bully. The statements made it clear that Sophia hadn't told her family about Costas's double life, but she'd confided in friends like Celeste.

Celeste said they had seemed very much in love when the relationship started, but had argued over Sophia having a pet cat that Costas thought was dirty and hated. Costas was possessive too, and they were always 'in each other's faces', mostly verbally. The relationship deteriorated.

Celeste said that she and Sophia had once gone out for a drink, only for Costas to repeatedly call, telling Sophia to come home. Celeste was also with Sophia a few days before the murder when, in a drunken call, Costas told Sophia he had finally made a decision to get a divorce and make things right with her.

But it was too late. Sophia had waited long enough, and was trying to break off the relationship. She told Celeste she wanted to get the flat keys back from him, and had even considered going to the police, but hadn't wanted to get him into trouble.

I carried on through the witness statements.

Costas's wife, Lina, described a good marriage initially, but said they had argued frequently. Her husband would disappear for days on end, either without any explanation or saying that he was working back-to-back shifts. He had left the family home about two days before his arrest, but called Lina, sounding drunk, to say that he didn't love her any more and was fed up with being married.

I realised the train was pulling into Derby station, so I shoved the bundle of papers into my rucksack and hurried off.

I don't recall the details of Derby Crown Court that day; I think it was a routine sentencing hearing. I do, however, remember a prolonged wait on another hard, plastic chair, where I sat to read more papers. I asked reception to tannoy the barrister to meet me outside court. I had to shift focus, forget Costas for an hour or so, and get my head into the case I was here for, to mentally prepare to give evidence. Hectic, yes, but, in truth, that's probably the way I like it. For me, there is one thing worse than deadline pressure, and that is boredom.

Maintaining interest has always been essential, as some days I'd think about giving it all up and trying something different. But in medicine, as you pursue a specialist path, doorways to other careers rapidly close, and you have to make the best of your decisions. Although I'm not in academic medicine, I kept my interest up by teaching, doing policy work (on public protection, for example), and writing or collaborating on the occasional paper on such topics as Holloway prisoners, terrorist detainees or the mind of the fraudster. But the interplay between brain, mind, biography and behaviour is too interesting to let you get jaded for long. What could better pique one's curiosity than tearing open a fresh murder case bundle? The intellectual challenge of psychiatric and legal puzzle-solving keeps you going, even when the CPS call you up a week before your summer holiday.

I was on a tight schedule with Costas's report, having accepted instructions on a ridiculously short deadline for a murder case. But I didn't mind on this occasion. It was an interesting case and I was happy to get back into the papers on the train journey back to London.

Reading on, I found nothing else to suggest organic brain disease or obvious mental disorder. Usually an explanation for the killing emerges at some point as you work up a case.

Immersed in the papers, making sure there was no other passenger in eyesight, I flicked through it all, skipping over the repetitive police statements proving preservation of the crime scene and the custody chain of evidence.

There was the police custody record, CPS unused material and the lengthy transcript of the tape-recorded interview, full of 'no comment' answers. As the train rolled through the outskirts of north London, I was getting ready to pack up the papers again.

Then I reached the statement of Oscar Novak.

Sophie had begun seeing Oscar without telling any of her friends or family, perhaps because she was ashamed of starting with someone new before she had resolved the situation with Costas. Oscar's number was on Sophia's phone record, as he had called her several times in the week before the killing, and so police had taken a statement from him.

The police say that every murder investigation ruins a relationship or two. Why? A cop once explained to me that anyone connected to the victim, or found to have been near the scene, will have to give a detailed and truthful statement (under penalty of perjury) to account for their whereabouts at the time of the killing. And, of course, some people turn out not to have been where they told their partner they were.

In Costas's criminal case, the overworked and underfunded solicitors must have missed Oscar's statement, as they hadn't mentioned it in my brief instructions. But here was an account which not only revealed the actual movements of the victim on the night in question, but also provided evidence of what was on Sophia's mind – and all from a man who had started a new relationship with her just before she died.

Oscar said that in the short time he'd known her, Sophia rarely spoke about Costas, but confirmed that she'd been trying to break off the relationship, and had told him Costas still had a key to her flat. He said she had considered involving the police to get it back, but didn't want Costas to get in trouble or lose his job. Oscar and Sophia had been on a date the day before she died, and she'd been receiving repeated texts and phone calls from Costas. They'd taken a room at a Premier Inn because she was worried Costas might cause another argument, and she told Oscar that last time she'd seen Costas, he had tried to look at the call history on her phone.

So, there it was. I had a 'normal' motive. It looked like, after dithering for years, Costas had finally said he would leave his wife, but it was too late. Sophia had found someone else. When she returned to her flat at 3 a.m., having been with her new boyfriend, she found Costas waiting for her. Perhaps he'd been wondering where she'd been so late at night. So in a drunken state, he confronted her, and they argued. Buying the petrol suggested premeditation – predatory violence, in other words. But sometimes you get a combination of predatory and affective violence. He may have been thinking about scaring her, burning her, threatening to burn himself, or both of them together, but the final argument, fuelled by alcohol, had taken him over that tipping point to the fatal conflagration. As mentioned previously, murderers sometimes know, or are reckless to the possibility, that alcohol or cocaine will give them the Dutch courage they need.

Still, you don't torch someone to death just for leaving you. To provoke such a response, in my view, you need to throw jealousy into the volatile mix.

Costas's alcohol consumption was so heavy that his initial amnesia early after the offence may well have been genuine. He said that his memory had started to recover, and at that first interview with the police, as well as later with me, he had always reported patchy islands of memory, which suggested alcohol memory blackout was more likely to be true. Ultimately, I thought it likely that, even if the patchy amnesia was genuine to start with, he had begun to remember more about the murder than he was letting on, although he denied being aware of Oscar. I had my doubts. But he preferred to maintain, after his arrest, that he was unaware of a rival, so he could imply to the court that the murder had been spontaneous rather than pre-planned.

This had been a full-blown psychiatric fishing expedition. The solicitors had asked me to comment on his amnesia, the possibility of brain damage, post-traumatic stress disorder, perhaps a brief psychotic episode, insanity, diminished responsibility and fitness for trial. Maybe, as he had tentatively suggested to the police, he'd planned to burn himself instead of, or at the same time as, Sophia. Or maybe the petrol was a way of distancing himself from the murderous act. He didn't have to strike or stab her, just toss the fuel and light a match. In the end, this looked like a classic intimate partner homicide, another man experiencing the narcissistic injury of losing a love object. The rage towards the departing lover had been inflamed by the jealousy of her starting to see someone else.

I wrote up my report, setting out all the alternative explanations for the amnesia. I said I thought that the alcohol memory blackout with patchy recall was probably genuine, at least early on after the murder, but I could not determine whether he was lying about his continued inability to recall. I had ruled out brain damage and psychosis, so there was no insanity or other defence. Voluntary alcohol consumption, by law and as a matter of public policy, is not an excuse for murder, even if you can't remember what you did. Whether Costas remembered or not, he chose not to challenge the evidence and pleaded guilty to murder, thus avoiding a trial.

Verdict: murder. Life imprisonment; twenty-one-year minimum term.

Severe alcohol problems don't explain Costas's offence, but they certainly contributed to it. Had he sought treatment for his drinking before, he might not have been so intoxicated that night. But even had he asked for help, treatment for drugs and alcohol addiction has become much harder to obtain on the NHS.

Detox and rehab services must surely be a worthwhile investment, as the health and social costs of untreated addictions are huge – especially when you take into account the violence and murders associated with the illicit drugs trade. In 2018, 332 homicides – forty-four per cent of all homicides in England and Wales – were drug-related.

But there are no longer any NHS-run detox and rehab programmes left in the country. The 2012 Lansley reforms, now widely accepted to have been a massive public policy failure, made sure of that. Funding for addictions treatment was hived off and the responsibility pushed on to cash-strapped local authorities, which have priorities other than drunks and drug addicts.

The funding for addictions services, which are now all contracted out to private or charity providers, spirals downwards every year. So if a politician says that the solution to the rise in knife crime is to improve drugs programmes, ask them why they shut them down in the first place. Or not so much 'shut them down' – just cut off their central NHS funding and cynically left them to wither on the vine.

Nevertheless, there are beacons of excellence left. One voluntary sector non-profit rehab facility at East Knoyle, just outside the Dorset border, is Clouds House; a world-class residential drug and alcohol rehab facility in an Arts and Crafts period country house. The programme is still available if you can afford it – or if you can persuade your local NHS Clinical Commissioning Group to pay £8,900 for the shorter twenty-eight-day programme.

This is way cheaper than a fully private option available for the well-heeled like Elton John, who gives a striking account of the benefit of drugs detox, rehab and enduring recovery in his autobiography, *Me*.

I visited Clouds in 1995 on a fact-finding trip to help with an upgrade of the programme at the Maudsley alcohol unit (before the decision was taken some years later to close it). There is a bin at the end of the drive to throw away your last cans and bottles. Once inside, you get a full detox and are dry within a week or so. Then there's a searching group- and individual-based analysis of the underlying issues that have led to the drugs or booze, and a plan is made to avoid relapse triggers.

Alcohol detox and rehab is not the only attraction of East Knoyle village. On some weekends, after a week dealing with cases like Costas and Sophia, I like to head west to Dorset to visit family, and for a forty-eight-hour respite from London, often with my daughter and sons in tow.

On my usual route I turn off the A303 and cut through Hindon, past an old coaching inn called The Lamb. As I turn on to the A350 to Shaftesbury, I always nod to the white road sign to 'Clouds House'. Below it, to my recurring amusement, is a brown signpost to an alternative attraction, or maybe a last port of call on the way to rehab at Clouds: The Fox and Hounds.

I haven't made it to The Fox and Hounds, and plan to avoid ever needing a Clouds House rehab. But I sometimes slope off to one of the Dorset locals, like The King John at Tollard Royal, for a pint of Sixpenny Gold.

While having a pint, I try not to think about Costas or my AL3 patients, or the scientific details of how the alcohol affects the brain, such as the dopamine release or the modulation of inhibitory neurotransmitters. Neither do I reflect on the ancient cultural serendipity that must have led early humans to discover the properties of fermented fruit juice. Instead I just appreciate the calming effects and the social bonhomie that goes with a drink.

I admit that, by the end of a weekend in Dorset, I'll be starting to miss the buzz of the city. But one thing I've always liked about that area, and other rural parts of England, is the relative scarcity of serious violent crime, and the almost complete absence of murder cases.

Well, in theory, anyway . . .

Financially Motivated Murder

Case Study: Who Killed the Colonel?

23

At 04.57 on 8 January 2004, the Hertfordshire ambulance control room took a 999 call. It came from Braughing, a small village which lies between the River Quin and the River Rib, about three miles from the village of Furneux Pelham. The male caller requested that an ambulance be sent to Hollyhock Cottage, but he didn't say why or what had happened. The anonymous caller misspelt the name of the village as 'Furneaux Pelham' with the same extra 'a' that appears in an old village sign, which is also misspelt. But he pronounced it 'Furnix', just as a local would – the Anglo-Saxon version is preferred to the Frenchified pronunciation. The caller also said to the ambulance controller, 'That's near Buntingford.' He pronounced the last syllable of Buntingford as 'fud' in a heavy rural accent. (And when the police later had the recording analysed, the caller was thought to be a local, possibly as old as sixty, according to the linguistics expert.)

Despatched to Furneux Pelham, the ambulance crew drove around the village looking for Hollyhock Cottage. But it was the middle of the night, there was no sign of any activity in the village, and they couldn't find a house called Hollyhock Cottage, so they returned to base.

The following morning, Josette Swanson, a housekeeper, attended Hollyhock Cottage to help her elderly and infirm client, Colonel Riley Workman, at the start of his day. She found him slumped across his front doorway, unresponsive.

Unsure what to do, Mrs Swanson called a neighbour, Edward Davidson, a barrister and churchwarden who lived nearby. Davidson made his way to Hollyhock Cottage and would later say that he was struck by the look of dread on the old man's face. Meanwhile, the paramedics arrived, checked his vital signs and determined that he was indeed dead. Given the Colonel's age, it was presumed he had died from natural causes – a heart attack or stroke – although the exact diagnosis was left for a subsequent post-mortem. Some hours later undertakers arrived, and while moving the body on to a gurney for transfer to the hearse, they noticed bloodstains around a very neat exit wound, probably less than an inch wide, on his back, which looked as though it must have come from a firearm.

Police were summoned. This death had suddenly become a murder investigation. But by now the housekeeper, the neighbour and the paramedics had trampled all over the place, and it was too late for perimeter security to ensure effective preservation and forensication of the scene. Post-mortem and ballistic analysis determined that the Colonel had been killed with an unusual form of ammunition, namely a 'buckshot' cartridge fired from a 12-gauge shotgun. A normal 12-gauge shotgun cartridge, used for shooting pheasants or pigeons, contains between 170 and 270 tiny pellets, weighing around two grams each and made of lead mixed with antimony for hardness.

A buckshot cartridge, on the other hand, contains around eight large pellets, almost a centimetre in diameter and weighing over fifty grams each. Famed for its stopping power, it's used primarily in the USA for police and 'home defence' tactical shotguns. A buckshot entry and exit wound would be narrow and concentrated, unlike a standard shotgun blast wound, hence why it was missed at first.

In the UK, buckshot cartridges are generally restricted for use by gamekeepers culling large 'ground game' like foxes. The nearest shop selling this type of ammunition was in East Barnet village, over fifty miles away from Furneux Pelham.

Whatever its origin, ballistics experts were able to determine that the cartridge had been discharged from about ten feet away. Incontrovertibly, this was deliberate murder. What's more, nothing was missing, not even the Colonel's valuable silver collection, so it had to be a cold-blooded execution: maybe a grudge killing of some kind.

Mrs Swanson had last seen the Colonel the night before at around 7.35 p.m. Police house-to-house enquiries – in what remained of the 'golden twenty-four hours' for evidence gathering – revealed that a number of witnesses had heard a bang at around 8.20 p.m. the night before. However, evening gunshots are commonplace in an environment as rural as Furneux Pelham, and thus no alarm was raised.

Aged eighty-three when he died, Colonel Workman was a Second World War veteran. Oxford-educated, he had joined the army straight after university, and during the war had served for the Oxfordshire and Buckinghamshire Light Infantry, which later became part of the Green Jackets Brigade. He spent much of his time engaged in the war against the Japanese in Burma. During his subsequent army career, he was stationed in Canada, Nigeria, Germany and Cyprus, and travelled widely in the United States. He was described by army contacts as a first-class officer.

Workman had retired from the army in the mid-1960s. After working in the antiques trade for a while, he settled in the village of Furneux Pelham. The ambulance crew's confusion had arisen because of different names for his house. Although his wife, Joanna, liked the name 'Hollyhock Cottage', the Colonel preferred 'Cock House', as he had a weather-vane depicting a cockerel on the roof.

After Joanna became disabled in later years, Workman was said to have been her carer, visiting her in hospital constantly during her last illness. She had eventually died in 2003 and was cremated, her ashes mingled with those of their pet dog, Tara.

Workman used to buy cigars and take a drink at his local, The Brewery Tap. However, after Joanna's death, he was seen less often in the pub and became something of a recluse, spending his time in the cottage re-reading *The Lord of the Rings* and the Harry Potter series. The year before his death, he had engaged Mrs Swanson as carer to help him cope around the house. It was her, of course, who found his body that morning.

This was a stone-cold whodunnit. The police had no leads.

A recording of the 999 call was posted on the Hertfordshire police website in a bid to identify the caller. Detectives took the handset from the village phone box in nearby Braughing, from where the call had been made, and eventually removed the entire phone box, leaving just a hole in the ground. Around 200 people contacted Hertfordshire police about the anonymous call, but there were no concrete leads.

Robert Nokes, the local vicar, asked why anybody would shoot Workman, 'an old man making the best of life'. Meanwhile, speculation grew. It seemed inconceivable that this cold-blooded, calculated murder could have been committed by someone in the local community. Was it a case of mistaken identity? Perhaps the killer was a resentful soldier from his former army days?

One line of enquiry was whether there had been a financial motive for the murder and, if so, how the police could identify the culprit. Workman was a relatively well-heeled resident of Furneux Pelham and potentially a target for acquisitive crime. He lived in a cottage whose value had increased substantially over the years. He had the generous index-linked final-salary pension of a senior army officer, along with a valuable antiques and silver collection acquired from his years in the trade, so a financially motivated murder had to be high up the list for the investigating detectives.

The questions multiplied. Was he the victim of a fraudster? Or had there been an attempt at blackmail, with threats of publicising either true or false information about the Colonel unless financial demands were met? Might it have been extortion of money or property, forcing him to change his will? Or had he become involved in a dispute with somebody from the antiques trade?

The case had all the hallmarks of TV drama, but murder stories from fiction and TV tend to overemphasise calculated premeditated killings for money. Financially motivated murder is surprisingly rare. Of 726 homicides in 2018, only forty-seven cases (six per cent) were committed in furtherance of theft or financial gain, whereas 373 offences (fifty-one per cent) resulted from a quarrel, a revenge attack or a loss of temper.

This overall figure is replicated in the United States, where financially motivated murders also accounted for only 851 (six per cent) of 14,123 murders in 2018. Of these, 548 were robberies gone wrong, 75 happened during a burglary, 23 during theft, 6 were over gambling disputes and 199 – or 1.4 per cent of the total number of murders – occurred in an argument over money or property. Of course, in a robbery homicide, the initial motive is acquisitive, not homicidal. The killing happens because the weapon used to intimidate the victim causes serious injury, or the victim resists, or the robber is just reckless and impulsive – it's still murder, of course. By the same token, burglary homicides usually start as burglaries, which then go wrong if, for example, the burglar is disturbed (unless it is a fetish-burglary-rape-homicide, of course – see chapter three).

So this means that, once the robbery, burglary and gambling homicides are accounted for, cold-blooded financial murder must make up only a fraction of that remaining 1.4 per cent of homicides.

Premeditated murder of an intimate partner for money is very rare indeed. As we've already seen, murders of intimate partners are much more likely to be carried out in the heat of the moment. The police don't have to look far to find the perpetrator when one half of a couple is killed. Those contemplating bumping off a spouse for the insurance money or inheritance, or in the midst of a dispute over divorce settlement must be at least dimly aware of this, but not always, it seems.

Consider the recent case of Emile Cilliers, an army fitness instructor who was convicted of two counts of attempted murder of his wife. Leading a double life, he had run up debts, used sex workers and was having an affair with a woman he had met online. After investing in his wife's life insurance, he tried to kill her by tampering with their home's gas supply. When that failed, he went to the airfield – where they were both keen recreational parachutists – and sabotaged her parachute. She suffered spinal injuries and broke her leg, collarbone and ribs as a consequence of the tangled chute, but she survived this second attempt on her life.

After two criminal trials, which included expert evidence from an experienced parachute instructor, Cilliers was convicted on both counts of attempted murder and sentenced to life imprisonment with a minimum term of eighteen years.

No psychiatric evaluation of Cilliers has been referred to in the press, although it has been suggested in press coverage that, given his likely motive and behaviours, Cilliers must have had psychopathic traits. You will have to judge whether that is reasonable conjecture.

Cilliers's case aside, it is clear from other case studies that psychopathic traits like conning, manipulative behaviour, glib and superficial charm and a lack of empathy can be found amongst those in apparently normal, law-abiding walks of life, such as in corporate environments. You may have encountered someone who fits this description. Robert Hare, an expert in the field, examined 'corporate psychopaths' in his book *Snakes in Suits*.[52] He argues that the destructive nature of the corporate psychopath may be overlooked because of their tendency for charming behaviour.

But the psychopathic fraudster can also turn out be a psychopathic murderer. One notable feature of financial fraudsters is their tendency towards narcissistic personality traits, and it is the combination of narcissistic traits and psychopathic traits that can provide the link from fraud and deception to murder.

The concept of narcissism – as described by psychiatrist and psychoanalyst Jessica Yakeley[53] – has developed from descriptions of a personality trait to do with vanity and self-love to a full-blown psychiatric diagnosis in the form of narcissistic personality disorder. Narcissistic traits are thought to exist on a sliding scale. At one end of the spectrum, a healthy or normative degree of narcissism can be adaptive: that is, it can protect the individual from feelings of low self-esteem.

But at the other extreme, the features of narcissistic personality disorder include grandiosity and self-importance: persistent fantasies of success or power, and beliefs about being special, along with a sense of entitlement. These traits can be accompanied by a tendency to exploit others, a lack of empathy, and envious or arrogant behaviour. It has also been suggested that there are two subtypes of narcissism, namely the arrogance and self-assuredness of the 'thick-skinned' narcissist versus the overly sensitive, insecure, defensive and shameful anxiety of the 'thin-skinned' narcissist. Sometimes the thick-skinned form is a psychological defence against the thin-skinned. For example, narcissists are notorious for their ability to dish out cutting derogatory jokes at others' expense, while being unable to take such ribbing themselves. It has been suggested that some prominent politicians on the global stage combine excessive self-regard and over-confidence with intolerance of criticism in this way.

A narcissistic personality disorder can lead to problems at work and in interpersonal relationships, as well as in financial affairs. Narcissists tend to require constant attention and excessive admiration, and they expect to be recognised as superior. They exaggerate their own achievements and are preoccupied with fantasies about success, power, and beauty. They can be exploitative or manipulative to get what they want, and they have an inability or unwillingness to recognise the needs and feelings of others above their own. They may insist on having the best car or the best office; they may demand the most comfortable bunk in the prison cell; or they may become angry if they're not the first patient to be seen in the secure psychiatric unit ward review.

People with narcissistic personality disorder also have trouble handling anything they perceive as criticism, and they may have difficulty regulating emotions and behaviour. It has been suggested that narcissists lose sight of their 'true self', replacing it via grandiosity with a 'false self', which has the function of shielding themselves from narcissistic injury through feelings of omnipotence.

This means that the narcissist may take what they think they deserve through fraud or deception, lacking compunction or guilt, and disregarding the impact of their behaviour on others. When thwarted or challenged, they might then react impulsively, killing while enraged or to cover their tracks.

Narcissism is intimately connected to the concept of the psychopath, as the narcissistic traits of grandiosity and lack of empathy are items on the psychopathy checklist, and it has been said that if you take a narcissist and add antisocial behaviour and sadism, then you end up with a psychopath. Narcissism is also a thread that runs through many areas of forensic psychiatry, as it helps us to understand the behaviour of fraudsters, con men, murderers of intimate partners, stalkers, querulants and spree shooters.

In extreme examples, the false self of the narcissist can be expressed through pathological lying ('Walter Mitty Syndrome'), and adopting a completely new identity as an imposter.

One further personality trait of relevance here, and one which overlaps with narcissism, is the concept of Machiavellianism, although it is a bit of a fringe notion and not an official psychiatric diagnosis. Machiavellianism refers to the use of self-interested strategies, such as deceit, flattery and emotional detachment, to manipulate social and interpersonal interactions. The combination of Machiavellianism, narcissism and psychopathy is referred to as the 'dark triad' of personality traits and is thought to be associated with adverse workplace behaviours and financial misbehaviour.

24

Alongside my assessments of homicide cases, I've also been asked to assess a number of fraud defendants, initially for both sides, but as I grew more experienced, mostly for the prosecution. The mind of a fraudster was the subject of an academic paper I co-wrote, in which we made the case for a typology of mental disorder in fraudsters.[54]

My introduction to fraud and malingering had been when I was asked to assess Diane Whitworth, one half of a couple who had set up a Ponzi scheme. The crime involved persuading vulnerable pensioners to invest £5,000 each in an investment scheme with an interest rate that was too good to be true. Instead of investing the premiums they collected from unsuspecting investors – over £600,000 – Whitworth and her husband spent the money on a luxury car and lavish foreign holidays. Later, while under investigation by HM Revenue and Customs and then the police, Whitworth feigned seizures in police custody. The defence tried to argue that she was mentally unfit to be tried. When I examined her at her home – an expensive rural property with a Bentley parked outside – she was completely mute. She then appeared at court, claiming to be blind and paralysed down one side. In my naivety, I postulated that she might have an arterial spasm in an extreme form of migraine or a stroke to account for her symptoms. But after a robust 'trial of fitness', which is a sort of trial-within-a-trial with a separate jury, she was found to be fit to plead and stand trial. One of the clinchers, as highlighted by the prosecution QC, during his withering cross-examination of a psychiatrist in private practice who had treated her, was that she had repeatedly malingered illness to make bogus travel insurance claims. It became clear that this was 'barn door' malingering. She and her husband were then convicted of fraud and sentenced to four and six years' imprisonment respectively.

I have seen many examples of this type of behaviour, some of them comical in the absurdity of the fraud and the claimed amnesia that follows it. Barrister John Wilmot tried to claim a £17.5 million VAT rebate for a bogus business deal involving non-existent Boeing jet engines. He was found to be 'fit to plead' despite proffering mental disorder, which he was thought to be malingering, and he was jailed for five years. After I had given evidence for the CPS in a series of high-value fraud cases like this, I was asked to provide training to the Serious Fraud Office about the fitness-to-plead issues usually raised in these trials. What emerged from my case series was that individuals who deceive during their fraud offence may subsequently try to deceive the court process, and the assessing psychiatrist, by malingering amnesia in order to pervert the course of justice.

I soon encountered a case that demonstrated the callousness, lack of empathy and parasitic lifestyle of a likely Machiavellian, and possibly psychopathic, financial fraudster spilling over into homicidal behaviour. This was the case of Anand Varma.

Anand Varma, twenty-six, had been playing the financial markets and spread betting online. He passed himself off as a futures trader, when in fact he was a problem gambler who had lost in excess of £100,000.

To cover his debts, he borrowed money against his parents' home and, without their knowledge, took out loans in their names. All told, he defrauded over £270,000 by forging his parents' signatures and also those of his solicitors. The money was used to pay spiralling spread-betting debts.

He must have been confronted, as on 26 October 2003 Anand Varma strangled his father, fifty-nine-year-old Dinesh Varma, before packing his body in a suitcase and hiding the case in the boot of his car, a Ford. The day before the killing, he had looked up the phrases 'murder poison' and 'murder kill' online. He then reported his father as a missing person.

What he did next was quite extraordinary, and in my view is explained partly by the mindset common to many fraudsters, who have a tendency to deny the truth, not only to their victims and the police, but also to themselves. 'I'll raid the pension fund, but it's okay, I'll repay the money,' they might say to themselves. And I think it must have been this process of psychological denial that lay behind Varma leaving his father's body to decompose in the boot of his Ford for two months.

Out of sight, out of mind.

After the disappearance of his father, Varma joined in the searches. He claimed to have sold the Ford and bought himself a BMW 5 Series as a replacement, but there was no paperwork to back up that version of events.

Incredibly, Varma kept returning to the car containing his father's decomposing body to remove parking tickets, which he placed in the glovebox of the abandoned vehicle. The tickets were all timed and dated and had his fingerprints on, so the CPS could show clear evidence that he had repeatedly returned to the car.

It seems that Varma's compulsive drive was so powerful that he prioritised gambling while neglecting the body disposal, evidenced by his dissociation from the very existence of the corpse.

I did a series of psychiatric assessments of gamblers for a specialist clinic, although it soon became clear to me that forensic psychiatry has no useful role in assisting the courts in these cases.[55] I was struck both by the intense nature of the addiction and its ability to drive quite extreme and sometimes fraudulent behaviour. But although gambling impulses may be very powerful, even irresistible at times, the gambler has the capacity to desist, and thus the criminal courts will always hold gamblers responsible for their actions. This was a lesson I learned after a particularly difficult court hearing when it became clear that a gambler had told me a pack of lies. Nevertheless, although Varma was in control of his actions, it's useful to note that brain scan research has shown activation of the ventral striatum (the brain reward centre) during simulated gambling experiments. Gamblers are not addicted to winning: they are addicted to the fleeting uncertainty of the moment before finding out whether they have won or lost. They call it 'being in the game'. It is masochistic but highly addictive, and may have been a factor in tipping Varma over the edge to murder. After police discovered the body, Varma was arrested and was awaiting trial at the Old Bailey. An open-and-shut case, surely, if you'll forgive the pun.

However, while on remand in Belmarsh, Varma came up with another fraudulent plan to suggest that someone had bought the car. His cellmate, Nagu Murphy, was a man with crack cocaine addiction and low IQ who was in prison on minor charges and soon to be released.

Varma charmed and manipulated his cellmate into helping him, saying he'd make him rich by teaching him how to trade online. Murphy agreed, but a short time after his release from Belmarsh, he was arrested in connection with an unrelated minor criminal matter. Police found him in possession of prosecution papers relating to the murder case involving Varma, along with documents written by Varma setting out a proposed false statement that he intended would be turned in to police by a third party. The documents gave details of how the statement should be made and the payments that would be received.

In a police interview, Murphy confessed the whole plot.

I became involved as there was a dispute over Murphy's fitness for police interview. But after the trial-within-a-trial, Murphy's confession was allowed to go before the jury. The pair were convicted of perverting the course of justice and Varma was convicted of the murder of his father.

Verdict: murder. Life imprisonment; fourteen-year minimum term.

So, Varma was probably one of those fraudster-murderers we're talking about, you might think. Which brings me back to the Colonel Workman murder, because one possibility in that case was that a fraudster-murderer, blackmailer or extortionist – perhaps one with psychopathic traits – had murdered him after he'd threatened to report them to police.

It certainly must have been one avenue of investigation, though it appears that police were unable to generate any leads to a financial motive. As you would expect, this type of investigation usually involves an analysis of bank records, looking for any unusual transactions and an analysis of phone records, et cetera. But nothing like this seems to have been found. Not at first, anyway.

The next key area of investigation was to try and track the shotgun used to shoot Workman on his doorstep. The police were facing two questions here: Why had a gun been used in this murder? And how?

Firearms killings in the UK are rare, thanks to some of the world's most stringent gun laws. An application for a shotgun licence takes several months and involves a requirement for evidence of lawful purpose, such as access to game shooting, the need for agricultural pest control or membership of a clay pigeon club. Unlike in the USA, there are background checks, including of medical and criminal records, and

Firearms Enquiry Officers conduct an interview at the home of the applicant before a final decision is made. Once approved, a secure gun safe must be installed and tested by a firearms officer before a certificate is finally issued, and all registered shotguns have an indelible serial number engraved into the stock and barrels.

Despite these safeguards, there are over a million shotgun owners in the UK, many of them clay-pigeon shooters, and there are also more than 500,000 firearms owners (that is, owners of hunting or target rifles), which require even more stringent checks, because of their longer range. In all, there are just under two million gun owners in the UK, which is not a great deal when you consider that in the USA, with a population approximately five times larger than the UK, there are a staggering 265 million legally held guns.

As for their use in crime, in England and Wales in 2018 there were twenty-nine murders by gunshot, slightly above average, as over the previous six years there had been between twenty-one and thirty-two. Of these, only a handful were by legally owned guns, most of them being gang-related shootings with illegal handguns and sawn-off shotguns. By contrast, in the USA in the same year there were 10,265 homicides by gunshot, accounting for almost three-quarters of all unlawful killings. The USA had 986 police-involved fatal shootings in 2017, whereas in the UK there were only six, including the four terrorists from London Bridge and Westminster, who had been intent on 'suicide by cop'.

So one question that had to be answered in the Colonel's case was whether the murder weapon had been an illegal weapon (that is, a sawn-off) or – much more likely in a rural area – a legally held shotgun. There was no cartridge case left at the scene, and it is not possible to do any useful ballistic analysis of shotgun pellets, as shotgun barrels are smooth and leave no tell-tale rifling patterns.

Police enquiries turned up nothing among local legal gun owners, and the case remained a mystery. Despite being featured on BBC television's *Crimewatch*, there were no further leads and the case went cold.

Although I had spent over twenty years living in London (apart from some overseas stints), I was familiar with this rural milieu. The village of Furneux Pelham was not unlike the village in Dorset where I had first gone to school. Once my boys and my daughter were old enough to run around, Dorset was a perfect antidote to the restrictions of London life on children. They relished trips there, where they could run around without traffic worries and collect free-range eggs or feed the rabbits. This is Thomas Hardy country. It was farmed on a feudal basis for more than half a millennium and is now prime dairy farmland. There are prestigious partridge shoots on the hills of nearby Cranborne Chase, and in winter many farmers use their downtime hunting pheasants for the pot or rough shooting for pigeon and to control vermin on the farm. In short, guns are an integral part of the way of life.

Given my familiarity with this environment, I was naturally curious when, in July 2004, I was asked to see a local rat-catcher and keen country sportsman, Christopher Nudds, who had been one of those questioned after the shooting of Colonel Riley Workman earlier that year.

Nudds, then in his mid-twenties, lived with his parents in Stocking Pelham, not far from Furneux Pelham. As a self-employed pest controller, he was regularly seen around the area in his four-wheel drive. He cleared moles from gardens, and helped local farmers deal with vermin such as rats, mice and foxes. Nudds had previously worked for the Colonel, having cleared wasps' nests in the three years running up to 2003 for a fee of £30.00.

When Nudds had attended the police station on another, minor matter, shortly after the murder, he had been questioned about it. He admitted to the police that he'd visited and spoken to the Colonel about the wasps' nests some three months before his death, but said he had not been in contact since. Not a shred of forensic evidence linked Nudds to the crime scene. There was some shotgun residue in his vehicle, but this would have been a common incidental finding in the area. As a result, and without any apparent motive or evidence to link him to the murder, he was released without charge. However, after his police interview, his picture had made the local papers. With the consequent publicity, he found it difficult to keep working and lost many clients.

Had the police unfairly targeted him because of his status as a somewhat socially isolated individual, and a rat-catcher to boot? In other words, in the absence of any other suspects, was he one individual who seemed to stand out a bit in the local population?

I suspected there was speculation that his work exterminating animals had somehow been transferred to the extermination of humans. Do animal hunters ever switch their gun sights on to human quarry, as suggested in the 1924 Richard Connell short story, *The Most Dangerous Game*? Well, there was one prominent case in the USA, that of Robert Hansen. Hansen had abducted seventeen women in order to sexually assault, cuff and transport them in his two-seater light aircraft to the Alaskan wilderness. Once there, he released them, sadistically allowing them a moment of hope that they were free. But he then mercilessly hunted and killed them, as depicted in the 2013 film *The Frozen Ground*, starring John Cusack as Hansen. Girls at high school had rejected Hansen, who became a loner, channelling his resentment into hunting animals. He was slightly built, socially awkward and was teased for his stammer. His desire for revenge on those who mocked him saw his behaviour escalate from hunting animals to stalking human quarry. Sentenced to life, he died in prison in 2014.

Could Nudds, also a loner, have similarly switched from animals to humans, with his professional role exterminating garden moles, rats and other vermin having inured him to inflicting death, or maybe even given him a taste for killing? Or had he tried to defraud the Colonel in some way?

I was asked to see him before a court appearance in relation to some unrelated minor charges.

I won't reveal what we discussed at my confidential interview in July of 2004, but the descriptions of Nudds in the press at the time reminded me of some of the innocuous country folk I had encountered in Dorset – those who made a living in and around the world of farming, shooting and fishing, like the local fisherman who would exchange fresh sea trout from the River Frome for fresh eggs from my mother's chickens.

But Nudds didn't have a shotgun certificate, and therefore no access to a registered 12-gauge capable of discharging the heavyweight buckshot that had killed the Colonel. I heard no more about the case and presumed Nudds had gone back to rat-catching and other country pursuits. The investigation went quiet and the murder of Colonel Workman remained unsolved.

The next thing to happen was that, not long after bonfire night, on 30 November 2004, a young man called Fred Moss, a member of the travelling community, went missing from his home.

I didn't pick up the reports, as they only featured in Essex local news. Fred had a very keen interest in country sports, including hare coursing with his pet lurcher Nellie. Hare coursing uses sighthounds, fast running dogs like greyhounds or cross-breed lurchers, who chase their quarry by sight rather than by scent. Coursing was a precursor to greyhound racing, where the dog chases a simulation hare. It is now illegal in the UK, but not in the Republic of Ireland. It is popular in the UK travelling community, despite the prohibition. Fred ran a road tarmac business and had bought two plots of land with the proceeds, where he was planning to build a permanent residence.

Fred Moss was last seen on the morning of 30 November at his aunt's home in Stansted Mountfichet, Essex. He left with Nellie in his yellow Astra van – and then seemed to disappear off the face of the earth. When he was still missing thirty-six hours later, his family offered a £125,000 reward for information about Fred, and 500 volunteers from the travelling community were involved in searching for him. When Nellie was found near the village of Newton, the search party switched their attention to that area. It had started as a missing person investigation, but as the days passed, there was increasing concern that Fred may have been victim to some form of foul play.

By Friday, 3 December 2004, when Fred's van was found apparently abandoned in a car park, the case was being treated as a murder investigation. So, the police in the adjoining areas of East Herts and West Essex had a second rural murder mystery on their hands inside a year. Were the two connected?

Police said they had questioned a man on the afternoon of Sunday, 5 December, but the officers would not reveal where he was being held, only that he was not a farmer, a landowner or a member of the travelling community. And that man was none other than the rat-catcher Christopher Nudds.

It turned out that, as a matter of routine, police had been checking all known associates of Fred Moss, and they had found out Moss and Nudds knew each other. Nudds would trap rabbits for Moss to use when training his lurcher in preparation for coursing bigger and faster hares. Nudds was brought in for questioning about Fred's disappearance and readily admitted that they were friends, but he denied any knowledge of where Moss had gone or what had happened to him.

Fred Moss's body had not been found, but the police began a thorough investigation and started to piece together the evidence. Mobile phone cell-site analysis showed Moss's phone in the Buntingford area. Analysis of Christopher Nudds's phone indicated that he had also been in the Buntingford area at the same time as Moss, and the police concluded that the two must have met there. At 1 p.m. on 30 November, Moss's van and a dark green Range Rover – consistent with the appearance of Nudds's car – were seen on CCTV, travelling in convoy through a nearby village. By 1.15 p.m., Moss's mobile placed him in the area close to Highfield Farm near Littington. Highfield Farm is an isolated area of farmland where the tracks are accessible only by four-wheel drive. Moss's mobile phone disconnected with the network sometime between 3.15 and 3.37 p.m.

Police enquiries had ascertained that Nudds regularly shot pests at Highfield Farm. He had been given shooting rights by the owners, and would go there up to twice a week, sometimes lamping at night, as he liked to shoot rabbits. In other words, Nudds knew the area like the back of his hand.

The mobile phone analysis clearly showed Nudds's movements to and from the farm, as his mobile connected and disconnected to the separate radio masts in the surrounding area and beyond. Something I observed in many murder cases around the early 2000s was that killers were often unaware of the devastating impact of this new investigative tool. Mobile phone evidence has been a critical element in a high proportion of successful murder convictions. Nudds's account was inconsistent with this early evidence of his movements around the time of the killing, and he was charged with perverting the course of justice and remanded in prison custody. In the absence of a body, there was not enough evidence to formally charge him with murder. But if Nudds had been with Moss at the farm when Moss and his phone just disappeared, what had happened to Moss? Surely Nudds was the only person who could answer that question. And why had Nudds repeatedly returned to the spot? Was he looking for Moss? If so, why not come forward? Nudds had been unable to provide an innocent explanation for all this evidence.

Gradually, the police collected more evidence, but the question remained: what had happened to Fred Moss's body?

The answer came from Nudds himself. Remanded at Bedford prison, Nudds told a cellmate that he had killed Moss with a low-calibre gun, adding that the killing was 'a hundred per cent personal', and that he had dismembered the body with a knife and hacksaw, then transported it in the back of his vehicle to a spot where he burned the remains.

Nudds was said to have been nonchalant and sarcastic, telling his cellmate he had done Moss's family a favour, as at least they wouldn't have to buy him a coffin. The cellmate gave this information to the prison staff, who relayed it to detectives investigating the murder.

The police then turned to forensic evidence, and a search of Nudds's car revealed a DNA profile matching Moss's. Nudds had also given his cellmate information which led police to a hacksaw stained with blood. Further DNA analysis showed that the blood also matched Moss's profile.

The police case gradually being compiled for presentation to the CPS was that Nudds had lured Moss to the remote spot, shot him dead and cut his body into several parts with a knife and hacksaw. Moss's remains were thought to have been moved by car, placed on wooden pallets and set on fire so that nothing was left. Nudds had tried to cover his tracks by dropping the lurcher dog at a spot nine miles away to throw the family off the scent.

*

It took some time for all the evidence to be prepared, and the trial didn't proceed until well over a year later, in early 2006 at Northampton Crown Court. The prosecution presented their case, screening CCTV and explaining the complex mobile phone evidence painstakingly compiled by the forensic telecoms expert. On 23 February, the defence case opened and Nudds gave an entirely new account.

He tried to persuade the jury that there was some complicated explanation involving Moss being involved in a drug deal gone wrong. He claimed he hadn't mentioned this to the police before for fear that he would be implicated in drug dealing.

But Nudds admitted that his statement to the police about finding Moss's van a few days after he'd gone missing had contained a series of lies. Regarding the blood with Moss's DNA found in Nudds's car, he claimed that Moss had accidentally cut himself while a passenger in the car on an earlier occasion.

Nudds had only come up with this version of events well over a year after his arrest, once he had had a chance to see exactly what evidence the police had against him. Remember, Moss ran a successful tarmac business, and there was no suggestion from any other source of him being involved in drugs. And a drugs deal near a secluded farm? In a situation like this, the judge will have given a direction to the jury that they were entitled to draw an adverse inference from Nudds's failure to come up with his exculpatory story at an earlier stage.

The bloodstained hacksaw – connected to Nudds – with the victim's DNA on it, along with the reported confessions by Nudds to his cellmate, seem to have persuaded the jury.

On 27 February 2006, Nudds was convicted of the murder of Fred Moss and sentenced to life imprisonment with a minimum term of thirty years.

So how do you think I felt about this?

I had interviewed Nudds in late July 2004, and he had killed Moss on 30 November that year. The truth is that I felt uncomfortable. However, I wasn't treating Nudds, and I had not been in a position to influence the situation one way or the other. There had been no faulty post-mortem this time, as there wasn't even a body.

On the other hand, I have to admit that I felt a bit duped, but it took me back to the lesson learned in the Hardy case. Cold-blooded killers don't tend to speak of what they do unless, or until, they're caught, or unless they turn themselves in.

Nudds's crime contained features that seemed wholly incompatible with what had been presented to me, namely a misunderstood rat-catcher, a bit of a loner. If we accept the jury's conclusion (and I'd say that mobile phone analysis is pretty incontrovertible) that he had lured Moss, a close friend, to a secluded area in order to kill him and dispose of the body, then this apparently cold-blooded murder seemed to suggest a wholly different set of personality traits and behaviours: conning and manipulative behaviour, and a lack of remorse or guilt.

Why had he killed Moss? And had he also killed the Colonel? Were the cases connected? Was this my second case of a killer who had gone on to kill a second time – after I had done an assessment? These are very difficult thoughts for a forensic psychiatrist. We are supposed to be able to at least identify high-risk psychiatric states, even if we can't entirely predict the future. To repeat my long-range weather forecast analogy: had I, for the second time in my career, identified a Beaufort scale force-three gentle breeze when in fact there was a raging force-ten storm? If I do a psychiatric assessment of an individual who doesn't disclose a previous killing for which they have not been caught, then my assessment will be based on the information I have. But that assessment will be rendered worthless and inaccurate if they are later found to have committed an undetected murder in the period before I saw them.

Put another way, psychiatric assessments of serial killers halfway through their series might as well be shredded and thrown in the bin if the killer doesn't tell you what they're up to.

In Hardy's case, of course, it later transpired that he had killed Sally White before I interviewed him, and he'd gone on to kill his two other victims not long after my assessment (and after the assessments of several of my equally unsuspecting colleagues).

In May 2010, Nudds's appeal against the conviction for the Fred Moss killing was heard at the Criminal Court of Appeal on the Strand, London. The evidence against Nudds was said to be compelling, and his murder conviction was upheld. Meanwhile, police had continued to investigate the killing of Colonel Workman, and a new witness had come forward, albeit rather late in the day. Gary Chambers, a self-employed gardener, had been living in Furneux Pelham at the time of the Colonel's killing. On 7 January 2004, he had been at home helping to get his son ready for bed when he heard the 'bang of a shotgun'. Shortly afterwards, while out in his car in the village, he spotted a Range Rover driving near the scene of the shooting. He noticed that part of the number plate spelled out SOHO. At the time of the murder, Nudds was living nearby in Stocking Pelham and was known to drive a Range Rover with the number plate N50 HO. Other evidence came to light: Nudds's uncle, Peter Ward, had seen a sawn-off shotgun hidden under the seat of his nephew's car before the murder of Workman.

And, finally, a financial motive did indeed emerge. During the course of the investigation, it was discovered that Workman had led a double life in the 1960s. A respectable army officer, he had been secretly visiting gay bars in London, homosexuality still being illegal at the time.

In custody, Nudds was placed in a shared cell with a known informant. Nudds told his cellmate and one other prisoner that he had had an affair with Colonel Workman. His motive for killing Workman remained unclear, but it was believed Nudds had been extorting money from him.

Colonel Workman's case was reviewed in December 2007 after the cellmate informant provided details of Nudds's cell confession. Nudds had by now changed his name to Christopher Docherty-Puncheon and was in a civil partnership with a fellow prisoner. Nudds had told his cellmate that he had hatched a murder plot when Workman threatened to talk to police about the extortion. He subsequently killed Moss because the traveller knew too much about the Colonel's death. Nudds said that it was all about the Colonel's money – he was extorting Workman by threatening to reveal his secret gay life, or possibly details of their affair.

Nudds was charged with Colonel Workman's murder in July 2010, following the cold case review. There was a further criminal trial in November 2012.

Mr Latham QC presented the crown's case: '[Nudds told his cellmate] that he had known Colonel Workman since 1998, and that the two men had engaged in sexual activity with each other.' He had described the Colonel as both well heeled and generous. Nudds told his cellmate that it was he who had made the mystery 999 call in the dead of night. Further evidence from Nudds's landline proved he had not been at home on the night of Workman's murder. It transpired that he had dialled into his landline from his mobile to receive answerphone messages at a time when he had claimed to be at home. This was another example of the investigative power of phone records in Nudds's cases, and also the widespread ignorance of this technology at the time.

Of course, nowadays most habitual criminals know they have to use 'burners' to avoid having their location traced – but it still catches out some killers, who act in the heat of the moment and then forget to chuck out their SIM cards.

The jury of six men and six women were sent out and deliberated for seventeen hours and thirty-one minutes. Nudds was dressed in a dark suit and a striped tie. He remained expressionless as his fate was read out: guilty.

Verdict: murder. Life imprisonment; forty-year minimum term.

The real motive must have been financial all along. Blackmail or extortion is what the police case inferred – possibly the Colonel had refused to pay up and threatened to involve the police, leading to Nudds's switch from extortion to murder to cover his tracks.

Nudds will be eligible for first parole review in around 2045, when he's past retirement age. You can follow his campaign to prove his innocence online. Perhaps Nudds's sense of power over the life or death of animals had been translated to humans after all. If, when I am walking in the Dorset woods and fields, I happen to encounter a gamekeeper armed with a 12-gauge automatic shotgun, I can't help but cast my mind back to Nudds – although I suspect I won't encounter another gamekeeper like him.

Terrorism

Case Study: Mustafa Kamel Mustafa

25

When you start out in forensic psychiatry, you have to earn your stripes working on those minor criminal cases that we generally refer to as 'gas-meter-bandits', by which I mean acquisitive offences like theft, burglary or robbery. But having graduated from those cases to murder, and a year or so after 9/11, I started receiving referrals about criminal offences more serious than any I had dealt with before. In 2006, a set of case papers arrived under the distinctive bald eagle insignia of the US Department of Justice. The charges were of conspiracy to use weapons of mass destruction, providing material support and resources to terrorists, and conspiring to damage and destroy buildings. This was the gas limousines and financial buildings plot, which I will return to shortly. Around that time, I was also asked to interview a number of prisoners with alleged links to Islamic extremist terrorist cells. But amongst all these referrals, there was one that turned out to be more interesting than I anticipated.

In June 2005, like most Londoners, I wasn't thinking about Islamic terrorism. I had stopped off at Konditor & Cook on the Grays Inn Road and was checking my emails. In the subject line of one was a name, Mustafa Kamel Mustafa. Could I prepare a psychiatric report in relation to Human Rights Act Article 6 issues, namely the right to a fair trial?

When I read through the papers later, I realised that Mustafa was in fact none other than radical preacher Sheikh Abu Hamza, famous for his fiery rhetoric at Finsbury Park Mosque. Abu Hamza has been an influential man. His sermons have been linked to Richard Reid, the shoe bomber;

Zacarias Moussaoui, the missing 9/11 conspirator; Kamel Bourgass, the ricin plotter; and one of the 'gas limos' bombers, which I will discuss shortly.

Here's a snapshot of some of the things Abu Hamza has said:

'Every place of iniquity, every brothel, every video shop which is selling [porn films] is a target.'

'[The] nation of Muhammad must regain their dignity and this dignity would not be regained unless with blood . . .'

'Don't go to the man who is selling in a wine shop and tell him, "Please why you selling the wine?" Make sure that the man who gave him the licence for that wine shop does not exist any more on the Earth. Finish him up.'

'Killing a kafir [infidel or non-believer] who is fighting you is okay. Killing a kafir for any reason, you can say it is okay – even if there is no reason for it.'

The charges against Abu Hamza on both sides of the Atlantic were extensive. In the UK, he was charged with incitement to murder by virtue of his speeches at Finsbury Park Mosque. The US indictment alleged that in December 1998 he had conspired to take a number of hostages in the Yemen; that he had provided funds, knowing they would be used for terrorism/jihad in Afghanistan; that he conspired to set up a terrorist training camp in Oregon; and various other allegations. I added Abu Hamza's name to my to-do list of prison visits and resolved to read the papers once I had a spare moment.

To explain how I ended up being asked to see high-level terrorists, I have to rewind the clock to 1985 when, after finishing exams on all the core science subjects at medical school, there was an opportunity for a natural break before starting clinical studies at the hospital. I figured I was ready to see the real world for a bit. What's more, it was a time when Ethiopia and neighbouring Sudan were in the middle of a crisis. Michael Buerk's TV reports of malnourished Ethiopian refugees had ignited public concern, which was crystallised by the December 1984 Band Aid fundraiser song 'Feed the World' and the Live Aid open-air concert in July 1985. Spurred on by these events, not to mention motivated by naive ideas of solving the world's health problems, I decided I would spend my year off learning something about emergency disaster relief and tropical medicine, with the added bonus of spending a year in East Africa.

I was insufficiently qualified to get an aid agency post via head offices in the UK, but I had been told that the situation in Khartoum was chaotic and fast-moving, and that expat English teachers were being hired on local contracts. There had been drought and crop failures across the region and armed conflict had compounded the problems. There was an airlift and trucking operation to feed the west of Sudan, and numerous refugee camps had been set up to deal with the influx of tens of thousands of refugees from Chad and Ethiopia.

Thanks to a succession of agricultural summer jobs, I'd saved enough travel money to last a month or so, but I knew I'd need to find paid work when I got there. I decided to enter Sudan via the overland route in order to acclimatise, and so in late summer of 1985, I made my way through Egypt to the Aswan Dam in the south.

The only cheap hotel near the boat dock was full, so I ended up sharing a twin room with one of only five foreigners making the trip: Tim Lenderking, who was a graduate from Wesleyan University on a one-year travelling fellowship.

This trip (Cairo to Khartoum) was definitely not on the regular student backpacking trail – and still isn't. The overnight boat ride across Lake Nasser to Wadi Halfa in Sudan, followed by the two-day train ride across the Abu Hamed desert, introduced us to the heat, dust and thirst that would colour the next twelve months. Some of our fellow passengers were Sudanese herdsmen, who were returning home having delivered camels to Egypt via the Forty Days Road through the Sahara. The slow-moving train to Khartoum was so crowded at night that – following the example of some of the more agile Sudanese – Tim and I climbed up the gap between rattling carriages on to the roof of the train. On top of the flat-roofed 'restaurant car', which served pan-fried Nile perch with rice, it was possible to find a place to doze. (Some things you only do because, in late adolesence/early adulthood, your brain still has an underdeveloped prefrontal cortex, impairing the assessment of threat.)

Arriving in Khartoum after the arduous trip from Egypt, we had a very welcome shower and experienced out first taste of Sudanese hospitality when, after a meal in a local restaurant, we were told that the other diners had paid for us out of the respect due to rare foreign visitors. A few days later, a bus driver also refused to accept my payment, waiving the fare

Tim and I met up several times for iced water with limes in the Acropole Hotel during that month in Khartoum while I was looking for work, and again later that year. Tim must have found the experience of Khartoum as instructive as I did, because he went on to a career in Arabian Gulf international relations with the US Department of State.

After touting my CV around Khartoum, I was hired on a modest local salary of around £125 per month, plus board and lodging, by a disaster-relief NGO (non-governmental organisation). I was assigned to a refugee camp on the border between Sudan and Ethiopia, where 25,000 people were living in makeshift huts covered in plastic to protect them from the rain. The United Nations High Commissioner for Refugees (UNHCR) supplied the general ration of flour every ten days, and also dished out the plastic sheeting for the huts.

Boreholes had been drilled to provide fresh water, and healthcare was provided by independent aid agencies funded by grants and charity.

I joined a medical team with doctors and nurses from Europe and a large contingent of local staff, both refugees and Sudanese. There was a reed and grass thatched field hospital, and we provided an extended vaccination programme and supplementary feeding for the most malnourished of the children.

As you can imagine, it was a tough introduction to the realities of life, death and very basic healthcare in sub-Saharan Africa. The refugees were subsistence farmers who had fled Tigray after crop failures and civil war between the Soviet-backed Ethiopian government and Tigray separatists. I saw endemic medical conditions that I would never see in the UK: neonatal tetanus, malaria, tuberculosis of the spine and parasitic Leishmaniasis. These were compounded by severe malnutrition, dehydration, and the effects of spitting cobras and lethal carpet viper bites. The carpet or saw-scaled viper – an aggressive type of pit viper – kills more people than any other species of snake. The bites cause extensive necrotic tissue damage, spontaneous systemic bleeding and a lethal condition called disseminated intravascular coagulation. Without anti-venom, the mortality rate is ten to twenty per cent – and we didn't have the anti-venom.

I also witnessed the results of murderous attacks. I helped with the burial of an entire family, who were wiped out, I was told, by bandits. I assisted with the care of a refugee who'd survived an axe wound to the head, and that of a nomadic camel herd who'd turned up with injuries sustained in a sword fight (yes, the Beja nomads still carried traditional swords).

It turned out that my year in Sudan came at a pivotal moment in its history. Earlier in 1985, the dictator Jaafar al-Nimeiri had been deposed in a military coup, partly because his September 1983 introduction of Islamic Sharia law was unpopular with some. There followed a year of relatively liberal rule by a transitional military council, which was then followed by an election in 1986. In contrast to the austere culture of the recently deposed regime, the love songs of local singer Hanan Boulu Boulu were popular that year.

But Sudan was undergoing the changes which were becoming evident all over the Islamic world. On the morning of Wednesday, 15 April 1986, I walked into the market square for a thimble of spicy Sudanese coffee. The temperature had not yet reached the standard forty degrees centigrade and, appreciating the relatively cool air, I mulled over whether to have my coffee with ginger, cardamom or cloves. But I was interrupted by my first taste of the growing conflict between the Islamic world and the West.

An imposing Sudanese man began remonstrating with me, threatening me with his heavy walking stick, as thick as a cow's thigh bone. His companions restrained him and apologised to me, but it soon became clear that his gripe was quite specific. He was saying that the British were no good because Prime Minister Margaret Thatcher had allowed USF-111 bombers to take off from RAF Lakenheath in Suffolk.

I had not yet heard the news, but the locals had been listening to the Arabic language BBC World Service and Riyadh radio. Earlier that day, at 2 a.m., the US Marine Corps had conducted Operation El Dorado Canyon, with air strikes against Libya in retaliation for the 1986 West Berlin discotheque bombing. There were forty reported Libyan casualties, including, it was claimed, one of Gaddafi's daughters.

It pays to keep up-to-date with current affairs if you are living in the Islamic world, and I was six hours behind the curve regarding the latest news from Suffolk.

I noticed a change in the atmosphere that summer. Government officials who had co-operated with Operation Moses – the

Israeli government airlift of Ethiopian Jews – were on trial, and during a concert the singer Hanan Boulu Boulu had rocks thrown at her by Islamist hardliners. Towards the end of the year, the Muslim Brotherhood – the puritanical political-religious movement originating in Egypt – were campaigning for election. My Sudanese colleagues told me that the Muslim Brothers were handing out money in exchange for votes, and indeed, it later turned out that Saudi Arabia had been heavily investing in pushing Sudan towards a more puritanical and Wahhabist form of Islam.

At the same time, the refugee crisis in East Sudan was coming to an end, and the Tigrayans in the camp had decided they were ready to return home. After a night of celebratory songs, all 20,000 or so packed up and marched over the border for the long walk back to their farms – a frankly biblical scene.

Meanwhile, the aid agency was dealing with another refugee crisis on the opposite side of Ethiopia. They were short-staffed, so for the last three months of my year in Africa I was posted to northern Somalia (now the independent Republic of Somaliland). My job was to support a medical team dealing with another camp of Ethiopian refugees, this time housed in *M*A*S*H*-style tents on a dusty plain not far from the Ogaden desert. This was another culture, a new language – Somali – and another specific set of medical and political problems.

I was based in the regional capital, Hargeisa, where I attended weekly meetings with other agencies like UNHCR, UNICEF and the International Rescue Committee, in between running supplies from Djibouti – two days' off-road drive away – to the refugee camp.

There was an epidemic of relapsing fever – a louse-borne bacterial infection – requiring an emergency consignment of antibiotics via Djibouti. Also, the midwives and doctors were confronted with the terrible gynaecological and obstetric complications of female genital mutilation, which was, and remains, widespread in the region. (Although Nimko Ali is nowadays campaigning to change this, with the support of the local government.)

One afternoon, Somali government soldiers in fatigues went around the various aid agency offices to hand-deliver invitations to a drinks party being held by General Morgan, the local military commander. There weren't that many social occasions. With no mains electricity, most evenings were spent reading by Tilley lamp, or listening to the World Service while sipping mint tea or a rare glass of illicit whisky. So, out of sheer curiosity, and to my later regret, we decided to drop in on the party.

It was a bizarre and, with hindsight, chilling spectacle. It turned out that the party was at a sort of makeshift military club. We passed through the cordon of General Morgan's praetorian guard from the Somali National Army's 26th division, who were armed to the teeth with US-supplied weapons. We then walked into a marquee where all the guests, many of them young women, sat expectantly at tables, murmuring quietly. We took a seat and realised that in front of us was a collection of unopened soft drinks, which nobody dared to touch while we waited for the general to dishonour us with his presence.

After a delay, and unnerved by the military presence, my boss – who had travelled up from head office in Mogadishu – kicked me under the table. We both realised we'd made a terrible mistake in coming, and got up to make our excuses. I later found out from our local staff, and from reading a subsequent Africa Watch report, that many of the young women present had probably been coerced into attending by soldiers for their officers' amusement, and to take part in grotesque fashion parades and dancing competitions – a way of humiliating the local population by dishonouring their women.

But just as we were picking our way between the tables to the door, General Morgan swept in with his bodyguards and plonked himself down on an extravagant sofa at the front of the room, to the sound of hissing bottles of lukewarm pop being opened by the thirsty guests.

And so, astonished by this narcissistic spectacle, I found myself stooping to shake the hand of a man who would turn out to be the most prolific murderer of all the murderers I have ever met: General Mohammed Said Hersi Morgan.

Morgan, a former bodyguard and son-in-law of the dictator Siad Barre, was to become a perpetrator of genocide and would be dubbed the 'Butcher of Hargeisa' during Somalia's brutal civil war, when troops under his orders attacked that town. Devastation from shelling and bombing was followed by the house-to-house murder, rape and looting of the Isaaq people, 300,000 of whom fled to camps in Ethiopia. Over 50,000 were murdered (some estimates suggest 200,000) and the bodies were bulldozed into mass graves, while Hargeisa – the Dresden of Africa – was reduced to rubble in a few weeks.

This civil war happened at the dog-end of the Cold War, after the superpowers had switched allegiance, with the Soviets dropping Somalia to back General Mengistu's government in Ethiopia. This deprived Somali insurgents of their safe haven across the border and tipped the simmering conflict over the edge. Once the war had engulfed Mogadishu, Somalia became famous as a conflict zone and later a failed state, but the Hargeisa massacre, coming as it had so early in the war, didn't receive much press attention at the time or since. The term 'ethnic cleansing' had not yet been coined, and these awful events came to be known as the forgotten genocide.

After the collapse of the Barre regime in 1991, General Morgan became a warlord in the south of Somalia and his militia were responsible for causing a famine that led to thousands of deaths, as well as committing further murder, rape and looting for many years to come. Morgan is still prominent there: in 2019, he stood for election in the coastal region of Puntland. Resentment about his wartime atrocities is said to be one of the many aspects of inter-clan conflict, which remains – along with terrorist group Al-Shabab – a major block to lasting peace in Mogadishu.

I later returned to Somaliland on two fact-finding mssions. I saw the aftermath of the obliteration of Hargeisa, and visited mass graves in nearby Burao. The bedroom in the house where I had slept now had an enormous hole in the wall from a rocket-propelled grenade.

But in October 1986, with the terrible events of the 1988 genocide and the civil war still two years away, my time in East Africa was up.

I returned to London to resume my studies. Although my feet were back on UK soil, my head and heart took a while to follow – I was only one year older, but several years wiser. I had also equipped myself with some cultural and geopolitical knowledge, very rudimentary Arabic, and even more rudimentary Somali phrases.

In the subsequent years, as I worked my way through those junior doctor jobs, I would occasionally use these basic language skills with patients, as well as for greetings and pleasantries while ordering a kebab at Ranoush Juice or when meeting Somalis who had come to the UK after the civil war – including some who now work at my secure unit.

So when I entered forensic psychiatry, I had enough cultural awareness and – by then very rusty – language skills (along with French from school and Spanish from an elective in Ecuador) to break the ice with numerous bewildered, non-English-speaking prisoners and psychiatric patients. They included the Venezuelan drug mules at Holloway, a psychotic

Ecuadorian kitchen porter, a young Somali with khat-induced psychosis at Pentonville prison, and a suicidal Frenchman who was fished out of the Thames by the river police.

As you can imagine, you don't need to know many ice-breaker phrases to tilt the dynamic of an interview with a disorientated foreign patient or prisoner in a psychiatric ward or a windowless segregation cell.

During the 1990s, while I kept an eye on developments in the Middle East and East Africa, such as Osama Bin Laden's expulsion from Sudan in 1996, followed by the Kenya and Tanzania embassy bombings in 1998, my focus was on the psychiatric cases in front of me. But after the 9/11 attacks, and still processing the shock and grief from the deadliest terrorist attack in modern history, I thought back to my earlier exposure to the rising influence of Islamic fundamentalism. And I also turned, inevitably, to the mindset of the perpetrators.

As all the 9/11 hijackers (bar one) had perished as a result of their mass murder-suicides, the only way to get inside their heads would be to conduct a psychological post-mortem – or to interview other Al-Qaida conspirators caught before carrying out their plans. My colleague, Reid Meloy, produced a briefing paper in which he examined, in granular detail, the physical and biographical evidence relating to Mohamed Atta, one of the ringleaders of 9/11.[56]

Cross-referencing with an analysis of Timothy McVeigh, the white supremacist and anti-Federalist Oklahoma bomber, Meloy noted some features of what he dubbed the 'Violent True Believer'. Atta's background lay in a very strict and religious Sunni Muslim household in Egypt. He was a serious student and had travelled to Germany for postgraduate qualifications. It seems that Atta had a distrust of and alienation from women, and had an introverted temperament combined with superior intelligence.

Meloy noted that Atta seems to have been socially and geographically adrift, living as he did isolated from his student peers in Hamburg. He also attended a militant mosque in Hamburg (Al-Quds) and had been converted to extremist movements – initially the Egyptian group Gama'a al-Islamiyya (the Party of Islam) and later Al-Qaida. He experienced humiliation and rejection from his chosen career path because, despite his high-level education, he was convinced there would be bias against him in Egyptian society as a result of his political and religious views. In 1996 Atta became ever more immersed in hostile thoughts towards America, along with murderous ideas of causing civilian deaths in pursuit of his grievance. He later attended a terrorist training camp. The 9/11 attack was orchestrated over a long period of covert activity in an organised terrorist cell, with connections to a wider network.

Did Atta's profile fit in with existing theories about the mindset of terrorists – in this case Islamic violent extremists?

The prevailing theory in the 1970s was that terrorists were psychopaths, drawn to terrorist activity because it provided an outlet for their aggressive impulses. But once the concept of psychopathy was more closely defined by Hare in the psychopathy checklist, this fell out of favour. Later psychoanalytic theories suggested that terrorists have pathological narcissism – which makes them grandiose, with contempt for others – and pathological aggression. Yet in the years after 9/11, authors such as psychologist John Horgan argued that terrorists were more likely to be psychologically normal, in order to be able to plot targeted and carefully planned violence and work with others within a terrorist cell, while simultaneously maintaining secrecy.

The argument was that those with mental illness would be seen to pose a liability to the terrorist cell, and would therefore be excluded during the recruitment process. But terrorists in a cell may have different functions. From the ringleader to the quartermaster or suicide bomber, each role may be better suited to a different mindset.

Not long after 9/11, I was given the chance to form my own view about the mindset of people who we call 'group-actor terrorists' when I began assessing a series of terrorist detainees and prisoners.

26

It is hardly surprising that responses by the USA and coalition partners to the 9/11 attacks were swift, robust and decisive, given the collective global shock and grief at the mass civilian casualties (2,996 dead, from 90 countries; 6,000 injured, and countless bereaved, widowed or orphaned.) But with the benefit of hindsight, we can now see that there have been substantial unintended adverse consequences of the response.

Colonel Andrew Milburn, UCL philosophy graduate and former US Marine Corps Chief of Staff of Special Operations Command in Iraq, has described the military fallout of the war against terror in Iraq and Afghanistan and the fight against ISIS in his book *When the Tempest Gathers*. Likewise, the legislative, judicial and extra-judicial measures used to combat terrorism have sometimes backfired in unexpected ways. The British government introduced the Anti-terrorism, Crime and Security Act in 2001. As a result, a number of foreign nationals were imprisoned without trial on the grounds that they were a threat to national security. These detainees couldn't be tried in a criminal court: much of the evidence against them was based on intercepted intelligence, and to present it in court would have prejudiced national security. So the secret evidence – of which I saw only the two-page 'gist' – was enough to ensure detention indefinitely without trial at the special immigration appeal court.

In 2003, two years later, prolonged detention without trial had contributed to significant psychological and psychiatric problems in those subjected to it. I was among those asked to conduct psychiatric assessments of inmates who had presented with depression, suicide attempts, post-traumatic stress disorder and even psychotic breakdown.

The following year, in 2004, after appeals by the 'Belmarsh Nine', these provisions were overturned when the 'Appeal Committee at the House of Lords delivered a judgement that found detention without trial to be incompatible with human rights law. Lord Hoffman opined that 'it calls into question the existence of an ancient liberty [. . .] freedom from arbitrary arrest and detention.'

But the effect on the detainees over this three-year period had been significant.

The first man I saw – in 2003, while the controversial law was still in operation – was Adel, a French-speaking prisoner. He was from a country in the Maghreb, North Africa, where he had been accused of allegiance to extremist Islamic groups. Counter-terrorism police had arrested him in 2001 (pre 9/11) while his wife was pregnant. She suffered a mental breakdown and was later sectioned, while Adel's son was taken into foster care. Adel made suicide attempts at Belmarsh prison and had been cut down from makeshift ligatures.

In order to appreciate Adel's situation, you have to understand the security arrangements for terrorist detainees at Belmarsh. Given the appalling scale of 9/11, and later 7/7, it's not at all controversial that these prisoners must be detained in a high-security environment. It also needs to be impossible for them to communicate with accomplices, eliminating chances of tipping off, directing or coordinating further attacks.

Of 117 prisons in England and Wales, Belmarsh is one of the eight high-security prisons. Within it, there is what's been dubbed Britain's modern-day Alcatraz, which Muslim detainees call, in Arabic, the 'Sidgin tachil sidgin' or 'prison within the prison'. Officially known as the 'High-Security Unit', it has its own perimeter wall with extra fencing and underground rumble sensors in case anybody tries to cross the divide between the unit's interior block and exterior wall. Despite the fact that all staff and visitors have already been searched and X-rayed to get into the main prison, there are further searches at the entrance to the unit and special measures so that all items, even food trays, are X-rayed in and out. Every prisoner has their cell tossed and is moved to another one at random, without notice, no less than every twenty-eight days, to discourage – futile – tunnel-digging attempts or cell tampering.

Exercise is taken in a small roofed area, which means prisoners lose the ability to focus on distant objects. Some of the cells on the lower level have no natural light. It was common, at that time, for prisners to spend twenty-two hours per day behind the door, and association was limited to a three-hour period twice weekly, when phone calls to family had to be crammed in, along with reading a shared single newspaper, and so on.

Every prisoner has a full body cavity search on their way to and from their legal visits. So for a morning and afternoon session with defence solicitors, the term 'double-legal' means 'quadruple-rectal'.

'So what?' I hear you say. 'With such high-risk prisoners, special measures are clearly justified.'

This is true, but the prisoners claimed that they were placed under enormous pressure as a result of their public-enemy-number-one status. For example, they thought that prison officers were selling stories to the tabloids leaking their personal and medical information. This was later confirmed by Operation Elveden in 2015 when Grant Pizzey, a former Belmarsh prison officer, was jailed for two years for misconduct in a public office. He had made nearly £20,000 from tip-offs to tabloid papers, including stories about radical cleric Abu Hamza and another terror suspect.

My intervention with Adel involved documenting his psychological state for use in the deliberations about his fitness for deportation, as well as monitoring how the prison conditions caused him difficulties, and liaising with prison healthcare staff to ensure his suicidal risk was being dealt with adequately. There were no live issues around criminal responsibility or fitness for trial because there weren't any criminal proceedings, this being detention without trial.

His case eventually progressed to the point where, with all appeals exhausted, he was about to be extradited to France. But Adel had to be medically cleared for deportation, and he was on the waiting list for routine day-case surgery. This could have further delayed his enforced exit from the country, so a high-security transfer to hospital was arranged to sort out this last remaining glitch. Adel explained to me a few days later that he had been blue-lighted with an armed escort without notice (to prevent a planned escape) to Kings College Hospital. But the authorities had neglected to book a translator. Once there, with a phalanx of impatient armed police, Adel realised he might not get another chance, so he gave the surgeon the nod to go ahead with the procedure under heavy sedation – but he still didn't know what had been done. I pulled Adel's surgical discharge summary from his inmate medical file and was able to translate the details and results of the (as it happens, successful) surgical procedure.

Basic medical and psychiatric care becomes more challenging in the context of special security arrangements, and I can see how the surgeon must have fudged his usual consent procedure when faced with the unnerving sight of a corridor full of armed police. In forensic psychiatry, we are more accustomed to this, so we can put the security apparatus out of mind and not let it distract us.

Years later, Adel was released in France and reunited with his wife and son. He does not appear to have committed any further terrorist offences to date. Perhaps Belmarsh taught him a lesson.

Shortly after, I saw another detainee, Omar Salah, who had established links to more than one Salafist (jihadi) group. He had been raising funds to buy computers and frequency-hopping satellite phones for Chechnya, which he claimed were for non-military use.

He arrived at Belmarsh in April 2002, but by the time I saw him – two years after his arrest – he had become severely depressed, had psychotic symptoms, including delusions of poisoning, and was on an intermittent hunger strike. Again, my rudimentary cultural and language skills seemed to help break the ice and I earned his trust. Prisoners like Adel and Omar Salah had become mistrustful and paranoid about the prison healthcare staff. After having made some progress with these two tricky cases, the solicitors asked me to see the next terrorist case. And so, by chance, I found myself instructed to see a steady stream of terrorist prisoners over the following years.

Salah ended up being transferred out to a high-secure psychiatric hospital via a high-speed trip, with armed police escort, down the M3 to junction three and the Bagshot turn-off to Broadmoor.

After around forty assessments of similar cases, by myself and a group of colleagues, we wrote a paper for a psychiatric journal about the psychological impact of indefinite detention, which received media attention at the time.[57] In an exchange of views via academic literature, my colleague Simon Wilson pointed out that our profession was still failing to raise moral concerns and was instead cowering behind a veil of medicalisation. Forensic psychiatry is legal and medical – the clue is in the name – but we tend to tread carefully when it comes to moral considerations.

But special times need special measures, and in that post-9/11 war on terror, although the prison conditions were tough, it was clear that the British authorities had a difficult task in managing the risks to society posed by this group.

In light of the successful appeal against detention without trial, alternative legislation was hastily enacted to introduce a form of house arrest called a Control Order, which included electronic tagging, restrictions on phone calls and internet use and, in some cases, forced relocation.

As a consequence, Salah was released straight from high-secure hospital to house arrest under a Control Order. He later ended up being re-arrested and returned to high-security prison, from where he went back to Broadmoor. He ended up being transferred from one high-security establishment to another. This tends to happen with challenging prison cases – in prison slang, the process is known as the 'ghost train'. The last I heard, he was in high-security prison again.

Clearly thought to pose a risk to national and international security, cases like Salah's raise the difficult question of how we manage high-risk individuals who cannot be imprisoned or deported.

Control Orders were used on thirty-three individuals between 2005 and 2011, and were then replaced with Terrorism Prevention and Investigation Measures (TPIMs). TPIMs are a more focused and less intrusive system of measures, for use where individuals cannot be tried (because of the source of intelligence) or deported (because of risk of torture or execution).

In light of the attacks of Usman Khan and Sudesh Amman in 2019 and 2020, Lord Carlile, the former Independent Reviewer of Terrorism Legislation is suggesting – not unreasonably, you might think – that a similar form of restriction on movement and association, or even house arrest, is needed to manage those who have reached the end of their sentence for terrorist offences. Speaking not as a psychiatrist but as a concerned citizen, London Underground passenger and frequenter of London Bridge's Borough Market, such measures seem like the least-worst option. But however long you extend the prison sentence, or place other restrictions on liberty, the issue remains: what can we do with this group to try to change their mindset in order to reduce the risk they pose?

After 2004, I continued to see more terrorist detainees and prisoners, and ended up doing psychiatric assessments on special immigration appeal court and Control Order cases, including a suspect in an Al-Qaida conspiracy linked to Madrid; a former Bosnian jihadi turned Al-Qaida internet specialist; two sons of radical preachers on criminal charges – one a school contemporary of 'Jihadi John'; and several alleged terrorist fundraisers (by luxury car theft, a fraudulent retail refund scheme and bank robbery).

I need to make clear that radicalisation, in itself, is not a psychiatric issue unless it is in the context of vulnerability as a result of mental disorder, as set out in the position statement of my professional body, the Royal College of Psychiatrists.

This brings me back to the year 2006, and the eight men charged with conspiracy to use weapons of mass destruction; conspiracy to damage and destroy buildings used in interstate and foreign commerce; and possession of detailed reconnaissance materials relating to targets in the USA. The defendants, including Mohammed Naveed Bhatti, Abdul Aziz Jalil, Dhiren Barot and others, were know as 'the Luton cell', and their plans was later dubbed the 'gas limos project' and the 'financial buildings plot'. When armed police closed in to arrest the group simultaneously, the ringleader was sitting in a barber's chair having his hair cut. Although they were arrested in the UK, this was an international conspiracy, with clear links to those involved with the planning of 9/11. On 12 July 2004, police in Pakistan had arrested a computer expert with links to Al-Qaida and Khalid Sheikh Mohammed, the mastermind of 9/11. On his computer were proposals for attacks on targets in the USA and UK. This included a plan for an arson attack on the New York Stock Exchange, featuring information from studies of the building's fire security system, ventilating systems, security cameras, X-ray screening systems and construction materials. Other plans were to explode car bombs outside Citigroup buildings in Manhattan and Queens, and also the International Monetary Fund and the World Bank in Washington DC.

The planned UK attacks, meanwhile, were part of the thirty-nine-page 'gas limos project' document, which proposed to use propane, butane, acetylene and oxygen to blow up limousines in underground car parks at London hotels, including the Ritz. Other proposals were for a dirty bomb using small quantities of isotopes found in smoke detectors, and attacks on the Heathrow Express train and a Greenwich-bound train that passes under the Thames, in order to cause chaos via explosions, flooding, drowning and so forth.

All eight had been remanded in custody at HMP Belmarsh, but the defence team were concerned about one of them in particular, and thus I was asked to assess his psychological status and fitness for trial. I was later involved in the cases of two further members of the cell. I can't go into the details of the individual cases for reasons of confidentiality, but in broad terms the psychiatric issues revolved around the ability of the defendants to prepare adequately for their trial in the context of the tough conditions at Belmarsh, and the boxes full of evidence that they needed to consider. No matter how serious the charge and how compelling the evidence, every defendant has a right to a fair trial, and adjustments had to be made to the prison processes to ensure this.

The prospect of extradition to the USA – and likely multiple whole life sentences – must have concentrated the mind. All pleaded guilty to the UK charges and were given life sentences, with minimum terms of imprisonment between eighteen and forty years each (reduced to thirty on appeal). It is tempting to think of prison sentences like that as 'job done – end of story', but I picked up their stories afterwards, as they worked their way through the high-security prisons and into the de-radicalisation programme.

Later in 2006, another major conspiracy to blow up a series of flights from the UK to the US was broken up. This case led to the restrictions on taking fluids of more than 100 ml in hand luggage on board flights – something we have all endured ever since, although the details of the plot are often forgotten. I was asked to assess one of this high-profile group during three trials at Woolwich Crown Court.

The plot had come to light when a man with Al-Qaida connections came through a London airport with suspicious items in his luggage. Subsequent surveillance led to discovery of a group who had a bomb factory at an east London property. They had been stockpiling hydrogen peroxide for use in improvised explosive devices, which they planned to smuggle on to transatlantic flights disguised as soft drinks. When surveillance revealed they were recording suicide videos (martyrdom tapes) they were arrested. The ringleaders were convicted of conspiracy to murder airline passengers with liquid bombs, and were sentenced to life imprisonment, with minimum terms between thirty-two and forty years each.

In forensic psychiatry, it's often said that, if you deal with more than three cases of something, you become an expert on the subject.

Although there was no suggestion of psychiatric issues affecting criminal responsibility, these assessments gave me an opportunity to understand a little of what is in the mind of a terrorist who conspires to commit the mass murder of airline passengers. These men had been thwarted in their plans and so, unlike Mohamed Atta, one of the ringleaders of 9/11, they remained alive to be interviewed.

The gas limos project was disrupted at a relatively early stage, when ideas for targets and methods were still being scoped. The plane bombs plot, by contrast, was much closer to being actioned, as ingredients for the bombs had been stockpiled, specific flights had been listed and the suicide videos had been taped. In both cases, however, the intentions of the conspirators were clear – mass murder, with or without suicide, motivated by an extremist Islamic ideology.

According to my case series, the profile and mindset of these group-actor terrorists was, broadly speaking, as follows: most were educated or had at least some stable employment. Many had been to formal training camps in the Pakistan tribal areas, destroying passports on their return to apply for 'clean-skin' replacements. Pre-arrest, they employed tradecraft such as counter-surveillance techniques. They were organised with command-and-control connections to a wider network, in this case Al-Qaida. In some cases, individual conspirators didn't know each other, but were connected via a ringleader in a wagon-wheel cell structure where only the ringleader knew the full picture.

The ideological motivation seems to have come from grievances against the West for its perceived mistreatment of Muslims. The grievances of Bin Laden were wide-ranging. In his lengthy screed addressed to America – one year after 9/11 – he railed against military bases in the Middle East, the support of Israel and 'the immorality and debauchery that has spread among you'. He stated that he rejected the 'immoral acts of fornication, homosexuality, intoxicants, gambling, and trading with interest'.

He also said, 'What happens in Guantanamo is a historical embarrassment to America and its values, and it screams into your faces, you hypocrites.'

My experience of the group I interviewed suggested grievances about similar issues, particularly: the perception that Europe failed to intervene against Serbian genocide of Muslims; resentment about US and UK military presence in Saudi Arabia and other parts of the Middle East; anger about the atrocities committed by Indian forces against Muslims in Kashmir; and post-2003 civilian casualties in Afghanistan and Iraq.

But how does a religious, historical and geopolitcal grievance lead to the taking of terrorist action? This is currently being studied by Professor Paul Gill at UCL, who is using sophisticated statistical analysis to try to understand why potential terrorists act the way they do in certain situations, and to what extent they are influenced to move in and out of radicalising environments – like the banned organisation Al-Muhajiroun or extremist chat rooms on the dark web.

The following is a composite of reasons based on my interviews and experience of those group-actor cases.

'I grew up at the time of the National Front and experienced racism.'

'I was shocked by 9/11, but then I became more aware of injustice in the Muslim world . . . I started researching conflicts on the internet.'

'I developed a deep hatred for the West . . . why was Blair so influenced by Bush?'

'I went to talks by Abu Hamza.'

'When I saw the prisoners in Guantanamo Bay, that was the [tipping point].'

'I was carrying out Allah's will [by this conspiracy]. It must be Allah's will that I was caught [before blowing up the planes] so as to spread the message via the coverage of my trial.'

And in a neat illustration of the cognitive distortions or 'comfort stories' along the pathway to terrorist action:

'I thought I would just help out any way I could.'

'I thought he was doing something criminal, but I didn't realise what.'

'I started to think that explosions [would be acceptable] to cause disruption [but not to injure anyone].'

'I didn't care what happened.'

In order to try and tackle these beliefs and reset the mind of these murderous conspirators, there are de-radicalisation courses, such as the Al Furqan programme and the Healthy Identity Intervention. The Al Furqan programme (meaning distinguishing truth and falsehood) uses an in-depth study of Islamic texts and the life of the Prophet Muhammad (peace be upon him) and tries to challenge misinterpretations of Islamic texts and the single narrative interpretation of world history that supports Al-Qaida- and ISIS-influenced extremist violence.

The Healthy Identity Intervention was developed on the back of research looking at what works to help all types of offenders desist from their behaviour and develop good lives. The HII is an extended psychological treatment where progress is monitored by a checklist of the twenty-two-item Extremism Risk Guide (ERG22+). Although controversial, the ERG22+ identifies risk factors that can be modified, such as 'a need for identity and belonging', 'susceptibility to indoctrination', 'the need to redress injustice and express grievance', 'political and moral motivation', and 'the need for excitement, comradeship or adventure'.

One prisoner said to me that it was extremely difficult to engage in the programme, and stay out of trouble, when surrounded by more hard-core radicalised prisoners. Maintaining a clean behaviour record with provocation all around is no mean feat if your sentence is twenty years long.

And of course the other challenge is to know if a participant is really engaging with prison de-radicalisation rather than covertly pseudo-complying. This was emphatically illustrated by the two lone-actor attacks in 2019 and 2020 at London Bridge and in Streatham. These were both carried out by individuals recently released from prison. In the case of Usman Khan, he was thought to have engaged in the de-radicalisation programme in prison. Had he been lying and biding his time, or was he rapidly re-radicalised?

Given these challenges, what are the appropriate judicial measures for those suspected of involvement in terrorism but who are not yet convicted? Twenty-four-hour armed surveillance; house arrest; detention in high-security prison without trial; water-boarding in a CIA black site; or humiliation in an orange jumpsuit at Guantanamo Bay?

And for those convicted of terrorist conspiracies, or of involvement in actual or aborted terrorist attacks, do we impose a determinate prison sentence; imprison them for life with up to forty years' minimum term; throw away the key with a 130-year sentence at a US Federal supermax prison; subject them to extra-judicial scalding with boiling oil; or execute via lethal injection?

All of these measures have been used against terrorists, with varied degrees of success and public support.

As Nelson Mandela – paraphrasing Fyodor Dostoyevsky – said at the United Nations, 'No one truly knows a nation until one has been inside its jails. A nation should not be judged by how it treats its highest citizens, but its lowest ones . . .' To which I would add, '. . . and by how it treats pub-lic enemy number one, namely Islamic extremist and extreme right-wing terrorist detainees and prisoners.'

But in considering these issues, I suggest that the moral imperatives of human rights concerns and bleeding-heart lib-eral sensibilities are best put to one side. It is better to judge this on a purely practical, empirical and consequentialist basis. Namely, have the various measures employed had the desired effect of combating Islamic violent extremism on UK soil and de-radicalising those already imprisoned? Yet, having looked at this issue from a utilitarian angle, if we go beyond harsh but legal criminal penalties by allowing extra-judicial punish-ments, this does constitute an infringement of fundamental human rights, such as the US constitutional Eighth Amend-ment guarantee against 'cruel and unusual punishments' and the prohibition of 'punishment without law' in the Human Rights Act 1998.

A sentence by a British judge for a terrorist offence will nec-essarily involve lengthy imprisonment, which means prolonged loss of liberty, with restrictions on movement, association, shower access, food, exercise and visits, along with the monitor-ing of communications, a lack of internet access and shopping only allowed from the Argos catalogue. Surely that contravenes the Human Rights Act?

But we don't have the death penalty and – as I have said before – substandard or negligent medical care is not meant to be part of the punishment. The sentencing council guide-lines also don't allow for punishment by permanent maiming and scalp removal with boiling oil.

This is what actually happened to Dhiren Barot (now named Easa Barot), the ringleader of the gas limos project, in add-ition to life with a minimum term of thirty years.

Barot was 'kettled' with boiling oil, which was thrown over his head by fellow prisoners. He suffered ten per cent full thickness burns, permanently losing nearly all of his hair. When transferred to the burns unit for short-term skin grafting, he needed intravenous fluids and his pain required morphine. Initially he had been left lying in a segregation cell, treated with simple painkillers prescribed by a prison doctor, and was only transferred to hospital after his solicitor initiated judicial review proceedings. His eventual transfer required a press blackout request, secret identity to protect hospital staff, round-the-clock armed police cordon security and helicopter surveillance.

Deliberate kettling, also known as jugging, usually with a mixture of boiling water and sugar (a sticky mixture that burns the skin longer than water), is a form of punishment meted out by fellow prisoners and is generally used to settle grudges or as a punishment for sex offenders. Sex offenders are segregated in vulnerable prisoner units to protect them from this. So it could be argued that Barot was merely being subjected to something that happens in prison all the time. But boiling oil is much more damaging than sugar water.

Given the seriousness of his offences, it's understandable that there has been little public sympathy for Barot's maiming. But I would suggest that if we are going to successfully de-radicalise terrorist offenders in UK prisons, then we must ensure we are not seen by those prisoners to have condoned or turned a blind eye to acts of violent reprisal. Otherwise we risk further fuelling the flames of resentment, humiliation and grievance. There are a lot of impressionable young Muslims in British prisons (around 400 out of 900 inmates at Belmarsh, currently) and some will take notice of what happens to men like Barot.

In failing to protect one of the highest profile terrorist prisoners and an obvious target for attack, we have abandoned the moral high ground. In much the same way, the moral high ground was abandoned in the very public humiliation of orange jump-suited detainees at Guantanamo Bay – to say nothing of the torture in which some American psychologists actively participated.

James Gilligan, NYU professor of psychiatry and law, has argued that humiliation can be a powerful motivator for further violence. These orange jumpsuit tropes have certainly come back to haunt us via the sadistic ISIS beheading videos and staged immolation, which have proved such a powerful tool in both provoking horror and recruiting sympathisers in equal measure.

Did the public humiliation of Guantanamo Bay push the radicalised down the pathway to violence? As described above, at least one convicted terrorist from the gas limos plot has said as much. But to fully understand what influences the mind of a terrorist, we need to evaluate not just the source of their own grievances, but also the minds of those who inspire them.

27

After considerable delay while security matters were negotiated with the prison, it was agreed that I could interview Mustafa Kamel Mustafa, aka Sheikh Abu Hamza. My mental image of him had been coloured by re-reading the extracts of his sermons, and so it was with these utterings in mind that I headed back to the High-Security Unit at Belmarsh. What was I expecting?

Based on the press photos – often that image with his hook hand framing his eye – I thought it was going to be a difficult interview with a gruff and inscrutable terrorist extremist. After all, he had been charged in the UK with incitement to murder and racial hatred on several counts.

It took me at least an hour to get through the various procedures and into the High-Security Unit.

I was asked to wait yet again, and so spent another fifteen minutes twiddling my thumbs in the prison-within-the-prison which houses the most dangerous terrorist prisoners in the land. There I watched as a well-built prison officer joked with a male nurse. He broke into song and started waltzing around the room with the nurse, who was half his size. It was a very surreal moment indeed.

Finally, I was ushered to an interview room.

Still no sign of Hamza.

I sat alone in the room, feeling somewhat apprehensive, I'll admit, about whom I was about to meet. My job was not to assess his culpability in relation to terrorist crimes; it was merely to deal with the medical and psychological problems that were impeding his preparation for trial. Even so, I could feel the familiar flutter of nerves in the pit of my stomach.

At last, the door to the room opened and Hamza was led in by an officer. In my mental image of him, formed from the press shots, he wore his usual preacher garb. But not in prison, of course. He was in a simple loose cotton shirt, and gone was his fearsome-looking hook. Instead, his arms ended in stumps.

He took a seat, but didn't speak until the officer had left and the door was shut.

Far from being a difficult interviewee, he was precisely the opposite. Speaking softly, he told me how grateful he was that I had taken the time to visit him. He was very sorry about any delays coming into the prison and he wished he were able to offer me a cup of tea. He presented as an intelligent and charming man. He was unfailingly polite and positively avuncular. He is highly educated, after all – he has a PhD in Civil Engineering, and once worked on the refurbishments of the Kingsway underpass and Royal Sandhurst Military College. He told me that he is a Koran memoriser and described a little about how he had become a preacher.

His double amputation was said to have occurred in a de-mining accident in post-Soviet Afghanistan. Although some have doubted this, no other concrete explanation has been put forward. As has been reported in recent press coverage, the stumps of both arms are subject to regular outbreaks of bone infection. Blind in one eye, he also suffers from diabetes and psoriasis, and has to take at least two showers a day because of a neurological condition that causes excessive sweating.

To prepare for his trial there was a great deal of footage of his sermons, plus numerous documents to consider. He said that he was finding the 'double-legal' body cavity searches, on the way in and out of meetings with his lawyers, both uncomfortable and oppressive. Without hands, he was having a particular problem in his cell activating the push-button taps on the sink. He had not been allowed his hook due to concerns about him using it as a weapon. His lack of hands also meant he was struggling to take his medication, as well as having difficulty applying his skin creams. The creams were going into his eyes and his glasses were getting dirty, preventing him from reading the papers in the case against him. The defence were looking for a reason to delay his trial from the hot summer of 2005 until the autumn, a request that, on the back of medical evidence, was granted by the Old Bailey judge.

But almost immediately after this, on 7 July 2005, four terrorists detonated homemade bombs in quick succession on three London Underground trains and a double-decker bus. Fifty-two UK residents of eighteen nationalities were killed and over seven hundred were injured. These bombings emphasised the stark reality of what the UK was up against with Islamic extremist terrorism, a reality that subsequent events has done nothing to allay.

Although the 7/7 cell were never directly linked to Hamza, his conviction later that year for incitement to murder must have been straightforward for the jury.

He was sentenced to seven years' imprisonment, and I assessed him a number of times over the following years for issues around the psychological impact of physical health problems in an ultra-high-security environment and for deportation issues. My psychiatric opinions and details of Hamza's medical conditions are described in some detail in various High Court judgements, including the judgement setting out the reasoning behind the final rejection of his appeals against extradition in 2012. He was always polite and pleased to see me. He said that personal details about his situation were being published in the tabloids and he found this humiliating. On the last occasion before his extradition to the US in

2012, he wished me well and thanked me for my interventions. 'Dr Taylor, when I write my book, I will mention you.'

What have I learned from this?

My colleagues say that I was simply hoodwinked by his charm. Maybe so. His demeanour was certainly disarming given the extreme nature of his stated beliefs. But I suggest that by the lazy stereotyping of picture editors – who always choose that image of him on a bad hair day with a hook over his eye – we fail to accurately portray him, and therefore neglect to understand his influence and that of other radical clerics. Don't choose that image with a hook. Show the one of him with a neat black turban and aviator shades outside Finsbury Park Mosque. He is polite, intelligent and charming – and no doubt persuasive – and this is surely part of who he is and what he did.

In May 2014, after extradition to the USA, Hamza was convicted of eleven terrorism-related charges, including his involvement in the 1998 kidnapping of sixteen tourists in Yemen, providing material support to terrorists, and attempting to create a terrorist training camp in Bly, Oregon (of all places), in 1999. According to media reporting, Hamza's defence to the kidnapping charge was that he had been trying to help negotiate release of the hostages via a satellite phone, as opposed to being involved in or directing the kidnapping – one man's hostage taker is another man's hostage negotiator, in other words. The jury were clearly not persuaded, and after conviction he was sentenced to two life sentences, plus one hundred years' imprisonment with no possibility of parole.

After conviction in Manhattan Federal Court, Hamza was sent to serve out his sentence at ADX Florence federal supermax prison, which also houses Richard Reid, the shoe bomber; Zacarias Moussaoui, from the 9/11 plot; Ramzi Yousef, the 1993 World Trade Center bomber; Dzhokhar Tsarnaev, of the Boston Marathon bombing; Ted Kaczynski, the Unabomber; and drugs kingpin 'El Chapo' Guzman. It previously held Timothy McVeigh, the Oklahoma bomber, too, but he was executed in 2001. Hamza is appealing that the conditions amount to a 'cruel and unusual punishment'. A recent prison photo leaked to the press shows him white-haired and emaciated. He has requested a return to Belmarsh, where (having made a legal appeal regarding the regime on the unit), he had at least been able to mingle with other inmates, and have access to a daily healthcare aide.

Michael Bachrach, one of Hamza's appeal lawyers, is quoted as saying: 'He would go back to Belmarsh in a second if he could,' adding, 'We strongly believe that the conditions of his confinement violate the expectations of the European Convention on Human Rights and the promises that were made by the US.'

ADX Florence is a secretive installation; low and sprawling by the foothills of the Rockies, one hundred miles south of Denver, it contains over forty convicted Al-Qaida terrorists. This is the place America sends the prisoners it wants to punish the most, and those too dangerous to house elsewhere. Prisoners spend up to twenty-three hours a day in their tiny cells, eating every meal there. The cell windows are blocked so they can't see the mountains. They can watch a 12-inch black-and-white television or read books to pass the time. If they behave, they may get limited exercise in a one-man recreation pen.

So maybe conditions in the unit at Belmarsh are not so harsh after all. I think the best description of ADX Florence comes from former warden Robert Hood.

'In our system, there are 122 federal prisons. And there's only one supermax. It's like the Harvard of the system. It replaced Alcatraz.'

When asked to describe ADX Florence further, Hood said:

'It's the ultimate of all prisons. It has has twelve gun towers and a lot of razor wire. There is absolutely no contact with other inmates. Even family visits can be banned under special administration measures. Any newspaper supplied will be at least thirty days old and the TV will be restricted to programmes like the History Channel, with no chance of current affairs. There will be no relent in these isolated conditions.

'It's a kind of death sentence. It's a clean version of hell. I don't know what hell is, but for a free person, [ADX Florence] is pretty close to it.'

For the most high-profile of terrorists, this really is throwing away the key.

28

Abu Hamza and his Al-Qaida-inspired followers were group-actor terrorists.

But the murderousness of terrorism has shifted away from organised group actors to the much-harder-to-disrupt lone actors. Paul Gill and his team at UCL studied over one hundred lone-actor cases (not just Islamic extremists) and made a number of interesting findings.

Firstly, in contrast with group actors, lone actors are much more likely to have a mental disorder, and they also tend to have a personal grievance in addition to a political, religious or historical one. The false dichotomy between mentally ill terrorists vs non-mentally ill terrorists has also been challenged. Gill found a higher prevalence of schizophrenia, delusional disorder and autistic spectrum disorders in lone actors, but mental disorder is not thought to be the single cause of the extremist behaviour. The explanation is rather that the route down the pathway to terrorist action is multifactorial, so mental disorder is merely one risk factor that, combined with others, such as exposure to a radicalising environment, may lead to terrorism.

Two of the most devastating lone-actor attacks of recent years were motivated by extreme right-wing politics. Brenton Tarrant, who murdered fifty-one and attempted to murder a further forty during his March 2019 attacks on mosques in Christchurch, New Zealand, was motivated by white supremacist and alt-right ideology. His automatic weapons were painted with words and symbols (some of them in Cyrillic and Greek) relating to the conflict between Christianity and

Islam. There has been no suggestion that he was mentally ill, although he clearly has very extreme views.

By contrast there has been international controversy about the mental state of Anders Breivik – another extreme right-wing lone-actor terrorist – who, in July 2011, killed eight people by detonating a van bomb in Oslo. This was a diversion for his main target, which was a summer camp of the Workers' Youth League on the island of Utøya. Wearing a paramilitary uniform, he posed as a police officer to gain access to the island, where he proceeded to hunt and kill sixty-nine young students – reportedly laughing while he did so. Breivik had two thorough psychiatric assessments after his arrest. The first concluded that he was delusional and potentially legally insane. The second concluded that he was not delusional but was just an extremist – albeit with a personality disorder – and therefore was fully responsible for his actions.

Given the appalling nature and number of his crimes, there was understandably intense public pressure for a criminal conviction rather than an insanity finding. In addition, Breivik was determined to avoid his ideas and actions being labelled in any way mentally abnormal.

Having visited Oslo for a seminar on terrorism, where I saw the bomb-damaged building and met one of the psychiatrists involved in this dispute, I have given some thought to the mind of mass murderer Anders Breivik.

In one sense it doesn't make much practical difference as to whether he is imprisoned or detained in a high-secure psychiatric facility, as it seems highly likely he will never see freedom again. But having at first been convinced that Breivik was not delusional but was a political extremist, what I've heard and read has forced me to change my view.

Another factor, it has been argued, is that after hearing he had been diagnosed as delusional in the first report, Breivik sought to downplay his bizarre beliefs in the second psychiatric assessment. That second assessment was therefore probably invalid, even though the diagnostic conclusion chimed with public opinion.

In the first evaluation, Breivik described himself in striking terms.

He said that he was the leader of the Knights Templar, which was, 'a military order, a martyr organisation, a military tribunal, judge, jury and executioner'. He compared himself to Tsar Nicholas of Russia and Queen Isabella of Spain. He believed he would be the new ruler of Norway following a *coup d'état*. He said he was able to decide who should live and who should die in Norway, and he believed that a considerable proportion of the Norwegian population supported his deeds. He claimed that if he became the new regent of Norway, he would be given the responsibility for deporting several hundred thousand Muslims to North Africa. He thought the events he was a part of could start a nuclear Third World War.

I am persuaded that these are grandiose delusions which are so idiosyncratic and extreme as to be outside the sub-cultural beliefs even of Scandinavian neo-Nazis. Breivik was highly organised and he took years to plan his attack – for example, renting enough farmland to justify his purchase of fertiliser to make his bomb – but purposeful behaviour does not preclude delusional thinking.

In London, there has been an example of a more spontaneous and chaotic lone-actor attack by a man with a mental disorder. On 5 December 2015, twenty-nine-year-old Muhaydin Mire, a British Somali man, used a bread knife to attack three people at Leytonstone Underground station in east London. One of the three victims was seriously injured. A junior doctor who was passing the scene controlled the victim's bleeding, probably saving his life, while the other two victims sustained minor stab wounds.

During the attack, Mire had declared, 'This is for Syria, my Muslim brothers . . . all your blood will be spilled.'

He had a history of psychotic episodes and delusions that he was being followed by MI5 and MI6. Around a month before the attack, Mire's family had tried to get him sectioned, but he was found to pose no risk to himself or others.

Mire was convicted of attempted murder and four counts of attempted wounding, and was sentenced to life imprisonment with a minimum term of eight-and-a-half years. He was later transferred to Broadmoor hospital for psychiatric treatment. Although mentally ill at the time of the attack, his delusions had become wrapped in religious ideology.

ISIS calls on Muslims to engage in violence to regain the honour of Islam, with use of the term 'caliphate' conjuring up images of a culturally superior Islamic world. Initially many young Europeans travelled to Syria to become jihadis, but once ISIS territorial gains had begun to reverse, ISIS started instructing followers to commit low-technology attacks, thus weaponising this form of lone-actor extremist violence to devastating effect. Online publications such as *Dabiq* magazine, and gory murder cult videos, gave direct encouragement to take a knife or a vehicle to kill the non-believer. The simple act of the perpetrator scrawling an ISIS symbol on a piece of paper is enough for ISIS to claim the attack. The symbol is the first part of the Islamic declaration of faith, or *shahada* – 'There is no God but Allah' – then, below that, a circle, which signifies the image of the prophet's seal and contains the second part of the declaration: 'Muhammad is the prophet of God.'

Recent years have seen many lone-actor attacks using knives and vehicles, and also the highly unstable home-made bombs of Manchester Arena and Parsons Green. This is ISIS-inspired lone-actor terrorism as opposed to ISIS-directed terrorism. In other words, there is often no evidence of any command and control or communication between the perpetrator and an ISIS handler.

Lone-actor terrorists seem to have wrapped personal grievance about an unfulfilled life in a cloak of religious protest. Personal grievance may arise from a feeling of disadvantage and social exclusion, fuelled by incomplete education, illicit drug use, antisocial behaviour and failed employment and relationships. Khalid Masood, the Westminster Bridge attacker of 2017, is a case in point. Masood killed four and injured more than fifty with a rented grey Hyundai Tucson car, before stabbing PC Keith Palmer to death at the entrance to the Palace of Westminster. He had a violent history, but there was no evidence of any contact with ISIS handlers. In a WhatsApp message, sent just minutes before his attack, he sent an emoji kiss and asked for forgiveness, but also said he was waging jihad in revenge against Western military action in the Middle East.

His final attack may have represented a desire to go out in a blaze of glory, with death as a result of suicide by cop as part of the script. This has some parallels with what is colloquially known as 'running amok'. In fact, amok is a behavioural syndrome described in the Malay Archipelago as long ago as the sixteenth century and recorded by seafaring explorer Captain Cook. It has equivalents in other cultures, including 'berserkers', a Norse term referring to those who fight in a trance and a word which has also entered the English language. Amok usually involves a man with no history of violence who, after a prodromal period of withdrawal or depression, acquires a weapon – usually bladed – and then suddenly engages in a paroxysmal homicidal attack with apparent loss of self-control. The episode ends with the attacker being killed by bystanders or taking their own life. Those who run amok were once thought to be psychotic or in a trance-like state, or just at the end of their rope. ('Going postal' would be the modern American equivalent.) But amok may also be a useful description for the behaviour of lone-actor terrorists or spree killers enacting a final homicide-suicide in response to personal grievances that may or may not be wrapped up in an ideological cloak.

Elevated rates of mental disorder have been found in other types of lone-actor attack, for example, in David James's study of twenty-four lone perpetrators who carried out serious attacks on European politicians between 1990 and 2004. A high proportion of the attackers – almost half – were found to be psychotic, but their delusional fixations on their target were sometimes mistaken for politically motivated beliefs.

The most recent study by Paul Gill's team in 2020 has found that lone-actor terrorists have a lot in common with another form of lone-actor attack, which is single-issue spree shooters (those who kill more than four victims in total, in different locations). So both groups can be considered variants of lone-actor grievance-fuelled violence (LAGV).[58]

One important additional finding is that lone-actor terrorists are more likely than spree shooters to leak details of their attack to a friend or on Facebook, but not to the target. This may provide an opportunity for intervention, for example by monitoring of open source communications – web postings, Facebook updates, et cetera. The moral of this story is that anyone who witnesses declared murderous terrorist intentions should always take them seriously, although some lone actors are becoming wise to this, posting online only minutes before an attack (as in the New Zealand mosque shootings) to minimise the chance of any law enforcement intervention.

Many recent lone actors have committed suicide by bomb (Manchester Arena) or by cop, by wearing fake bomb vests (Westminster Bridge, both London Bridge attacks and Streatham). But what is in the mind of those willing to kill themselves for their cause? Are they also suicidal?

Terrorist suicide attacks have long been thought to have an intensely religious or extremist motivation, along with a willingness to make the ultimate sacrifice. But it seems that some who are already mentally disturbed and suicidal may say to themselves, 'I feel like killing myself. I might as well wrap it up in a cause and make some use of it.'

Ariel Merari[59] was able to study suicide bombers who were on the brink of suicide by bomb but whose device had failed to ignite. Merari interviewed Palestinian suicide terrorists, a control group of non-suicide terrorists and a group of organisers of suicide attacks. The would-be suicides were more likely to exhibit personality traits which made them more susceptible to influence. Some of the potential bombers, but none of the control and organiser group, had suicidal tendencies, depression and histories of childhood abuse.

Further research comparing thirty female and thirty male suicide terrorists from various groups, such as Hamas, Chechen separatists, the Tamil Tigers and Al-Qaida, found that female suicide terrorists were motivated more by personal events, whereas males were motivated more by religious/nationalistic factors. The types of personal events in female suicide terrorists included a history of drug problems or drug overdose, suicidal thoughts and self-reported depression.

There has also been extensive research on the group dynamics of terrorist cells, and one formulation has been proposed by John Alderdice, a psychiatrist and senior politician in Northern Ireland. Lord Alderdice has suggested that terrorist activities involve the premeditated use of violence to create a climate of fear aimed at a wider audience than the immediate victims, and he suggests that terrorist acts may be a repetition and re-enactment of historical conflicts and traumas which go back many generations – if past traumas are unresolved, then they may be repeated and perpetuated in a vicious cycle of violence.

This analysis is relevant to the effects of Guantanamo Bay and prison kettlings discussed earlier. Experiences of disrespect and humiliation may drive violence as a revenge for social and cultural wrongs, and as a way to reverse this humiliation. Note that there have been no protests from the Muslim world about ADX Florence. It may be harsh and utterly austere, but it has judicial legitimacy and does not seek to publicly humiliate.

Where does all this lead us in terms of preventing future lone-actor attacks?

One man's returning foreign-trained-fighter is another man's potential lone-actor terrorist, so how do we differentiate joyful holidaymakers from jihadi extremists – and how can we identify who will be the next Westminster or London Bridge lone-actor attacker?

The shorter the period of prediction, the easier it is. A force-ten storm in the Irish Sea means imminent risk of windy weather in Liverpool. Likewise, trouble may reasonably be expected from a highly radicalised prisoner due for imminent release.

To tackle this essential yet difficult task, Reid Meloy has identified eight proximal warning behaviours and ten distal characteristics of the lone-actor terrorist, which are incorporated in a risk assessment tool, the Terrorist Radicalization Assessment Protocol-18 (TRAP-18).[60] The risk factors include: personal grievance and moral outrage; failure to affiliate with an extremist group (terrorist cell rejects, in other words); dependence on a virtual community found on the internet; the thwarting of occupational goals; the failure of sexual pair bonding and mental disorder. The TRAP-18 may help as part of a structured anchored professional judgement, not forgetting that hair-on-the-back-of-the-neck feeling.

*

More recently, I interviewed a very young man who was considered to be a high-risk terrorist prisoner, with aspirations to kill others during a suicidal lone-actor attack. What was his profile and mindset?

His father had physically abused and then disowned him. He had dropped out of education and used drugs. He had no work and no current intimate relationship. He had looked at the dark web out of boredom, found *The Anarchist Cookbook* and become addicted to ISIS beheading videos, saying he liked the powerful soundtrack of jihadi *nasheeds* (chanting).

'[Watching ISIS videos] made my heart sink. [I couldn't stand seeing] bombs dropped on innocent people.'

'I watched online videos of Abdullah al-Faisal and Anwar al-Awlaki [both radical preachers].'

'I followed Salafist [jihadi] thinking and I was reading the hadiths and studying Islam more intensively recently.'

'I was attracted to the idea of the Caliphate. I believed there should be a Caliphate.'

'I watched videos of white phosphorus burning people alive and videos of drone strikes. I was very angry with whoever was doing it.'

'I thought Assad in Syria is an idiot. The behaviour of the Assad regime is disgusting.'

'I believe in *takfir* [labelling people as kafir or unbelievers].'

'I believe that Apostates [those who renounce Islam] should be beheaded.'

'But I'm not sure, as the prison Imam told me that this is wrong.'

It is easy to see how an impressionable young man with these attitudes could be malleable enough, in the company of older, more experienced, ISIS-inspired prisoners, to be pushed along the pathway towards a murderous terrorist attack.

ISIS may have been defeated on the battlefield in Syria and Iraq, but a core group of battle-hardened veterans – the rump of the Caliphate's army – could easily be the nucleus of a resurgent ISIS. The international community's abandonment of young jihadi brides and their children at al-Hawl refugee camp plays into the ISIS narrative of mistreatment by the West. And, given the confusion caused by US and Turkish military actions in northern Syria, there must be a significant risk of a re-emergence of ISIS in the region.

Even if this doesn't happen, there is enough ISIS recruitment material circulating on the web to motivate those with an Islamic extremist mindset. Likewise, the manifestos and mass murders of right-wing extremists, such as Anders Breivik in Norway and Brenton Tarrant in New Zealand, may provide both an inspiration and a template that could push those with personal grievances and underlying mental vulnerability into murderous action.

Sentencing, Treatment, Recovery and Release

29

Most murderers spend a long time in prison. Prison is used for retribution and punishment; to keep the public safe; for deterrence of other would-be killers; and, last of all, for rehabilitation which depends on the jurisdiction and on how serious the crime. In the USA, what amount to whole-life prison terms are common, especially after convictions for first-degree murder – that is, intentional murder with pre-planning or malice aforethought. Amongst the 2.3 million prisoners in the US, over 100,000 prisoners convicted of murder are serving life imprisonment without possibility of parole, or sentences so long – in one case 750 years – that death in custody is certain.

At the same time, the proportion of offenders sent to secure psychiatric hospital after being found not guilty by reason of insanity is very low, and so there are many psychotic murderers in US prisons rather than hospitals, often receiving inadequate treatment.

When imposing a mandatory life sentence for murder, sentencing judges in the UK set the minimum term. Depending on the facts of the case, this minimum term has three potential starting points from which the sentence may then be increased or reduced, according to aggravating and mitigating factors. For adult offenders, a whole-life minimum term applies to double murder and to repeat murder offences by someone who has killed before (two strikes and you're out). Thirty years is the starting point for cases involving firearms or explosives. Those committing postcode drug-gang turf-war killings who bring a knife to the scene can expect twenty-five years. Otherwise, for an impulsive, unplanned killing of a single victim, fifteen years is the baseline. Years will added on if there are aggravating factors, such as: a significant degree of planning; an older or disabled victim; suffering inflicted on the victim before death; the killing of a public servant; and concealing or dismembering the body. Mitigating factors, which can take years off the minimum term, include: the lack of premeditation; the killer themselves being in fear of violence; and the killing being considered a 'mercy killing', for example of a terminally ill relative. The victim's family can choose to make a personal statement, which the judge will use to assess the impact of the crime and pass sentence accordingly.

A life sentence always lasts for the rest of the offender's life, no matter how long or short the minimum term. At the end of the minimum term, the offender can apply to the parole board for release on life licence, but will only be released if they are no longer a risk to the public. So life does mean life for many killers.

But for most 'lifers', a decision must be made at some point about safety for release, and this will be addressed by a panel of three, comprising of a judge, a lay person and a psychiatrist (or clinical psychologist). Second killings after release are extremely rare but even so, between January 2007 and May 2015, twelve people were murdered by convicted killers.

In the UK, the proportion of killers who are sectioned to a secure hospital has been declining (especially where illicit drug use is a feature). A hospital order (section) to secure psychiatric hospital is only available for around twenty to thirty cases initially charged with murder in an average year. Whether the perpetrator is sent to prison or to hospital, the principles are much the same in terms of the treatment, recovery and re-offending risk assessment of those who have killed.

*

The cases in this book have described the myriad nature and circumstances of those who kill, which leads us on to the question of how a murderer is made – and if we can unmake them. Some murderers are born, like those who inherit an increased risk for schizophrenia and who kill while psychotic, or the small group of children with inherited callous unemotional (CU) traits (like Lee Watson from chapter three). But even with schizophrenia, genes are only half the story. And for fledgling psychopaths, it is the environment that determines whether the adult outcome is sadistic killer or corporate snake – drug-ridden housing estate vs Winchester College, for example.

The fact is that most murderers are neither born nor made but a mixture of both. The current research findings[61] have shown that it is a complex interplay of genes and environment that leads to the antisocial behaviour and substance abuse that are found in the backstory of many killers. In the past, genetic and behavioural influences on child development focused on two possible mechanisms. The first of these is the suggestion that it is the individual child's own biological make-up which adversely influences the parent–child relationship. In other words, if an infant has a hard-wired problem with emotion regulation or temperament, this will have an adverse impact on the relationship between mother and child from a very young age. The notion of the hard-wired problem child that cannot be modified by parenting is illustrated by the eponymous character in Lionel Shriver's novel *We Need to Talk About Kevin*. It is the biological make-up of the child which influences that child's environment.

The alternative model is the reverse, by which I mean it is the environment that directly influences an individual child's biology. For example, a parent that fails to respond to a child's needs appropriately may cause psychological and emotional stress, which in turn provokes an increase in adrenaline, which adversely impacts on emotion regulation in the child. But these processes cannot be separated, and so current research focuses on how these Genetic and Environmental ($G \times E$) elements work together as each individual child develops.

Child development researchers, such as Marian Bakermans-Kranenburg and Marinus Van IJzendoorn in the Netherlands, have analysed data from long-term cohort studies, where the same subjects are followed throughout a long period of time (in this case, from childhood), with repeated sequential batteries of blood tests, interviews and collateral record searching. These studies have shown interactions between candidate genes and environmental factors such as caregiving setting and parental sensitivity. The interaction of genes with the childhood environment is thought to be mediated via the attachment relationship to the mother or other caregiver, which I will describe in more detail shortly. Specific genes may lead to variations in the levels of various chemicals that affect the brain and behaviour, such as dopamine, serotonin and oxytocin, but these biological predictors of behaviour may be moderated by the environment in which the child is raised. For example, research with children in institutional care[62] showed that those carrying the same gene variation as a control group of children in the more nurturing environment of foster care had a much a higher likelihood of disrupted attachment to parents. Conversely, for children in the same child-rearing environment, differing genetic make-up may predict an adverse outcome. But each child is individual, and even children in the same environment and with the same biology may develop along different pathways.

And so, whether genes associated with later antisocial behaviour are present or not, the outcome is modified by early experience: often as early as their interactions with the primary caregiver – the mother – during the first eighteen months of their life.

In other words, nurture can substantially modify nature – and vice versa.

This applies to young, antisocial men who kill each other with knives; men and women who kill their intimate partners; those who kill while drunk or high on drugs; and those who kill as a result of violent extremism. Many of them are likely to do what they do at least in part as a result of their early interactions with their mother. For this reason, the target of treatment for those who kill often involves trying to mitigate or reverse the effects of the adverse childhood experiences, while accepting that there may be underlying biological or innate and hard wired factors which make this treatment process more difficult.

My forensic patients often have interpersonal problems that don't fit into standard psychiatric diagnostic boxes, one of which is best described by the concept of attachment disorder mentioned above. If I had to pick one theme that connects many different types of murder, then this is it: studies have shown that violent offending is strongly associated with disordered attachment.[63]

Attachment disorder theories are based on the work of psychiatrist John Bowlby, who researched the positive and nurturing bonds created between infants and their mothers, which he called the secure base. His theories have subsequently been supported by extensive experimental research with young children by Mary Ainsworth[64] and others. Secure attachments to caregivers are said to be an evolutionary necessity, as they provide a safe haven for managing an infant's distress in response to threat. Early attachment bonds are reflected in adulthood relationships, having been found to affect how someone copes with stressful life events.

Infants who have experienced stable parenting become securely attached – they are able to use the caregiver as a base from which to explore the surrounding environment and as a source of comfort when distressed or threatened. Securely attached adults value relationships, seek out intimacy and support, and are able to explore unfavourable feelings. Conversely, in forensic patients – and in others with various mental disorders – there is often attachment disorder, illustrated by insecure emotional regulation and excessive sensitivity to being let down in relationships.[65] At times, this means that distressed patients can be indifferent to the attempts of treating staff to help them, as they've not been used to this kind of support in childhood.

There is a structured interview that can be used to tease out these issues and this can inform treatment. Questions include: 'Can you remember times when you were emotionally upset, physically hurt, separated or rejected, or suffered abuse or loss?'

'I am not sure that I can always depend on others to be there when I need them – yes or no?'

It is not difficult to imagine how Charlotte, who killed her abusive partner Lennie, would answer these questions in light of her experience of childhood abuse by her stepfather, with a mother who looked the other way and failed to protect her.

Many of the treatments for murderers apply to the ones who end up in prison as much as those in secure psychiatric hospital. But although both groups may have personality disorder and illicit drug abuse, the ticket for entry to psychiatric hospital is usually psychosis at the time of the offence.

All killers are unique to some extent, but I can divide my psychotic patients who have killed into three broad clusters. There are those who have led a 'normal' life before the onset of psychosis and who respond quickly to antipsychotic medication, recovering insight, engaging with treatment and progressing quickly – such as Jonathan Brooks from chapter seven.

Then there is a second group, whose psychosis is already long-standing before they kill. They are often resistant to treatment; their progress can be slow and tortuous, and for some, a return to the community is just not safe.

The final cluster is the triple diagnosis group, which is the most common. This group have what you might call a 'triple whammy' of diagnoses, by which I mean a combination of personality disorder, illicit drug use and psychosis.

These patients present with a combination of the abused and neglected childhood of Charlotte, the alcohol or drug use of Dennis Costas (who immolated his girlfriend) and the psychosis of Jonathan Brooks (who killed his mother). They are disadvantaged, neglected and abused young men and women with failed education and work histories. They tend to have maladaptive coping strategies which involve self-harm and/or antisocial behaviour. They've used illicit drugs and abused alcohol and, on top of all that disadvantage and their bad life choices, they suffer the onset of psychosis – that is, serious mental illness – during early adulthood. And this is when they kill. Psychiatrist and psychoanalyst Dr Robert Hale described this group in his paper 'Flying a Kite', which was based on over 2,000 cases.[66]

Recovery can be a case of 'two steps forward, one step back'.

Self-defeating behaviour patterns and difficulty forging relationships can lead to conflict with staff and other patients, with reversion to antisocial or self-harming behaviour, aggression, drug use and poor engagement with therapy.

Trying to treat this group is a core part of forensic psychiatric work. Many respond to antipsychotic drugs, meaning the psychosis fades into the background. The personality disorder and challenging behaviour then become the main focus of treatment and risk management.

A typical case of mine like this would involve a homicide in a patient's early twenties, in the course of a psychotic and/or manic episode. After transfer to secure psychiatric hospital, they might respond to antipsychotic and mood-stabilising medication, but the backstory usually confirms that I have a lot more to do than just treat psychosis with medication.

Typically, the father has been violent, hard-drinking and later absent. There will have been violent abuse of the mother and the child (later my patient). Often the mother may have been hospitalised with depression, for example, or just emotionally unavailable and focused on her own needs (drug use or placating multiple abusive partners).

This means that the opportunity for stable attachment will have been missed. There is often a history of being sent to live with extended family or grandparents, local authority intervention, foster care or children's homes. Those with a childhood disrupted by these unstable, delegated parenting arrangements will often go on to struggle in education. They might be disruptive in class and inattentive. They then get into fights, start truanting and end up suspended or excluded from school, resorting to alcohol and cannabis abuse at an early age and coming into contact with a delinquent peer group. There may be an attempt to reach out to absent parents, only to have the door closed in their face.

If the child develops an early pattern of conduct disorder, such as aggressive, deceitful or destructive behaviour, then this is more likely to lead to life-course-persistent antisocial behaviour, in contrast to later-onset peer-influenced or socialised conduct disorder. Typically, a delinquent peer group or gang can provide bonds which are absent in the family, and there may be early involvement at the lower end of the drugs trade. Postcode gang violence might also force them to seek protection in company.

I recently dealt with a young man who went on to kill at age eighteen in a 'joint enterprise' gang stabbing. (Verdict: murder. Life imprisonment; sixteen-year minimum term.)

He had been threatened by other lads at his pupil referral unit and absconded from London to Cardiff to seek sanctuary with his uncle and two cousins. Perhaps he envied his cousins' more stable existence. (My cousin Hannah had no doubt envied me, my brother and our other two sets of cousins for our stable, loving homes.)

What usually follows is the chaotic world of youth offending. In the UK, we have one of the youngest ages of criminal responsibility – age ten – and so young offenders will soon find themselves in and out of the courts, probation and custody. After community orders for offences like public disorder, robbery of a mobile phone and theft of a restaurant meal while drunk at Brixton Spudulike (in one case of mine), offending often escalates to possession of drugs with intent to supply. There are periods in custody, punctuated by incomplete attempts at further education or work. Prison sentences may lead to victimisation – like being slashed across the face with a prison shank (made from a razor blade melted into a toothbrush).

These experiences can contribute to paranoia, which is then made worse by smoking cannabis on a daily basis, especially the more potent skunk.

What can follow is early contact with psychiatric services after offences of violence linked to paranoia and intoxication. These episodes will typically be written off as drug-induced, although with hindsight, once we examine the history in detail at the forensic unit, we can see a pattern of more enduring psychosis emerging.

It is during this psychosis that the offence of murder is committed. This is often through use of excessive violence in response to a sense of threat, or may involve more systematised delusional thinking. A young psychotic man who believes his neighbours are listening in on him may burst through the door swinging a weapon. Or there may be more complex beliefs about global power elites trying to establish a totalitarian new world order. Such ideas are popular among conspiracy theorists, but Illuminati preoccupations can also become entwined with psychotic delusions.

There is often mood disturbance as well as psychosis at the time of the killing. For example, a few days before an attempted murder committed by Lloyd, one of my forensic patients, his girlfriend had come home to find the door of her ground-floor flat wide open. Her television, stereo, CD collection and clothes were missing, as was the furniture. Even the new mixer tap had been unscrewed and taken, the bathroom left with water leaking on to the floor.

The person responsible for the manic flat clearance, Lloyd, had a backstory much as I've described above. After emptying the flat, he had been found out on the street, speaking loudly and rapidly, telling passers-by to take what they wanted. Following this, he disappeared for a day, whereabouts unknown. Then, manic and paranoid, he attacked a fellow passenger on a train platform with a broken bottle. Although it was psychosis (schizoaffective disorder) that may have tipped him over the edge, his life trajectory was heading towards persistent adult antisocial behaviour and drug use.

So, how might this trajectory have been different? Would a firm hand from the absent father have helped? What treatment or intervention might have diverted Lloyd from his pathway to offending and ultimately to murder?

Research has shown that harsh discipline doesn't actually work as a child-rearing strategy, especially with the most antisocial kids. Fledgling psychopaths with callous-unemotional traits often make excellent bullies, choosing skilfully how best to hurt their victims without caring about the impact, and they are notably impervious to punishment.

More effective parenting strategies have been identified in research. Child psychiatrist Stephen Scott studied video recordings of child-parent interactions and found that really effective parents use far more carrot than stick. The best parenting approach is to increase positive child behaviour through praise and incentives, improve parent-child interaction through relationship-building, set clear expectations and use non-aversive (non-violent) management strategies as a consequence for non-compliance or problem behaviour. These principles have been further modified into the Helping Families Programme, a sixteen-session intervention using structured, goal-orientated strategies and collaborative therapeutic methods to improve parenting, and child and parent functioning. Current research led by clinical psychologist Crispin Day[67] is testing this intervention on a particularly vulnerable group of children at high risk of adverse developmental outcome: namely, children with significant emotional/behavioural difficulties who have parents affected by severe personality difficulties. Early feasibility studies have been encouraging, but the ongoing randomised controlled trial comparing this programme against a standard psychoeducation approach will be the only way to be sure. Unfortunately, in the UK, whenever the issue of adverse childhood development and youth antisocial behaviour comes up in public and political discourse, the discussion around appropriate interventions tends to involve populist and jingoistic rhetoric instead of empirical research evidence.

Judicial approaches like 'scared straight', boot camp, short, sharp shocks or youth imprisonment may seem plausible, and are often espoused by populist politicians looking to impress voters with their law-and-order credentials, but the evidence is that they don't produce any benefits.

Family interventions that take the other tack have been shown to reduce youth re-offending rates by a third to a half. These interventions aim to help parents develop the right carrot/stick combination, promote time with a pro-social peer group, sort out after-school activities and empower the family to be assertive in dealing with neighbourhood problems. Admittedly, that last item is a tough nut to crack on a London housing estate.

How much carrot and how much stick?

In research, the best foster parents – those who repeatedly turn around behaviourally disturbed kids – give positive praise or neutral feedback thirty times more frequently than negative criticism.

With this empirical evidence in mind, I have found myself consciously trying to use more positive re-enforcement of good behaviour than telling-off for bad with my own kids. I am uncomfortable around parents who lose self-control with explosive rage and shouting. I prefer to earn the respect of my children, rather than demand it.

But what do we actually do – in the UK especially – with troubled adolescents who offend? The answer is that we put them in local authority secure accommodation or Feltham Young Offender Institute.

Criminologist Loraine Gelsthorpe suggests that public discourse about criminal justice policy in the UK reflects social processes known as late modernity, as illustrated by the emergence of a culture of control and the politicisation of law and order. This means that discussions about punishment of young offenders tend towards the demonisation of young people who commit offences.[68] It has also been suggested that a neo-liberal economic model, coupled with a first-past-the-post political system, fosters a tendency towards populist law-and-order politics in common with other 'majoritarian' countries where political parties must target crucial swing voters.

By contrast, in corporatist or social democracies (those much-vaunted Nordic countries again), a disturbed eight-, nine- or ten-year-old child that commits a serious violent offence is seen as a tragic failing and problem for society to solve collaboratively, rather than an evil child to demonise and condemn.[69]

Young offenders will find themselves somewhere such as Feltham, a troubled place where violent incidents, high levels of self-harm and assaults against staff are rife. As a result, it's more intimidating than many adult prisons I visit, where many inmates just want a quiet life on a settled wing. One case that highlights how adverse an environment Feltham can be was that of Robert Stewart, who I interviewed before his trial and conviction for the murder of cellmate Zahid Mubarek. Zahid Mubarek was a teenager serving ninety days for shoplifting. On his last night in prison, he was in a shared cell with Robert Stewart, who had a catalogue of offences on his record. Stewart had expressed racist views and had a cross with the letters 'RIP' tattooed on his forehead. During that night, he took a broken table leg and beat Mubarek around the head, killing him. (Verdict: murder. Life imprisonment; twenty-five-year minimum term.)

The subsequent Mubarek inquiry reported a 'bewildering catalogue of shortcomings' that contributed to the death, with prison overcrowding and low staff morale playing a key role in Feltham collapsing as an institution in the run-up to the murder.

In my experience, Feltham often failed to set young offenders back on the right path. Imprisonment, especially during short sentences when there's not much opportunity for education or treatment, does little to avert the downward spiral of a return to further drug use and offending behaviour. This can then trigger that psychotic state and murderous behaviour which leads to secure hospital transfer and, frequently, a diagnosis of schizophrenia or schizoaffective disorder.

In cases of psychosis with seriously violent behaviour, we often have to medicate without consent (while adhering to stringent safeguards). This is one of the most difficult aspects of forensic psychiatry: forcing treatment on someone who doesn't want it. We do it because we know that, for around three-quarters of our patients, they will improve. Many – though, sadly, not all – later develop insight (that is, they realise that the treatment helps). But it's not something we do lightly or without considerable thought.

The mainstay of treatment for the mood component of schizoaffective disorder is a mood stabiliser like lithium (or various alternatives) along with the dopamine-blocking antipsychotics I have described in earlier chapters.

Lithium salts have been a tried-and-tested anti-manic ever since the evidence for their efficacy emerged via Danish studies as early as 1950. In the early 1960s, when my aunt Georgina was recovering in St James's Hospital in Portsmouth, lithium was available, as were the first generation of antipsychotics, such as chlorpromazine.[70] Georgina recently told me (over fifty years on) that various medications were tried, but they did not make her feel better. She was tormented by delusions of contamination or infestation (known as Ekbom's Syndrome), and no doubt guilt at what she had done in smothering her daughter.

It was after this treatment failure and several suicide attempts that she had readily agreed to pyschosurgery, and she remembers talking it through with her psychiatrist. Georgina gave fully informed consent and went on to have two lobotomies, several years apart. She didn't get full relief from the first operation, but felt much improved after the second.

To my surprise, I was recently able to track down Georgina's psychiatrist, Dr Ian Christie, a former medical director of two psychiatric hospitals and pioneer of novel treatments. Dr Christie told me that a number of his patients in those days had lobotomies, and in his experience many of them benefited. Some did not, but he did not observe any disastrous outcomes. He said the principle indication for psychosurgery was 'extreme distress' in the context of mental illness, and that certainly fits Georgina's own description of her state in that period.

By the time of Georgina's last operation, her surviving daughter Hannah was old enough to visit her in hospital. Georgina remembers young Hannah being upset and frightened by the sight of her mother with her head swathed in dressings. But the long-term adverse impact on Hannah was more than just having seen the scary bandages. Georgina was too unwell to be a consistently available mother, and so Hannah suffered that disrupted early attachment that is known to predispose adults to maladjustment.

By chance, Dr Christie's subsequent career illustrates the changing attitudes to psychiatric treatment in the 1960s and 1970s, as he went on to pioneer alternative approaches which are still used in forensic psychiatry today. In 1968 he and David Warren-Holland founded a therapeutic community in the 'Pink Villa Huts' of St James' Hospital in Portsmouth.

Inspired by residential visits to the Phoenix unit in New York, these two wooden buildings situated in the hospital grounds were the start of Europe's first concept-based therapeutic community (TC). The philosophy was to 'provide total rehabilitation for an individual . . . by challenging and reinforcing that which is positive and normal so that the ability exists to eventually overcome that which is distorted and sick in the personality'. This approach had also been developed at the Northfield Military Hospital during the Second World War, where the idea was that the hospital worked as a community, with every member sharing in decision-making. In addition, reality confrontation was used in large groups to help patients understand how others saw their behaviour.

Therapeutic communities remain the gold standard for managing serious offenders with personality disorder, and there are TCs, for example, at the Millfields Unit in east London, and at

HMP Grendon near Aylesbury, where many murderers on life sentences can seek treatment.

Treatment in forensic psychiatry involves a synthesis of these two opposing approaches: the manipulation of brain function with psychotropic drugs at one end, and social treatment via a community experience at the other, as well as more or less everything in between that has been shown to work – by which I mean the various group and individual therapies to address offending and other problem behaviours.

There are many different talking therapies for antisocial men and women and their problems with paranoia, anger and drug use, and they must be tailored for each patient, much as I described earlier with therapy for borderline personality disorder. These therapies are often cognitive behavioural, but we take an eclectic approach and use 'what works'.

Reasoning and Rehabilitation (R&R), which is used in prison and probation, and which targets offending behaviour, has been adapted for hospital use. It employs a problem-focused approach to address single-symptom issues, such as how to manage anger (without hitting someone).

Forensic patients may have difficulties in asserting themselves. They might bottle up frustration, only to explode with aggression later. Teaching them how to assert themselves verbally – in an R&R group – can reduce this tendency. It's a bit like learning how to politely send an undercooked plate of food back to the pub kitchen, rather than opting not to complain and repressing that frustration, only to end up letting it all out at the bar staff later on.

Working with a clinical psychologist, individually and in groups, on drug use, insight into mental health relapse, assertiveness, anger and the causes of aggression, we aim to help our patients gradually improve their understanding of the interaction between psychosis and its treatment, as well as personality traits such as paranoia and impulsivity, illicit drug use, and how all this links to violent behaviour.

Alongside therapies it is also important to try to divine the 'meaning' of the killing for each offender. This is because if we don't understand what the offence means, then we risk it being repeated. Second and third homicides of intimate partners in similar circumstances have happened – inexcusably – although this is extremely rare. By the same token, there is a risk that an incomplete offence may later be completed, like the case of one of my patients who had killed his mother-in-law while meaning to kill his wife, or another who had killed her aunt while meaning to kill her mother – an unconcious displacement.

In both cases, the intended victim remained at large and needed to be kept in mind.

Psychotic offences are often self-preservative. As far as one of my patients was concerned, at the material time when he attacked someone with a broken bottle, a conspiratorial and murderous Illuminati persecutor had become confrontational and abusive to him, so he had to defend himself.

We had to keep him free from psychosis with medication, and away from the drugs which could also increase his paranoia and aggression. And most of all, we had to help him learn to believe that people wouldn't always let him down; to reduce his impulsive aggression and equip him with better ways of resolving conflict. On top of that, our occupational therapy team then needed to give him life skills and help him find training that suited him, to ultimately bring him to a level of functioning well above anything he had achieved before. By that I mean getting him to a stage where he was ready to work, or at least to carry out a structured programme of useful activities. Sometimes, as suggested by Gwen Adshead,[71] it feels as if we're providing a second chance for the patient to experience the 'secure base' of supportive and consistent parenting, along with stable education and work training.

Once a sufficiently stable mental state and behaviour has been achieved, then we can begin to look at escorted leave outside of the hospital perimeter, always watchful for any relapse factors, violence risk or what we call offence-paralleling behaviours. In a homicide case, it is typical for the hospital stay to be at least five and up to ten years or more, so we sometimes end up working with a patient for a decade. When they do make progress, there can be a sense of achievement. Before we can contemplate release, however, we must consider the risk, and for that we have to use a combination of actuarial and clinical factors. Historical factors are mostly fixed – like previous violence at a young age. You can't undo the past. Lloyd, for example, had plenty of actuarial risk.

To help target strategies for managing this, we use a checklist developed in the Netherlands. It's a scale of protective factors that have been shown to lessen the risk of violence, which include employment, leisure activities, financial management, social network, intimate relationships and living circumstances. And they are all factors that we can help to change.

With our secure hospital patients, we only discharge them to supported accommodation, with a programme of work or training and close supervision by a full team, and (if necessary) long-acting injectable medication, which we know they are taking. In other words, we beef up those protective factors.

Incidentally, attention to these aspects would also improve the outcome for prisoners released at the end of a sentence. I visited Suomenlinna open prison in Helsinki, where the policy is that no prisoner is discharged without a place to live and a job or training lined up. In the UK, by contrast, we often release prisoners with a £46 discharge grant and a black bin bag for their possessions.

As well as using more of a Finland-style[72] planned discharge model for forensic psychiatric patients, we share information with other agencies, and the views of the victim's family will be sought. This may result in an exclusion zone to reduce their distress and to manage the danger of any future conflict.

Having ensured that all this support is in place, and after many years of intensive treatment, diligent risk management and cautious testing via gradually increasing periods of leave from hospital, we do eventually release our patients, although we have the power to recall them at a moment's notice.

I was walking my daughter to junior school a few years ago when, on the other side of the road, a man in his forties waved at me cheerily. 'Hello, Dr Taylor.'

I waved back politely. 'Hi, Eugene.'

Eugene had spent many years under my care, having beaten his father to death and set fire to him before sticking a meat thermometer into his abdomen. He was acutely psychotic at the time.

'Why did you do that, Eugene?'

'To see if he was done, I suppose.'

Eugene had recovered and, after a prolonged stable period and lots of testing, had been discharged under close supervision.

'Who was that, Daddy?'

'Oh, just someone I used to work with.'

30

As well as treating men in medium security, I worked for around twelve years in a low-secure hospital for women with complex needs and challenging behaviour. They often had histories of abuse and neglect, and (usually) borderline personality disorder, in combination with mental illness and illicit drug use, arson, violent behaviour and neglect of children, most often as a result of mental health problems.

Many had disturbing family histories. One severe self-harmer received a birthday card from a family member, but inside the card was taped a razor blade, an obvious pointer to the toxic family dynamics at play.

Meanwhile, the abusive partner of another patient, Jacquelyn (admitted after a suicide attempt), would call her on the phone to verbally abuse her. 'You fat slag . . . Go on, do yourself in . . . no one gives a damn.'

Jacquelyn had once been in medical intensive care, having taken a liquidised cocktail of stockpiled antidepressants. She was pregnant. Her previous child had been taken into local authority care, partly because of her mental health problems, but mostly because she couldn't extricate herself from her relationship with her abusive, hard-drinking and violent partner. Faced with a choice between child contact and her deadbeat boyfriend, she had been unable to make the sensible choice. Coercive control or battered woman syndrome seemed to apply with Jacquelyn, as it did with Charlotte.

The problem was that Jacquelyn had effectively attempted an extended suicide with her unborn child. Thus, treating her was complex and challenging, as antidepressant medication had to be adjusted to avoid any harm to the foetus, while still managing Jacquelyn's disturbed mental state and suicide risk. Liaison with antenatal care and social services was needed for pre-birth risk-assessment issues.

It was agreed that she would be safe enough to be allowed to hold her baby for a few minutes after delivery under the watchful eye of a midwife and social worker, even though she had tried to take her own life while pregnant rather than have another child taken from her.

At our review meetings, Jacquelyn used to give me that hair-on-the-back-of the neck feeling thanks to her thousand-yard stare and her habit of smiling incongruously, despite her desperate situation. But her depression gradually lifted. We had prevented suicide during a critical period in her life, and I felt a great sense of relief when, some months later, she was transferred for ongoing care and further parenting assessment in a psychiatric unit closer to home.

On the back of attachment research, current child protection procedures recognise the child's needs for a stable and caring environment during that crucial early period, so this consideration is placed above the mother's need for contact. This may sound tough from the point of view of the mother – and it is – but the aim is to try and avoid visiting the travails of one generation on to the next as far as is possible. Working with this troubled group of women and dealing with the issues around risk to newborn babies inevitably took my mind back to my aunt Georgina and cousin Hannah.

In light of her mother's previous infanticide, Hannah became, in the terminology of the early 1970s, a 'ward of court'. But unlike in Jacquelyn's case, the child protection law of the time allowed Georgina decision-making power over Hannah, and Georgina had not consented to Hannah's longer-term fostering or adoption. Nowadays, as I've said, the law is such that, acting in Hannah's best interests, this decision would be taken out of Georgina's hands.

While Georgina had another spell in hospital, there had been a happy interlude when Hannah – aged around six – lived with my family for almost a year in the rustic surroundings of Dorset. Hannah's father had by now left the picture, having divorced Georgina. But Georgina later insisted that Hannah must live near her, to allow for regular visits, so Hannah spent many years in and out of the children's homes of the 1970s, seeing her mum on day visits.

Reflecting on this now, it is clear to me that Hannah would have been much better off with stable adoptive parents. This would have been tough on Georgina, of course, but the effect of the unstable environment of the children's homes on Hannah was just as bad, and she was later to seek treatment for depression. Despite that, she managed to build a stable relationship, had children of her own and engaged in individual psychotherapy in conjunction with antidepressant medication.

But I lost touch with her. I was busy helping my patients – male and female – and raising my own kids. In fact, after one Christmas, as I threw out the tree at my parents', I noticed Hannah's present unopened in the corner of the room, out of sight, as we had not managed to catch up with her. I felt a twinge of regret and resolved to make time to see her.

During my twelve years at the women's secure hospital, I would often avoid the traffic in the Limehouse Link tunnel and instead burn off all that transferred distress from my Wednesday all-day ward round by cycling home along the Thames through Limehouse and Wapping. The following day, on Thursday mornings, I would then review my male patients and return to considerations of risk, leave and readiness for discharge. The appeal tribunal needs to be satisfied that a patient who has killed no longer poses a risk to themselves or others. The final decision is out of my hands – for which I'm very grateful – but my recommendations and oral evidence are carefully recorded for reference if it all goes wrong.

Even though a longing for freedom is normal, it is not uncommon for patients to put a spanner in the works of their own discharge. Gate fever is often observed. In other words, I often find that patients who feel safe in the heavily supervised and supportive environment of psychiatric hospital, may not acknowledge their anxiety about fending for themselves and, instead, deliberately fail a urine drugs test in the days before a discharge hearing (that always scuppers it).

In the discharge planning meeting shortly before he was due to be released, I asked one patient what he had learned.

'First and foremost, I realise I need my medication,' he told me, adding, 'I've put my drug use behind me. I've learned to walk away from people who get in my face. I feel terrible for what I did. I thought he was going to kill me. I can see now that it was all a delusion. I wish I could turn back the clock. I just want to get on with my life. Do something useful . . . work . . . keep my head down.'

After a planned conditional discharge, any change in mental state, failure to attend an appointment or breach of conditions by spending the night away could trigger a recall to hospital.

This brings me back to the anxieties I described at the start of the book. They all involve fatal outcomes. Firstly, I worry about my inpatients. Have they died while in my custody from an undetected medical condition, or as a result of side effects from a treatment I have prescribed? Next, I worry about suicide. But most of all, I worry about a serious further offence. Has someone I am treating, or have recently assessed or released from hospital, committed an act of violence, or worse, a homicide?

As it happens, my current work is split, so I spend half my time treating male offenders in secure hospital and the other half working in liaison-diversion and threat assessment. This involves assessing cases that have come into contact with various elements of the police and criminal justice system, and diverting those that need it into treatment. I still feel responsible for any adverse outcomes – that's just a fact of life in my work. I am always a mobile phone message away from a serious untoward incident.

On a New Year's Eve not long ago (with no thought in my mind of that fateful New Year's Eve in 2002 and Anthony Hardy's headless torso collection), I dropped off one of my boys at a party. I then drove back through west London and stopped at The Cow on Westbourne Park Road for a last half-pint before dry January. I had elected to stay in that night, and was planning to cook oven-baked fish with a Thai sauce. Thoughts of my forensic caseload and report deadlines were far from my mind.

The day after New Year's, I was once again travelling across the city to my women's low-secure unit, back to work during that slightly bleak first week after the holiday festivities. I braced myself for another challenging ward review.

I reminded myself that many of the women would have spent the break with only fellow patients and nurses for company. They are often isolated from family, so the holiday periods can be tough, with thoughts of their missing children who are at foster parents', or permanently adopted away. The failed attachment of their own childhood so often transmitted to the next generation. Enforced adoption of your child, plus once-a-year letterbox contact, is a tough pill to swallow.

I swiped my ID card on the gate sensor and edged my car into the over-full car park. Double-parking, I scrawled my mobile number on the inside cover of an old A-Z map to leave in the front window in case I was blocking someone in.

As I was making a cup of powdered instant coffee in the canteen, I felt a buzz from my mobile phone. I saw it was my mother, but didn't have time to call her back. There was no indication that it was urgent.

Later that morning, I stepped outside to call.

She picked up after three rings, sounding agitated.

'What's the matter?' I asked.

'I'm afraid I've got some bad news. It's about your cousin Hannah. She's dead, Richard. It happened on New Year's Eve.'

'How?' Hannah was roughly my age.

'She jumped off a roof. She has taken her own life.'

Hannah had apparently been in hospital briefly not long before and had been seeing a therapist, as well as taking anti-depressants. But the treatment had failed. She had written a note to Georgina, her mother, apologising, and then thrown herself off the top floor of a five-storey block of flats.

I hadn't seen her for a number of years.

I have never bought into the notion of suicide being a sum-mation of someone's life: suicide must be about how desperate someone feels in that moment. But Hannah's experiences must have cumulatively taken their toll. And, clearly, life had seemed more painful than death, because it would have taken huge courage or desperation to go like that.

So in the end, Georgina's third child also lost her life in tragic circumstances. And yet they were all linked, because there's no doubt in my mind that Hannah's suicide was a direct consequence of the death, by infanticide, of her older sister at the hands of her mother.

I literally felt gutted. I had been too busy looking after my own family. And, more poignantly, I had been too busy looking after my own patients, many of them damaged, dis-tressed and suicidal women. Week in, week out, I had been trying to keep them safe and help them recover and, in over twelve years at my women's low-secure unit, I never lost one.

But I had neglected my own cousin, and there was nothing I could do now.

You can't turn back the clock.

Sometimes the consequences of murder can't be undone with treatment, no matter how hard you try.

Afterword

I am not convinced there can ever be such a thing as 'closure' if you have lost a loved one to murder – that sort of grief must stay with you.

There certainly wasn't closure in my family. At least, not until all of Georgina's children, including my cousin, were dead. Who can survive murderous behaviour in their mother?

Meanwhile, I am left to wonder how much my family history is responsible for the path I took in life. For the fact is that I didn't start out intending to work with murderers and their victims. I knew I wanted to study medicine, of course, mainly because I wanted to pursue my interest in biological science and use that to relieve the suffering of others. But I had no thoughts of pursuing forensic psychiatry, which barely existed outside of Broadmoor and a few prisons anyway.

However, I can't think of a medical speciality better suited to my interests. I'm eternally grateful that forensic psychiatry found me.

So what have I achieved? What have I learned and what has been its toll on me?

Regarding achievements, all I can say is that I have tried – with the help of my team of clinical psychologists, OTs, nurses and social workers – to relieve the suffering of those psychiatric patients and prisoners I have treated, whether they have murdered or not. And although the suffering of the victims of murder and their loved ones is hard to imagine, I hope I've at least helped to shed some light on why a killing took place, and what should be done with the perpetrator.

Of course, the newspapers don't report that the plane has landed safely, and likewise it is not possible to know whether I have helped prevent any murders, although I can think of a few near misses. For almost twenty years, I have been an advocate for the involvement of psychiatrists in multi-agency public protection. In any event, psychiatrists, police, prisons and probation are all talking to each other more than they used to, and that cannot be a bad thing.

Regarding what I have learned, it should be clear after reading this book that murderers are mostly made, not born. Poor parenting, disrupted attachment, failed education and early substance misuse will be found in the backstories of many killers. And, in the right circumstances, anyone can become a killer; we are all just a psychotic episode away from murder. Another flashpoint is the break-up of an intimate relationship. Feelings of jealousy and entitlement are powerful and can drive otherwise normal people without a criminal record to harassment, threats, violence and murder – men in particular.

I don't have illusions that this book will effect any change or make any dent in the annual global toll of over 400,000 murders, but there are three issues that I think society should at least try to combat.

First, we have to cut down the rates of femicide. Intimate partner abuse is still a massive problem globally, and much has been done to tackle it, but we must do more.

I don't have any easy answers to the crisis. Toxic masculinity must be challenged via better relationship education for young men, and the social and criminal justice response to intimate partner violence must be improved, especially in patriarchal communities. This will sound controversial, but there is a major cultural issue with differing attitudes to a woman's right to make choices about her relationships. By this I mean that there is a clash between misogynist and paternalistic cultures – where women's needs are subjugated to men's – and other societies, which are mostly liberal or social democracies, where women have rights to autonomy and safety.

We also need to do more to protect young British women from culturally sanctioned misogyny, abuse and violence, including so-called honour violence, and this is more important than misguided concerns about offending cultural sensibilities.

There are stalking projects underway, which include collaborations of police, mental health services and victims' organisations. The hope is that these will help reduce those murders linked to harassment by rejected former intimates. If these projects can demonstrate their efficacy – and early reports suggest that they will – then they should be funded as a priority.

Secondly, to tackle knife crime we need to hand funding from local authorities for drugs and alcohol services back to the NHS. Substance abuse is too big a public health problem to be left to cash-strapped local authorities. It is illicit drug abuse that fuels turf wars, and the knife killings that follow. The austerity-hit youth employment and training programmes in our deprived inner city areas must also be a priority.

We must tackle the availability of knives using a public health approach as described by forensic psychiatrist John Crichton.[73] Young men should be targeted with educational programmes and appropriate penalties to reduce knife-carrying outside the home. Long, sharp-tipped knives are not essential in the kitchen and can easily be replaced by a different design. So high-risk households can be offered a free replacement set of kitchen knives, and impulsive knife homicides can be prevented, whether they are psychotic, as in the case of Jonathan Brooks, or related to domestic violence, as in the case of Charlotte Smith.

Finally, we have to improve access to psychiatric assessment and treatment for those becoming mentally ill for the first time, and for those relapsing. In my current work I am confronted with the Byzantine processes required to get the acutely mentally ill into assessment and treatment, and I'm often exasperated by the euphemism, 'discharged to GP follow-up'. How can we expect our overwhelmed GPs to deal with all complex mental disorders as well as everything else? Patients with serious and enduring mental illness should remain on the books, even if only for a twice-yearly review. That way they can be kept in mind – because if we, as psychiatrists, don't, then nobody else will. And let's have a genuine single point of contact for every catchment area in the country. We also need more short-term psychiatric inpatient beds. The cuts have gone too far so that only the most disturbed are allowed an inpatient stay and the least-worst are discharged rapidly. Psychiatrists cannot predict which mentally ill patients will go on to kill, but if we give all patients better treatment, by making referral easier and treating for longer, then we may prevent some psychotic murders (even if it's only a handful). And all patients will get better treatment in the process.

As for the toll on me, of course there have been stressful times. But these have been more than made up for by the enduring interest and intellectual challenge of the work and by the rewards of helping many – but sadly not all – patients to recover. My enthusiasm for my work – and some incredibly supportive colleagues and family – have kept me going through the harder times. When things are tough, it's no bad thing to be surrounded by forensic psychiatrists. They know how to be firm and honest as well as empathic and caring in equal measure. Perhaps that's the best description of what forensic psychiatrists do.

As my day job involves joint work between forensic psychiatry and law enforcement, my focus now is on managing those who make threats or who are thought to pose a threat in one way or another. We call it liaison and diversion, and although the main outcome is facilitating access to treatment, there is also an element of harm reduction and of homicide prevention. With over sixty active cases open at any one time, I am unlikely to be bored or my mobile phone to stay quiet.

Finally, I must say a word to any budding forensic psychiatrists: we have vacancies. Applicants need only possess the stamina to complete medical training, an inquisitive mind, an aptitude for the nuances of legal and psychiatric language, a capacity for empathy, the desire for a challenge and, of course, a strong stomach. Forensic psychiatry provides a unique opportunity to explore the darkest reaches of the mind through the offenders and patients you meet. And, through learning about what makes the mind of a murderer, you will reach a deeper understanding of what's inside the mind of your fellow human beings and, most of all, a deeper understanding of yourself.

Appendix

A note on the Rorschach Test

At the time of my aunt Georgina's hospitalisation in the late 1960s, the Rorschach test was popular. Although it has now fallen out of widespread use in the UK, it is worthy of mention as it tells us much about the history of psychiatry. Hermann Rorschach first published his set of ten inkblots in 1921. The interviewer shows the respondent ten standardised inkblots. The test uses our tendency to see patterns in the clouds. 'Pareidolia' is the technical term. The respondent is asked, what might this be? After that is done with all ten cards, the cards are looked at again. The respondent is then asked to explain why it looked that way to them. This is repeated for each card.

The test was so popular in the mid-twentieth century that in literature and culture the word Rorschach became a metaphor for unconscious thought processes – it still shows up in international discussions around the world to describe an ambiguous stimulus. The Rorschach was perceived to have poor coding reliability – a problem that has been corrected – but it still has its enthusiasts. In recent years, systems have been developed to improve reliability, first by John Exner, and more recently by others, through the Rorschach Performance Assessment System (R-PAS). The R-PAS aims to provide a simplified, uniform and logical system of terminology by comparing test takers' scores to a large international reference sample, and there is a growing body of research literature on the R-PAS.[74]

There is some interesting cultural variance in how the blots are perceived. For example, inkblot three is generally interpreted as two figures engaged in a collaborative activity, such as two dancers round a campfire or two waiters serving food. Rorschach-trained interviewers might say that a respondent who interprets card three as disembodied body parts or skeletal remains could be from a Latin American culture that celebrates the Day of the Dead.

Or they could be a potential sexual homicide perpetrator.

This may sound shocking, but not when considered in the context of other tests we often rely upon: one well-known neuroscientist points out how his brain image is very similar to the brain images of serial murderers. Biology is not destiny, and it is always mediated by social and psychological factors in humans.

The Rorschach test doesn't provide any clue as to the historical behaviour of the respondent, and it doesn't provide a diagnosis, but its proponents argue that it can quite accurately describe how their personality is structured. When a group of sexual homicide perpetrators were assessed, many of their perceptions – as measured by the Rorschach – were quite different from the perceptions of other, more normal groups of individuals. One example from a colleague of mine, who has done research in this area, involved a sexual sadist who had killed several victims. When he did the Rorschach, the subject was preoccupied with female genitalia, a very unusual finding. Artist Andy Warhol created a series of inkblots inspired by the Rorschach test by painting a canvas on one side and then folding it to create the mirror image. In fact, he had misunderstood the test, as he thought patients created the inkblots and that doctors interpreted them.

The cover of this book is an adaptation of Rorschach inkblots numbers one and three. Other than a skull or brain, what else can you see?

Acknowledgements

There are many people I need to thank for helping me bring my experiences to the page. First of all, thank you to Andrew Holmes for being such a great mentor; to Ella Gordon for such insightful editing and to Claire Baldwin and Sarah Bance for line- and copy-editing. Thanks to Alex Clarke and to all the team at Wildfire, Headline and Hachette for listening to my pitch and for giving me this terrific opportunity, and thanks to the Art Department for the ingenious cover inspired by the Rorschach inkblots.

I am incredibly grateful to Rob Bullock, whose encouragement has been instrumental in making this book a reality.

A big thank you to all those who read early drafts of parts of the book for their invaluable feedback, namely: Freda Litton, Hobie Walker, Graham Riche, Robbie Riche, Nimko Ali, Simon Wilson, Chris Walker, Frank Farnham, Lucy Davison, David Reed, Ian Christie, Claudia Diez, Mike Taylor, Tom Beretvas and Vivian Nazari. Thanks also to Tim Lenderking, fellow traveller to the Sudan; to Mayday hospital colleagues Charlie Easmon, Graham Berlyne and Rhys Thomas; to Reid Meloy for advice on the Rorschach test; and special thanks to Jessica for the support and for the psycho-analytic case formulations.

Thank you to those colleagues and friends who have either worked with me or helped me to survive forensic psychiatry. You are too numerous to name individually, however I must acknowledge in particular: Derek O'Sullivan QC, Sherine Mikhail, Scott McKenzie, Mehdi Veisi, Shamir Patel, Stephanie Bridger, Sara Henley, Alice Taylor, Lyle Hamilton, David James, Alan Reid, Dave Porter, Steve Cook, Tim Turner, Mike Watts,

Rob Halsey, Jim MacKeith, Tony Maden, Gísli Guðjónsson, Paul Bowden, Paul Mullen, Mark Scally, Judith Etheridge, Danny Sullivan, Cleo Van Velsen, Andrew Johns, Ed Petch, John Baird, Rory O'Connor, Caroline Garland, Renée Danziger, Simon Barry, and Brad Vincent.

I must also thank all those colleagues I have worked with in various secure hospitals, outreach teams, prisons – especially HMP Holloway – and at the MAPPA Strategic Management Board.

I would like to thank all those from various disciplines who have helped educate me over the years, especially: Chris Brown, who first taught me to think about ethics; Roland Littlewood at the UCL Department of Anthropology, who taught me transcultural psychiatry; and Michael Neve at the Wellcome Institute, for his seminars on 'Madness in Society'.

Thanks to all at the Royal Bethlem and Maudsley Hospitals and the Institute of Psychiatry, Psychology and Neuroscience, especially Christine Sachs.

Thanks also to all my classmates and staff at the Institute of Criminology, University of Cambridge, Applied Criminology and Penology MSt course, especially Alison Liebling, Ben Crewe, Loraine Gelsthorpe, Katrin Müller-Johnson, Lucy Wilmott, Glenn Carner, Amy Ludlow, Nitin Ramesh and Pedro Bossi.

I am grateful to all my current and former colleagues from the Metropolitan Police, especially Keith Giles, who got me involved as technical adviser to *The Critical Few*, Richard Walton, who invited me to the original New Scotland Yard MAPPA working party and everyone at FTAC and the Hub.

To all the barristers and solicitors I have worked with, thank you for the instructions, but not for the cross-examinations. I apologise unreservedly for the blown deadlines.

Thanks to Karen Lock, Charlotte Walton, Christine

Revell, Loraine Millan, Claire Wells, Marnie Pillow, Anil Thapen, Donna Morgan and Ann Gadsen for unfailing administration and typing support – often at very short notice – and thanks to all the staff at the British Library, and UCL Library's Scandinavian languages section.

Finally, thanks to all members of my family, without whose support and understanding none of this would have been possible – especially my father Bill and mother Freda, who both inspired a love of books.

Selected Bibliography

1 Douglas, J.E., Burgess, A.W., Burgess, A.G. and Ressler, R.K., 2013. *Crime Classification Manual: A Standard System for Investigating and Classifying Violent Crime*, John Wiley & Sons.

2 Canter, D.V., Alison, L.J., Alison, E. and Wentink, N., 2004. 'The organized/disorganized typology of serial murder: Myth or model?'. *Psychology, Public Policy, and Law*, 10(3), p. 293.

3 Schlesinger, L.B., 2003. *Sexual murder: Catathymic and Compulsive Homicides*. CRC Press.

4 Yakeley, J. and Wood, H., 2014. 'Paraphilias and paraphilic disorders: Diagnosis, assessment and management'. *Advances in Psychiatric Treatment*, 20(3), pp. 202–213.

5 Dietz, P.E., Hazelwood, R.R. and Warren, J., 1990. 'The sexually sadistic criminal and his offenses'. *Journal of the American Academy of Psychiatry and the Law*, 18(2), pp. 163–178.

6 MacCulloch, M.J., Snowden, P.R., Wood, P.J.W. and Mills, H.E., 1983. 'Sadistic fantasy, sadistic behaviour and offending'. *The British Journal of Psychiatry*, 143(1), pp. 20–29.

7 Revitch, E., 1957. 'Sex murder and sex aggression.' *Journal of the Medical Society of New Jersey*, 54, pp. 519–524.

8 Meloy, J.R., 1988. *The Psychopathic Mind: Origins, Dynamics, and Treatment*. Rowman & Littlefield.

9 Meloy, J.R. and Hoffmann, J. eds., 2013. *International Handbook of Threat Assessment*. Oxford University Press.

10 Meloy, J.R., 2000. 'The nature and dynamics of sexual homicide: an integrative review'. *Aggression and Violent Behavior*, 5(1), pp. 1–22.

11 Blais, J., Forth, A.E. and Hare, R.D., 2017. 'Examining the interrater reliability of the Hare Psychopathy Checklist – Revised across a large sample of trained raters'. *Psychological Assessment*, 29(6), p. 762.

12 Blair, R.J.R., 2003. 'Neurobiological basis of psychopathy'. *The British Journal of Psychiatry*, 182(1), pp. 5–7.

13 Marshall, J., Watts, A.L. and Lilienfeld, S.O., 2018. 'Do psychopathic individuals possess a misaligned moral compass? A meta-analytic examination of psychopathy's relations with moral judgment'. *Personality Disorders: Theory, Research, and Treatment*, 9(1), p. 40.

14 Taylor, P.J. and Gunn, J., 2008. 'Diagnosis, medical models and formulations'. *Handbook of Forensic Mental Health*, pp. 227–243.

15 Meloy, J.R., 2006. 'Empirical basis and forensic application of affective and predatory violence'. *Australian and New Zealand Journal of Psychiatry*, 40(6-7), pp. 539–547.

16 Larsson, H., Viding, E. and Plomin, R., 2008. 'Callous–unemotional traits and antisocial behavior: Genetic, environmental, and early parenting characteristics'. *Criminal Justice and Behavior*, 35(2), pp. 197–211.

17 Kolla, N.J., Malcolm, C., Attard, S., Arenovich, T., Blackwood, N. and Hodgins, S., 2013. 'Childhood maltreatment and aggressive behaviour in violent offenders with psychopathy'. *The Canadian Journal of Psychiatry*, 58(8), pp. 487–494.

18 Taylor, R. and Yakeley, J., 2019. 'Working with MAPPA: ethics and pragmatics', *BJPsych Advances*, 25(3), pp. 157–65.

19 Singleton, N., Meltzer, H., Gatward, R., Coid, J., Deasy, D., 1997. Psychiatric Morbidity among prisoners. Office for National Statistics London.

20 Blair, R.J.R., 1997. 'Moral reasoning and the child with psychopathic tendencies'. *Personality and Individual Differences*, 22(5), pp. 731–39.

21 Eastman, N., 1995. 'Assessing for psychiatric injury and "nervous shock"'. *Advances in Psychiatric Treatment*, 1(6), pp. 154–160.

22 Bunclark, J. and Crowe, M., 2000. 'Repeated self-injury and its management'. *International Review of Psychiatry*, 12(1), pp. 48–53.

23 Fazel, S., Gulati, G., Linsell, L., Geddes, J.R. and Grann, M., 2009. 'Schizophrenia and violence: Systematic review and meta-analysis'. *PLoS Med* 6(8), p.e1000120.

24 Wilson, S., Farnham, F., Taylor, A. and Taylor, R., 2019. 'Reflections on working in public-figure threat management'. *Medicine, Science and the Law*, 59(4), pp. 275–81.

25 Schug, R.A., 2011. 'Schizophrenia and matricide: An integrative review'. *Journal of Contemporary Criminal Justice*, 27(2), pp. 204–29.

26 Welldon, E.V., 2018. *Mother, Madonna, Whore: The Idealization and Denigration of Motherhood*. Routledge.

27 Friedman, S.H., Cavney, J. and Resnick, P.J., 2012. 'Mothers who kill: evolutionary underpinnings and infanticide law'. *Behavioral Sciences & the Law*, 30(5), pp. 585–97.

28 Mullen, P.E. and Pathé, M., 1994. 'The pathological extensions of love'. *The British Journal of Psychiatry*, 165(5), pp. 614–23.

29 Mullen, P.E. and Maack, L.H. 'Jealousy, pathological jealousy and aggression'. *Aggression and Dangerousness*, edited by Farringdon, D., Gunn, J. John Wiley Chichester, 1985, pp. 103–126.

30 Mullen, P.E., Purcell, R. and Stuart, G.W., 1999. 'Study of stalkers'. *American Journal of Psychiatry*, 156(8), pp. 1244–1249.

31 Mullen, P. E., Pathé, M., and Purcell, R., 2008. *Stalkers and their Victims*. 2nd edn. Cambridge University Press.

32 Farnham, F.R., James, D.V. and Cantrell, P., 2000. 'Association between violence, psychosis, and relationship to victim in stalkers'. *The Lancet*, 355(9199), p. 199.

33 Purcell, R., Pathé, M. and Mullen, P., 2004. 'When do repeated intrusions become stalking?'. *Journal of Forensic Psychiatry & Psychology*, 15(4), pp. 571–83.

34 McEwan, T.E., Mullen, P.E., MacKenzie, R.D. and Ogloff, J.R., 2009. 'Violence in stalking situations'. *Psychological Medicine*, 39(9), pp. 1469–78.

35 Schlesinger, L.B., Gardenier, A., Jarvis, J. and Sheehan-Cook, J., 2014. 'Crime scene staging in homicide'. *Journal of Police and Criminal Psychology*, 29(1), pp. 44–51.

36 Gelsthorpe, L. 'Female Offending: A Theoretical Overview'. *Women Who Offend*, edited by McIvor, I. G. 2004, pp. 13–37.

37 Birmingham, L., Gray, J., Mason, D. and Grubin, D., 2000. 'Mental illness at reception into prison'. *Criminal Behaviour and Mental Health*, 10(2), pp. 77–87.

38 Liebling, A., 2011. 'Moral performance, inhuman and degrading treatment and prison pain'. *Punishment & Society*, 13(5), pp. 530–550.

39 Chao, O. and Taylor, R., 2005. 'Female offenders at HMP Holloway needing hospital transfer: An examination of failure to achieve hospital admission and associated factors'. *International Journal of Prisoner Health*, 1(2/3/4), pp. 241–7.

40 Browne, A., 2008. *When Battered Women Kill*. Simon and Schuster.

41 Mezey, G. 'Battered women who kill'. [Conference presentation]: *Women as Victims and Perpetrators of Violence*. Queens College Cambridge, September 2004.

42 Smith, R., 1997. 'Don't treat shackled patients'. *BMJ: British Medical Journal*, 314(7075), p. 164.

43 Bateman, A. and Fonagy, P., 2016. *Mentalization-Based Treatment for Personality Disorders: A Practical Guide*. Oxford University Press.

44 Grosz, S., 2013 *The Examined Life: How We Lose and Find Ourselves*. Random House.

45 Shedler, J., 2010. 'The efficacy of psychodynamic psychotherapy'. *American psychologist*, 65(2), pp.98-109.

46 Downs, D.A., 1996. *More Than Victims: Battered Women, the Syndrome Society, and the Law*. University of Chicago Press.

47 McHam, S.B., 2001. 'Donatello's bronze David and Judith as metaphors of Medici rule in Florence'. *The Art Bulletin*, 83(1), pp. 32–47.

48 Parker, L., 1992. '"Pure Woman" and Tragic Heroine? Conflicting Myths in Hardy's Tess of the D'Urbervilles'. *Studies in the Novel*, 24(3), pp. 273–281.

49 Guðjónsson, G. H. and MacKeith, J. A. C. (1988) 'Retracted Confessions: Legal, Psychological and Psychiatric Aspects'. *Medicine, Science and the Law*, 28(3), pp. 187–194.

50 Taylor, R. and Yakeley, J. 'Women in Prison'. *Psychiatry in Prisons: A Comprehensive Handbook*, edited by Cumming, I. and Wilson, S. Jessica Kingsley, 2009, pp. 86–97.

51 Jelicic, M., 2018. 'Testing claims of crime-related amnesia'. *Frontiers in Psychiatry*, 9, p. 617.

52 Babiak, P., Hare, R.D., 2006. *Snakes in Suits: When Psychopaths Go to Work*, Regan Books.

53 Yakeley, J., 2018. 'Current understanding of narcissism and narcissistic personality disorder'. *Advances in Psychiatric Treatment*, 24(5), pp. 305–315.

54 Wallang, P. and Taylor, R., 2012. 'Psychiatric and psychological aspects of fraud offending'. *Advances in Psychiatric Treatment*, 18(3), pp. 183–92.

55 Yakeley, J. and Taylor, R. 'Gambling: addicted to the game'. *Addictive States of Mind*, edited by Bower, M. Routledge, 2018, pp. 125–50.

56 Meloy, J.R., 2004. 'Indirect personality assessment of the violent true believer'. *Journal of Personality Assessment*, 82(2), pp. 138–146

57 Robbins, I., MacKeith, J., Davison, S., Kopelman, M., Meux, C., Ratnam, S., Somekh, D. and Taylor, R., 2005. 'Psychiatric problems of detainees under the Anti-Terrorism Crime and Security Act 2001'. *Psychiatric Bulletin*, 29(11), pp. 407–9.

58 Clemmow, C., Gill, P., Bouhana, N., Silver, J. and Horgan, J., 2020. 'Disaggregating lone-actor grievance-fuelled violence: Comparing lone-actor terrorists and mass murderers'. *Terrorism and Political Violence*, pp. 1–26.

59 Merari, A., 2010. *Driven to Death: Psychological and Social Aspects of Suicide Terrorism*. Oxford University Press.

60 Meloy, J.R. and Gill, P., 2016. 'The lone-actor terrorist and the TRAP-18'. *Journal of Threat Assessment and Management*, 3(1), p. 37.

61 Golds, L., de Kruiff, K. and MacBeth, A., 2019. 'Disentangling genes, attachment, and environment: A systematic review of the developmental psychopathology literature on gene–environment interactions and attachment'. *Development and Psychopathology*, 32(1) pp. 357–381.

62 Van IJzendoorn, M.H., Palacios, J., Sonuga-Barke, E.J., Gunnar, M.R., Vorria, P., McCall, R.B., LeMare, L., Bakermans-Kranenburg, M.J., Dobrova-Krol, N.A. and Juffer, F., 2011. 'Children in institutional care: Delayed development and resilience'. *Monographs of the Society for Research in Child Development*, 76(4), pp. 8–30.

63 Ogilvie, C.A., Newman, E., Todd, L. and Peck, D., 2014. 'Attachment & violent offending: A meta-analysis'. *Aggression and Violent Behavior.* 19(4), pp.322–339.

64 Ainsworth, M.D.S., Blehar, M.C., Waters, E. and Wall, S.N., 2015. *Patterns of Attachment: A Pyschological Study of the Strange Situation*. Psychology Press.

65 Meloy, J.R., 2003. 'Pathologies of attachment, violence, and criminality', edited by Weiner, I.B., *Handbook of Psychology: Forensic Psychology*, 11, pp. 509–526.

66 Hale, R., Dhar, R., 2008. 'Flying a kite – observations on dual (and triple) diagnosis'. *Criminal Behaviour and Mental Health*, 18(3), pp. 145–152.

67 Day, C., Briskman, J., Crawford, M.J., Foote, L., Harris, L., Boadu, J., McCrone, P., McMurran, M., Michelson, D., Moran, P. and Mosse, L., 2020. 'Randomised feasibility trial of the helping families programme – modified: an intensive parenting intervention for parents affected by severe personality difficulties'. *BMJ Open*, 10(2).

68 Gelsthorpe, L. 'Criminal Justice: The Policy Landscape'. *Criminal Justice*, edited by Hucklesby, A. and Wahidin, A. Oxford University Press, 2013, pp. 17–33.

69 Green, D.A., 2012. *When Children Kill Children: Penal Populism and Political Culture*. Oxford University Press.

70 Healy, D., 2000. 'Some continuities and discontinuities in the pharmacotherapy of nervous conditions before and after chlorpromazine and imipramine'. *History of Psychiatry*, 11(44), pp. 393–412.

71 Adshead, G., 2001. 'Attachment in mental health institutions: a commentary'. *Attachment & Human Development*, 3(3), pp. 324–329.

72 Lappi-Seppälä, T., 2009. 'Imprisonment and penal policy in Finland'. *Scandinavian Studies in Law*, 54(2), pp. 333–380.

73 Crichton, J.H., 2017. 'Falls in Scottish homicide: lessons for homicide reduction in mental health patients'. *BJPsych Bulletin*, 41(4), pp. 185–6.

74 Meloy, J.R., Acklin, M.W., Gacono, C.B. and Murray, J.F., 2013. *Contemporary Rorschach Interpretation*. Routledge